Cough

From Lab to Clinic

Cough

From Lab to Clinic

Juraj Korpas
Autar S. Paintal
Ashima Anand

Anshan

ANSHAN LTD

Ane Books India

First Published 2007

ANSHAN LTD
6 Newlands Road
Tunbridge Wells
Kent.
TN4 9AT. UK
Tel: +44 (0) 1892 557767
Fax: +44 (0) 1892 530358
e-mail: info@anshan.co.uk
Website: www.anshan.co.uk

Published in arrangement with
Ane Books India
4821, Parwana Bhawan, 1st Floor
24 Ansari Road, Darya Ganj, New Delhi -110 002, India
Tel: +91 (011) 2327 6843-44, 2324 6385
Fax: +91 (011) 2327 6863
e-mail: anebooks@vsnl.com
Website: www.anebooks.com

ISBN-10: 1 905740 63 8
ISBN-13: 978 1 905740 63 5

British Library Cataloguing in Publication Data
A catalogue record for this book is available from the British Library

This edition not for sale in India, Pakistan, Nepal, Sri Lanka and Bangladesh

Printed at Gopsons Paper Ltd., Noida (U.P.), India

This Book is Dedicated to

Juraj Korpas,
(On his 80th Birthday)

Pioneer and world leader in our understanding of cough and its therapy. Not only has he made several novel contributions himself in this field, but has also set up an active school of experimental respiratory studies in the Jessenius Medical School at Comenius University Martin, Slovakia.

Ashima Anand
Sona Franova
Jan Hanacek
Kamil Javorka
Jan Jakus
Juraj Mokry
Gabriela Nosalova
Renata Pecova
Jan Plutinsky
Jurina Sadlonova
Martina Sutovska
Milos Tatar

List of Contributors

Ashima Anand **PhD.**	Principal Scientific Officer DST Centre for Visceral Mechanisms V.P Chest Institute, Delhi University Delhi, India E-mail: visc.mechs@mail.com
Sona Franova **RNDr., PhD.**	Associate Professor, Department of Pharmacology, Comenius University in Bratislava, Jessenius Faculty of Medicine, Martin, Slovakia E-mail: franova@jfmed.uniba.sk
Jan Hanacek **M.D., PhD.**	Professor, Department of Pathological Physiology, Comenius University in Bratislava, Jessenius Faculty of Medicine, Martin, Slovakia E-mail: hanacek@jfmed.uniba.sk
Kamil Javorka **M.D., PhD., D.Sc.**	Professor, Head of Department of Physiology, Comenius University in Bratislava, Jessenius Faculty of Medicine, Martin, Slovakia E-mail: javorka@jfmed.uniba.sk
Jan Jakus **M.D., PhD., D.Sc.**	Professor, Department of Medical Biophysics, Comenius University in Bratislava, Jessenius Faculty of Medicine, Martin, Slovakia E-mail: jakus@jfmed.uniba.sk
Juraj Korpas **M.D., PhD., D.Sc.**	Emeritus Professor, Department of Pathological Physiology Comenius University in Bratislava, Jessenius Faculty of Medicine, Martin, Slovakia E-mail: korpas@jfmed.uniba.sk

Juraj Mokry **M.D., PhD.**	Lecturer, Department of Pharmacology, Comenius University in Bratislava, Jessenius Faculty of Medicine, Martin, Slovakia E-mail: mokry@jfmed.uniba.sk
Gabriela Nosalova **M.D., PhD., D.Sc.**	Professor, Head of Department of Pharmacology, Comenius University in Bratislava, Jessenius Faculty of Medicine, Martin, Slovakia E-mail: nosalova@jfmed.uniba.sk
Late Autar S. Paintal **MD FRCP, FRS**	Programme Director DST Centre for Visceral Mechanisms V.P Chest Institute, Delhi University Delhi, India
Renata Pecova **M.D., PhD.**	Lecturer, Department of Pathological Physiology, Comenius University in Bratislava, Jessenius Faculty of Medicine, Martin, Slovakia E-mail: pecova@jfmed.uniba.sk.
Jan Plutinsky **M.D., PhD.**	Associate Professor, Head of 2nd Pneumology Department TB and Respiratory Diseases Institute, Nitra-Zobor, Slovakia E-mail: Plutinskyjan@nextra.sk
Jurina Sadlonova **M.D., PhD.**	Associate Professor, Clinic of Internal Medicine I., Comenius University in Bratislava, Jessenius Faculty of Medicine, Faculty Hospital, Martin, Slovakia E-mail: sadlonova@jfmed.uniba.sk
Martina Sutovska **M.D.**	Lecturer, Department of Pharmacology, Comenius University in Bratislava, Jessenius Faculty of Medicine, Martin, Slovakia, E-mail: sutovska@jfmed.uniba.sk
Milos Tatar **M.D., PhD.**	Professor, Head of Department of Pathological Physiology Comenius University in Bratislava, Jessenius Faculty of Medicine, Martin, Slovakia E-mail: tatar@jfmed.uniba.sk

Foreword

About 50 years ago, a remarkable research programme started in Slovakia (then part of Czechoslovakia). Teams from Kosice (eastern Slovakia) and Martin (middle Slovakia), led by Imrich Ivanco and Zoli Tomori and by Juraj Korpas respectively, began their collaborative study on cough and other defensive and protective reflexes from the respiratory tract. They began publishing papers on the topic in 1954, the first of a long succession of distinguished works. There had been a scattered literature on these subjects for over a century (indeed Hippocrates provided the first documentation of cough); but in spite of its physiological and clinical significance and importance to human welfare, the topic had been largely neglected apart from a few landmark research papers.

A Slovakian team, led by Juraj Korpas at Comenius University in Martin, evolved; they not only studied cough in a wide variety of species and in many different physiological and pathological conditions, but also extended studies on and named the 'expiration reflex'—the forced expiratory effort that occurs when the vocal folds are touched, and whose function is to prevent aspiration of foreign material into the trachea and lungs. In the University of Kosice, Zoli Tomori and colleagues were detailing the 'aspiration reflex'— the sniff- or gasp-like inspirations that are elicited by stimulation of the nasopharynx. In 1979 Korpas and Tomori wrote and published '*Cough and Other Respiratory Reflexes*',[1] a book that came to be regarded as the bible for workers in this field, and was probably the only detailed and serious major publication on the subject (apart from research papers) for the next 20 years.

The growing reputation of the Slovakian teams led to extensive international collaboration, with scientists from Martin and Kosice visiting and working at several research institutes outside their own country, and also visits in the opposite direction. One collaboration was between the Martin group and that of the late Professor Autar Paintal and Dr Ashima Anand in Delhi. It is therefore very appropriate that Dr Anand has not only contributed to this book but also played a major role in its publication.

The last few years have seen a surge of interest in studies on cough and related defensive reflexes, with a number of international symposia dedicated to cough[2-5] and at least one multi-author book.[6] It is no exaggeration to say that this flourishing world-wide research has been largely based on the solid foundation built by Korpas, Tomori and their colleagues in Slovakia. The present book consists mainly of contributions by workers at the Martin School, but its importance is enhanced by the fact that they cover extensively the relevant studies of their colleagues throughout the world. These colleagues, and others who want to learn about cough, should find the book of great value and interest.

John Widdicombe
Emeritus Professor
University of London

REFERENCES

1. Korpas J, Tomori Z. Cough and other respiratory reflexes. Progress in Respiration Research, vol. 12. Basel: Karger, 1979.
2. Widdicombe J, editor. Cough: methods and mechanisms. Pulm Pharmacol 1996;9:259–392.
3. Widdicombe J, editor. Cough: pharmacology and therapy. Pulm Pharmacol Therap 2002;15:185–338.
4. Korpas J, Widdicombe JG, editors. Cough: recent advances in understanding. Eur Respir Rev 2002;12:221–82.
5. Chung KF, Widdicombe JG, editors. Cough: acute and chronic. Pulm. Pharmacol. Therap. 2004;17:327–473.
6. Chung KF, Widdicombe JG, Boushey HA, editors. Cough: Causes, Mechanisms and Therapy. Oxford: Blackwell Publishing, 2003.

Preface

About twenty-five years after the publication of *Cough and Other Respiratory Reflexes (*Korpas J. & Tomori Z), the Slovak group from the Jessenius Medical School in Martin, has once again come together with their researches in a new book. With the arrival of its chapters for Professor Autar Paintal and me to edit, we were tempted to contribute one of our own. The etiology of dry cough though decidedly different from the one that occurs due to bacterial and viral infections or as an allergic response, necessitated it all the more to be juxtaposed with information on the latter. Having realised that in this collection there were not only basic laboratory studies but also advances that were meant for the physician to use in the clinic, Professor Paintal found it appropriate to give the book a title that would emphasise this.

Cough as one knows, is recognisable by its sound. The chapter on cough sounds or tussiphonography, provides distinct onomatopoetic clues about the underlying etiology of cough and this aspect emerges as one of the newest contributions of the book. The authors emphasise an objective recognition of cough sound as a diagnostic tool in current medical practice that continually looks forward to the emergence of precise and non-invasive diagnostic methods. Tussiphonography not only indicates the cause of cough; a worsening, an improvement but also the effectiveness of the therapy that a patient is undergoing. A careful analysis can also provide clues about the prognosis of the underlying disease.

Not only are the stimuli responsible for eliciting cough; numerous and varied, as has been described at length, but so are the types and subtypes of airway sensory receptors or associated nerve endings in the lung parenchyma that induce and modulate the cough intensity. From amongst these, the role of the slowly adapting pulmonary stretch receptors (SARs) is the least understood; whereas their direct stimulation neither gives rise to nor increases the intensity of cough, yet when their activity is blocked, the elicitability and the strength of the cough reflex is seen to be reduced. In this regard, further insights can be obtained from an interesting and uncommon reason for cough, that is thoracentesis and which refers to compression or a re-expansion of the lung parenchyma during bronchoscopy. This phenomenon is in fact being studied to generate new information to understand the genesis of cough during lung parenchymal disease.

Though a direct stimulation of either cardiac, splanchnic, oesophageal or nasal sensory afferent nerve fibres, does not give rise to cough, yet inputs from these extrapulmonary areas are found to have an important role in the regulation of the cough reflex. A stimulation of cardiac and splanchnic nerve endings, and block of peripheral chemoreceptor activity leading to a depression of breathing, is accompanied by a marked inhibition of the cough response when elicited in response to a mechanical stimulus. Conversely, in the presence of enhanced ventilation produced either by an increased peripheral chemoreceptor input or by a stimulation of the nasal sensory receptors an increased mechanically-induced cough response is seen. If hypoxia was to be prolonged, then the cough response is reduced, but ventilation remains increased. Similarly, during hypercapnia, the hyperventilation is accompanied by a reduced cough response. Thus, there is a distinct mechanism that is responsible for modulation of cough by extrapulmonary afferent inputs. It is likely that the central cough generator is less resistant to the direct inhibitory effect of hypoxia and hypercapnia, than are the mechanisms regulating central inspiratory activity.

One of the greatest challenges is to design experiments which will allow one to identify the neuronal substrate or the central control elements of cough; in other words, the hypothetical excitatory 'gate' mechanism or a cough suppressive neuronal network. This obviously indicates that further studies on the role of both non-respiratory and silent neurons in the control of cough, be undertaken. One could even consider a new hypothesis of a 'holonarchial supersystem' in the neurogenesis of breathing, coughing, swallowing, vomiting and other respiratory system-related motor behaviours. In this scheme,the functional control elements or holons could possess unique regulatory features for each of the motor activities mentioned—with the cough 'gate' being one such example. However, this requires a novel experimental approach.

During early ontogenesis, the development of vital body functions including control of breathing and defensive airway reflexes, show many peculiarities. For instance, newborns and children have an efficient neural and chemical regulation of breathing so as to make up for their rather demanding metabolic needs as well as to protect their vulnerable and delicate airways and pulmonary tissue. Certain visible morphological peculiarities are: a soft and compliant chest and a low tone of the intercostal muscles. Along with these peculiarities, position of the larynx and the soft tissues of the upper airways lead to difficulties in breathing through the mouth when required and the defensive airway reflexes are not as precise as seen in the adults. But nevertheless, premature newborns do possess an effective defense of the lungs. They have an active diving and Kratschmer´s reflex and are able to eliminate irritants from their airways by using intense expiratory efforts of coughing and sneezing. It is this ability which is less effective in newborns and especially in those who exhibit the respiratory distress syndrome. Thus an understanding of the physiological and patho-physiological differences in neonates and children, from those of adults and the clinical implications thereof, underlies appropriate clinical care that is to be imparted in neonatology and paediatrics.

The respiratory and cardiovascular systems form one functional entity; they adjust their activities according to their common mission i.e. to ensure oxygenation of as well as elimination of carbon dioxide from, the blood. In addition, they deal with special situations that arise during breathholding, coughing and sneezing which bring about massive increases in intrathoracic pressure. Much information about the effect of defensive airway reflexes on the cardiovascular has been obtained from experiments carried out on animals. But with the availability of advanced medical techniques that are both non invasive as well as provide beat-to-beat registration of heart rate, blood pressure and perfusion pressures have allowed one to study cardiovascular changes during coughing in humans as well. Besides one now has data that confirms experimental results with actual cardiovascular responses, for example one can now understand the events underlying cough syncope.

The capsaicin cough-test appears to reveal the presence of functional changes in afferent nerve-endings in the airways leading to cough. This is seen in response to those allergic processes that also produce an inflammation in the skin and nose. Although very little is known about the spread of atopic allergic processes into the airways, but utilising the capsaicin cough-test to detec t its presence could indeed be very useful. An advance that is awaited from such studies is being able to correlate functional changes of nerve-endings as markers for subclinical forms of pathological changes in the airways.

Antitussive drugs such as codeine and dextromethorphan are amongst the most commonly used prescription and over the counter drugs. A documentation of the cough-suppressive potential of agents from various pharmacological groups is essential to understand the precise mechanism of their antitussive action on receptors, such as opioid, dopaminergic, gabaergic, serotonergic, histamine and on ion channels (potassium, calcium and chloride).

In current clinical practice, the use of herbal agents with cough-suppressive properties is being preferred. So it is most appropriate that an evaluation of their activities as spasmolytics and local anaesthetics be known in addition to their antibacterial and antiviral properties as well as their influence on mucus production and its quality. The pharmacological entities imparting the antitussive and expectorant properties in herbal preparations are mostly, saponins, flavonoids, alkaloids, terpenoids, polysaccharides (mucilage, gums and pectins). This detailed information has been arrived at from studies carried out on the evaluation of the cough reflex not only in anaesthetised animals but also in conscious ones.

Ashima Anand

Contents

1 Causes of Cough

M TATAR

1.1 INTRODUCTION

The most common respiratory complaint for which a person seeks medical help is either shortness of breath or cough. Upper respiratory tract infections are the most familiar ones and a common reason for frequent visits to the physician, not only in the United States[1] but also all over the world. A cough is an explosive expiration that protects the lungs against aspiration of liquids and promotes movement of secretions and other airway constituents upward towards the mouth. It is a critical element in the self-cleansing and protective mechanisms of the lungs. A detailed description of cough components was published by Korpas and Tomori (1979).[2] Mechanisms of mediation and modulation of cough are described elsewhere in this monograph (see Chapters 4 and 9).

1.2 MECHANISMS

Two different mechanisms are responsible for producing a cough during pathological states. One is by the stimulation of sensory receptors directly by airway secretions, foreign bodies and tumours and another is by which an abnormal increase in the sensitivity of receptors leads to a persistent cough or it reduces the threshold for cough. The latter is also referred to as an enhanced 'cough sensitivity' and is a hallmark of many airway diseases; and most likely, it reflects plasticity in the neural circuits regulating this defensive reflex. Increased afferent nerve fibre excitability or changes in afferent nerve fibre anatomy or facilitatory interactions between sensory nerve fibre subtypes, are some of the important factors that could produce an enhanced 'cough sensitivity'.[3]

1.3 TYPES

1.3.1 Acute and Chronic Cough

For the sake of convenience, cough may be divided into two main types, but these cannot be considered mutually exclusive. Thus, there is 'acute cough' which lasts for less than 3 weeks and 'chronic cough', which could last for at least 3 to 8 weeks, or even longer.

While there are no published studies indicating the variety and frequency or causes of acute cough, yet overwhelming clinical experiences indicate that upper respiratory tract infections are its most common cause. Some of these infections are the common cold, acute bacterial sinusitis, and pertussis. It is also a principal feature of chronic bronchitis.

Most respiratory infections commonly give rise to acute cough or worsening of chronic cough in patients with chronic obstructive pulmonary disease, especially during exacerbation of this disease.

Acute cough can be the presenting manifestation of potentially life-threatening diseases such as pneumonia, congestive heart failure, pulmonary embolism, or those conditions that predispose to aspiration.

Cigarette smoking is another well-known cause of chronic cough in the general population, though generally, no medical attention is sought for relief from it. Chronic cough is a manifestation of almost all respiratory diseases, appearing as part of a symptom complex and usually indicating serious underlying pathology.

1.4 CAUSES

Cough can be caused by a multiplicity of disorders located in a variety of locations. Literally hundreds of diseases can cause cough. The following is a list of several well-known causes of cough and is based on information extracted from the book entitled, *Pulmonary Diseases and Disorders.*[1]

1.4.1 Infectious Diseases of the Respiratory System

- Infections of the upper respiratory tract
  - Common cold
  - Laryngitis
  - Epiglottis

  - Croup
  - Tracheitis
  - Otitis externa
- Acute bronchitis
- Bronchiolitis, with or without obliterans
- Pneumonia
- Atypical pneumonia
- Lung abscess
- Legionellosis
- Actinomycosis and nocardiosis
- Pulmonary candidiasis
- Endemic mycoses
- Cryptococcal infections
- Pneumocystic carinii infection
- Influenza
- Thoracic amoebiasis
- Pulmonary complications in malaria
- Chronic infections of lungs
  - Chronic bronchitis
  - Chronic obstructive pulmonary disease
  - Bronchiectasis
  - Tuberculosis
  - Fungal pulmonary infections
  - Cryptogenic adult bronchiolitis
  - Diffuse panbronchiolitis
  - Acute immunodeficiency disease (AIDS)
- Asthma
- Cystic fibrosis
- Angio-oedema
- Interstitial lung diseases
  - Sarcoidosis
  - Idiopathic pulmonary fibrosis
  - Hypersensitivity pneumonitis
  - Radiation pneumonitis
- Pulmonary manifestations of the collagen vascular diseases
  - Systemic lupus erythematodus
  - Rheumatoid arthritis

- Polymyositis-dermatomyositis
- Sjögren´s syndrome

- Eosinophilic pneumonias
  - Loeffler´s syndrome
  - Parasitic infections
  - Chronic eosiniophilic pneumonia
  - Allergic bronchopulmonary aspergillosis
  - Idiopathic hypereosinophilic syndrome
- Pulmonary amyloidosis
- Alveolar haemorrhage syndromes
  - Goodpasture´s syndrome
  - Pulmonary vasculitis and capillaritis
  - Idiopathic pulmonary haemosiderosis
  - Pulmonary histiocytosis
- Pulmonary alveolar proteinosis
- Pulmonary thromboembolic disease
- Acute pulmonary infarction
- Pulmonary oedema
  - Associated with high transmural vascular pressures
    * Cardiac dysfunction
    * High-altitude pulmonary oedema
  - Associated with reperfusion
    * Re-expansion oedema
  - Associated with aspiration or inhalation of foreign material
    * Gastric acid aspiration
    * Smoke and toxic gas inhalation
- Disorders of the pleural space
  - Nonmalignant pleural effusions
    * Parapneumonic effusions and/or empyema
    * Tuberculous pleural effusion
    * Parasitic infections of the pleural space
  - Malignant pleural effusions
- Pneumothorax
- Malignant mesothelioma and other primary pleural tumours
- Diseases of the mediastinum
  - Mediastinal masses
    * Congenital cysts (bronchogenic, enterogenous)

    * Lymphoma
  - Aortic aneurysm
- Blunt thoracic trauma
  - Tracheobronchial injuries
- Tumours
  - Laryngeal tumours
  - Non-small cell lung cancer
  - Small cell lung cancer
  - Primary lung tumours other than bronchogenic carcinoma
  - Pulmonary metastases
- Lymphoproliferative disorders
  - Benign lymphoid proliferation
  - Malignant lymphomas
- Foreign body
  - Immediate, while still in upper airways
  - Later, when lodged in lower airways
- Aspiration disorders
  - Neuromuscular mechanisms
    * Dysphagia due to neuromuscular disorders
    * Gastro-oesophageal reflux disease
- Mechanical etiologies of dysphagia
  - Retropharyngeal infection
  - Zenker´s diverticulum
  - Trauma
- Cancer
- Iatrogenic mechanisms
  - Enteral nutritional support
  - Tracheal intubation and tracheostomy
  - General anaesthesia
- Occupational lung disorders
  - Upper respiratory tract irritation (noxious gases and solvents in workplace gases)
  - Airway disorders
    * Occupational asthma (diisocyanates, anhydrides, wood dust, animal-derived allergens, latex)
    * Byssinosis (cotton dust)
    * Grain dust effects

    * Chronic bronchitis (coal)
- Acute inhalation injury
  - Toxic pneumonitis (irritant gases, metals)
  - Metal or polymer fume fever (zink or copper oxides, plastics)
  - Smoke inhalation (combustion products)
  - Pneumoconioses (asbestos, silica, coal, beryllium, cobalt)
- Outdoor and indoor air pollution
  - Sulphur dioxide
  - Ozone
  - Irritant aerosols and fumes
- Cigarette smoking
- Thermal lung injury
- Diving injuries and air embolism
  - Pulmonary barotraumas
  - Pulmonary decompression sickness
- Post-transplant respiratory complications
  - Bone marrow transplantation
  - Early complications (infectious pneumonia, idiopathic interstitial pneumonitis, lymphocyticbronchitis)
  - Chronic graft-versus-host disease (bronchiolitis obliterans)
  - Heart-lung transplantation, lung transplantation (brochiolitis obliterans is the main pulmonary complication)
- Cardiovascular disorders
  - Left ventricular failure
- Pulmonary toxicity associated with drug therapy
  - Chemotherapeutic agents
    * Cytotoxic antibiotics (Bleomycin, Mytomycin)
    * Alkylating agents (Busulfan, Cyclophosphamide)
    * Antimetabolites (Methotrexat, Cytosine Arabinoside)
    * Nitrosourea (Carmustine)
  - Drug-induced lung disorders due to nonchemotherapeutic agents
    * Drugs used to treat cardiovascular disorders (Amiodarone, angiotensin-converting enzyme inhibitors)
    * Tocolytic agents (Terbutaline, Salbutamol)
    * Antibiotics (hypersensitivity-induced pulmonary eosinophilia due to b-lactam, sulpha antibiotics, fluoroquinolones, Isoniazid, Ethambutol)
    * Nitrofurantoin toxicity

   * Anti-inflammatory agents (nonsteroidal anti-inflammatory drugs, Gold, Penicillamine)
   * Complication of illicit drug use (cocaine smoking)
   * Pulmonary pharmacotherapy (adverse effect)
   * Bronchodilators (Ipratropium bromide)
   * Anti-inflammatory agents (inhaled corticosteroids)
 – Oxygen toxicity.

1.4.2 Chronic Cough

The term 'chronic cough' is usually understood as the syndrome of cough in the absence of other obvious airway disease. Chronic cough can be seen in non-smokers who are not taking angiotensin-converting enzyme inhibitor (ACE) drugs and who have normal or nearly normal chest radiographs showing only inconsequential scars, normal basal spirometry with no pathological finding in physical examination of the chest. The complications of cough lead patients to seek medical attention. In them, the most common reasons are subjective perception of exhaustion and self-consciousness, and symptoms of insomnia, hoarseness, musculoskeletal pain, and urinary incontinence.

The most common causes of chronic cough amongst people worldwide, of all age groups that seek medical attention, are the following:

- postnasal drip syndrome from a variety of upper respiratory tract conditions (perennial rhinitis, post-viral upper respiratory infection, allergic rhinitis, vasomotor rhinitis, sinusitis),
- asthma, and
- gastro-oesophageal reflux disease.

1.4.3 Dry or Productive Cough in Adults

The less common but important causes of dry or productive cough in adults, are the following:

- unrecognised chronic bronchitis,
- eosinophilic bronchitis,
- bronchiectasis,
- post-infection cough,
- psychogenic and habit cough, and
- chronic interstitial pulmonary diseases.

1.4.4 Paediatric Patients

In paediatric patients, the common causes that could be considered are as follows:[4]

- congenital anomalies (involving the aortic arch and pulmonary, tracheobronchial tree and congenital mediastinal tumours),
- acyanotic congenital heart disease,
- foreign bodies (lodged in the airway, oesophagus, ear),
- chronic aspiration,
- passive smoking and dry air inhalation because of forced-air heating.

The European experience reveals a high incidence of idiopathic and post-viral cough. The majority of patients arriving for secondary care, may have one of the following three syndromes:

- a form of asthma where cough is predominant,
- gastro-oeosophageal reflux, and
- rhinitis.[5]

REFERENCES

1. Fishman AP, Elias JA, Fishman A, Grippi MA, Kaiser LR, Senior R. Fishman´s pulmonary diseases and disorders. 3rd ed. New York, St. Louis, San Francisco, Auckland, Bogotá, Caracas, Lisbon, London, Madrid, Mexico City, Milan, Montreal, New Delhi, San Juan, Singapore, Sydney, Tokyo, Toronto: McGraw-Hill Health Professions Division, 1998.
2. Korpas J, Tomori Z. Cough and other respiratory reflexes. Basel, Munchen, Paris, London, New York, Sydney: S. Karger, 1979.
3. Mazzone SB, Canning BJ. Plasticity of the cough reflex. European Respiratory Review 2002;12 (85):236–42.
4. Irwin RC, Boulet L-P, Cloutier MM, Fuller R, Gold PM, Hoffstein V, Ing AJ, MsCool D, O´Byrne P, Poe RH, Prakash UBS, Pratter MR, Rubin BK. Managing cough as a defence mechanism and as a symptom. A consensus panel report of the American College of Chest Physicians. Chest 1998;114 (Suppl.):133S–181S.
5. Morice AH. Epidemiology of cough. Pulmonary Pharmacology and Therapeutics 2002;15(3):253–9.

2 Cough Sounds

JURINA SADLONOVA, J KORPAS

2.1 INTRODUCTION

Cough is an unusual reflex. It can be a symptom of disease that may have a diagnostic significance. Usually, the cough reflex constitutes a defence mechanism that protects the respiratory system against aspiration of foreign material and removes excessive airway secretions. Coughing is recognisable by its characteristic sound. According to Sant´Ambrogio,[1] it has a clear onomatopoetic connotation, as the sound associated with it is reproducible.

Despite several attempts to highlight the objective registration of cough sounds, it is still unknown in medical practice as a diagnostic tool. As one of the main responsibilities of modern medicine is to search for new, precise and non-invasive diagnostic methods, it may be emphasised that tussiphonography, or detecting underlying disease from cough sounds, is an invaluable method in this field.

The study of 'recording of cough sounds' has an immense potential of diagnostic importance, as it enables the classification and quantification of one of the commonest phenomena of respiratory diseases. According to Widdicombe,[2] "The use of the tussiphonogram as a diagnostic tool is intriguing but introduces problems. It might be of considerable value in identifying the mechanisms of airway pathology present in respiratory disease. To establish this, there would have to be an extensive comparison of the tussiphonogram with pathological changes identified by biopsy. This kind of approach might also give information about the pathophysiological mechanism of coughing, by indicating the appearance of tissue in the airways, which leads to certain patterns of cough.

Tussiphonography may be of value in prognosis and might indicate the effectiveness of therapy and the progress of disease."

2.2 COUGH SOUNDS

Cough is one of the body's defence mechanisms that prevents the entry of noxious materials into the respiratory tract and clears potentially harmful debris from the lungs and airways.[3–5] Cough is not necessarily seen in healthy people, but if it is present or is persistent in patients, it assumes great clinical importance.

It is well known that coughing is expressed as a sudden expulsion of air accompanied by a typical sound. This sound is so characteristic that it allows identification of the cough and distinguishes it from other vocal manifestations. The word 'cough' has a clear onomatopoetic connotation since it reproduces the sound associated with coughing.[1]

The cough sound is a very important symptom of well over 100 diseases and other conditions of clinical significance.[6,7] Changes in the character of the cough sound can reflect pathological situations in the respiratory tract and this has been well known for a long time.[6, 8–15] The sound or timbre of cough can assist in distinguishing and diagnosing diseases such as pertussis, asthma, and laryngitis.

Ashurst et al[16] found that clinicians dealing with respiratory diseases can distinguish between cough sounds that are dry, moist or productive. They reported that subjects, when asked to identify gender, diagnosis and the three main properties of cough, that is, moist, productive, dry and wheezy from samples of 'recorded cough' that had been selected and classified by cough research workers, gender was identified correctly in 94 per cent cases, moist cough in 74 per cent, and dry cough in 87 per cent and wheezy cough in 58 per cent. However, a clinical diagnosis by listening to cough-sound recordings was only correct in 53 per cent of the cases. These results demonstrate that the ear can indeed recognise cough quality and thus it should be possible to develop a computerised algorithm to recognise the main characteristics of cough.

Even though cough as a symptom and some of its properties had been described as early as 2000 years ago by ancient physicians, such as Hippocrates, who thought that 'cough is the voice of the lung' and also by others, such as by Aulus Cornelius Celsus and Areteus of Cappadocia, yet a continued ignorance of cough sound registration prevented the development of further knowledge and significance of their change in disease. Attention was given for a long time mainly to normal and adventitious pulmonary sounds[17–19] and to find out the significance of cough counts, but no attempts were made to analyse the cough sounds themselves. Thus the objective recording of cough sound as a diagnostic tool is still absent from current medical practice in comparison with, say, the registration of the EEG, ECG, EMG.[20]

2.3 METHODS FOR COUGH SOUND RECORDING

The first few investigators,[21] who actually used cough sound recordings, were Kohts,[22] Hogyes[23] and Coryllos.[24] The methods used were different from those that are in use currently, and these were mainly based on chest movements and measurement of airflow at the mouth.[25–33] These were indirect methods for cough recording and therefore, not precise. A more exact method for cough sound analysis could be one based on recording the cough sound. It may be noted that since cough sound reveals its pattern only with high-speed recording 10–20 cm s^{-1},[34] the methods currently used for recording the cough sound with slow tape speeds are only suitable for providing evidence for the presence or absence of cough. Thus, the utility of this method is limited, as the record does not reflect the cough sound character; that is, its intensity or duration. Thus, this kind of recording can mainly be used for objective assessment of cough suppressants.

In current practice, cough sound properties are recorded using microphones, magnetic recorders, or telemetry systems. The cough sound is eventually collected by means of a sensitive condenser microphone (50 /mV/Pa) with a response frequency that must be linear, that is, from 5/5 Hz to 5/10 kHz or more.[35] The amplifier must have a maximum gain for the frequencies involved and the sound signal may be recorded in frequency modulation with the newer digital recorders.[7] Earlier, the sound record was visualised on the memory oscilloscope, at present it is visualised on a personal computer suitable for data acquisition, handling and processing. Subburaj et al[41] and others[3, 13, 36–40] have described the apparatus used for cough sound processing. These investigators have been developing methods to record cough signals from ambulatory subjects, telemetrically. A major challenge has been to develop an algorithm to identify automatically, the cough signals from recordings containing other signals such as speech, laughter, and throat clearing. The application of cardiograph recording as done by Kelemen and Cseri[42] seems to be unsuitable for precise registration of cough sounds (as the differences recorded is in Hz) and this distorts the real cough sound character or that produced as an effect of antitussive drugs. However, Korpas and Sadlonova[39] using a free-air microphone have achieved 90 per cent accuracy in cough identification. Further improvements in the system are underway to register cough counts, efforts, and latency.

2.3.1 Recording of Acoustic Pressure during Cough Sound

We consider that for cough evaluation in humans, the most precise method is the recording and analysis of the acoustic pressure during cough. This method is very simple. The subject to be examined sits in a quiet room at a standard distance (50 cm) in front of a sensitive microphone, that is, electrets condenser microphone which is a kind of microphone, with an optimal frequency response of 50 to 16,000 Hz. The subject either coughs spontaneously or when asked to. For the latter, he is instructed to do so after a deep inspiration. This cough can be repeated after 1 to 2 minutes. A signal is given and recorded on a tape recorder. For an evaluation of the cough, sound intensity serves as a sound integrator based on adding up the trace efforts. The quality of analysis depends on the speed of the paper on which it is being recorded. Finally, the cough sound record is analysed by a computer. The continuous signal from the tape recorder or directly from the microphone is digitised with an AD-converter (the optimum sampling rate was chosen as 11 kHz). The digitalised signal is analysed by using a computer either on- or off-line mode. The obtained traces allow an analysis of cough sound pattern by Fast Fourier Transform (FFT; visually or by software) giving the sound's intensity and duration. This method, developed by the authors has provided useful observations over the years,[20,40] and is now used widely.[10,43–44]

2.4 THE COUGH SOUND RECORD

The first cough sound (burst) seen on the record emerges at the moment of glottal opening. This is followed by a noisy interval on the record, which corresponds to steady-state flow with the glottis wide open. The glottis narrows at the end of the expulsive phase, which generates the second cough sound (burst). This appears as a double sound record (Fig. 2.1A). The cough record in some subjects shows only the first sound. This occurs when the glottis does not narrow down after having had opened wide during the expulsive phase. In this case, the record appears only as a single (mono) sound record (Fig. 2.1B). This

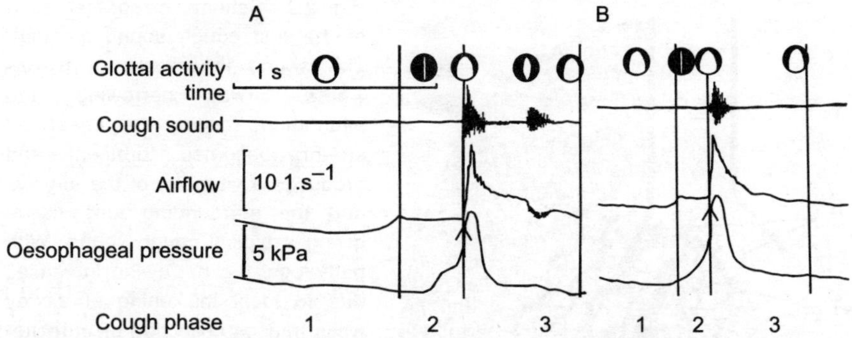

Fig. 2.1 Record of glottal activity, time, cough sound (recorded on a multiscriptor), airflow,and oesophageal pressure (inspiration downwards), during a single cough effort (↑) in a healthy person. Numbers 1,2,and 3 denote inspiratory, compressive, and expulsive efforts, respectively: **A,** cough with double sounds; **B,** cough with single sound. Note, a difference in the vibration of airflow curve as seen during the first and the second sounds indicates a difference in the origin of the sound burst. (Reproduced from Ref [9] permission from the Publisher).

may be due to a higher flow pressure in the region of glottis that stretches the vocal cords and prevents their oscillation. Another possibility could be fatigue or damage to the glottis muscles. It is possible that such an exhaustion can occur after several cough efforts, making the second sound disappear. The ratio of double sound to monosound is 1.4 : 1 in healthy subjects.

2.4.1 Interpretation of the First Cough Sound

The first cough sound in healthy subjects is created in places of constitutional airway narrowing and bifurcation, where the linear air stream becomes turbulent, and which produces vibration of the airway and the surrounding solid tissue[8,9,35,45] (Fig. 2.2). In pathological conditions, the airways narrow down (bronchoconstriction) either due to local thickening of their walls or due to the presence of inflammation, oedema or mucus collection, with the result that the first sound is more extended and folded.

This multiple local narrowing, behaves like a reed instrument, being necessary for the timbre of sound that arises as encountered in wide spread bronchoconstriction, provoked for example, by acetylcholine. After the administration of acetylcholine, the intensity of the cough sound decreases but its pathological character persists.[46]

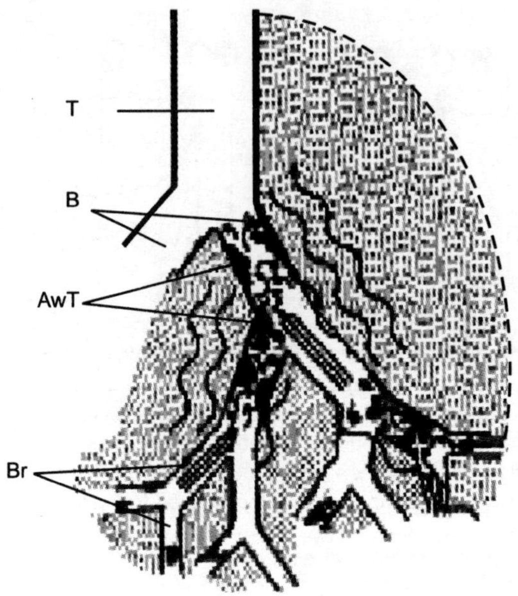

Fig. 2.2 Schematic representation of the first cough sound creation. The sound is created in places where airway narrowing and bifurcations occur: the linear air stream becomes turbulent and produces a vibration of the airways and the surrounding lung tissue giving a typical cough sound. With pathology, the narrowing increases due to local thickening of airway walls, mucus collection or broncho-constriction. T, trachea; B, bronchi; Br, bronchioles; AwT, airway thickening.

It is worth commenting that the administration of bronchodilatory drugs in healthy subjects and in bronchitic patients does not change the recorded character of cough despite the improvement in spirometric values. On the contrary, many patients show abnormal records because of greater mucus production due to the administration of derivatives of theophylline and ß-sympathomimetic drugs. The vocal cords do not take part in the creation of the first sound because they have been already widened to their maximum extent in order to provide a minimum resistance to airflow.

Therefore, despite their vibration during the expulsive phase of cough as observed by Leden and Isshiki,[47] no sound is created. It is possible that the creation of sound requires some degree of glottis vibration, which itself depends on the width of the glottis slot. The different vibrations of the airflow curve during the first and the second sounds testify to the different origins of the burst of sound. The first cough sound emerging in the ordinary way is louder than the second sound.

2.4.2 Interpretation of the Intermediate Cough Sound

The presence of an intermediate low-noisy part (the intermediate sound) between the first and second sounds indicates an inflammation of the trachea. A more significant record indicates a more intense inflammation. A small and thick increase in the intermediate noise indicates chronic tracheal inflammation[20,48] (Fig. 2.3).

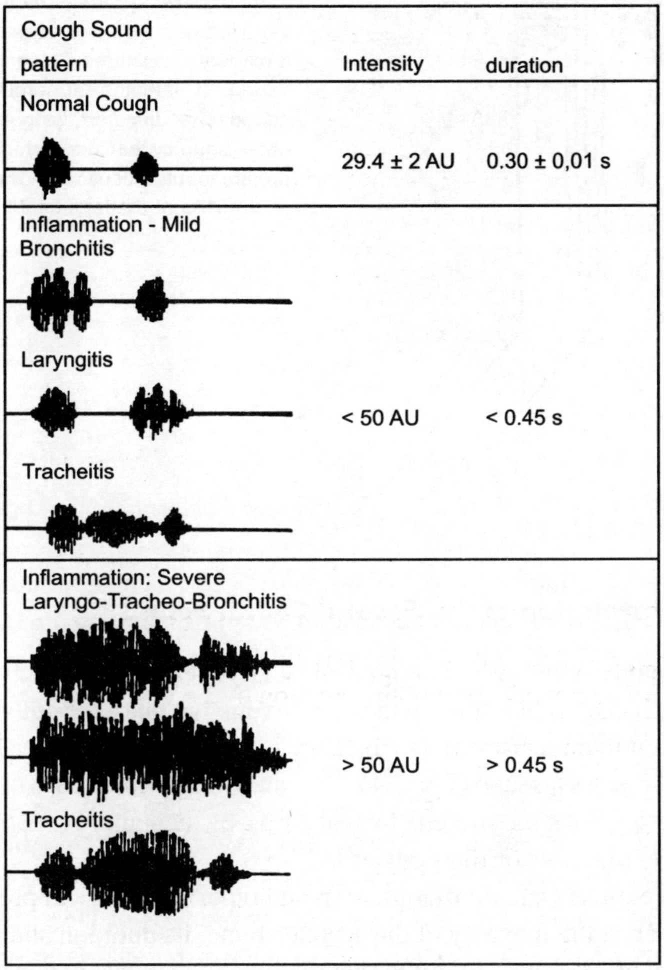

Fig. 2.3 Changes in cough sound pattern, intensity, and duration in healthy persons and in patients with mild or severe inflammation of the airways (recorded on a multiscriptor). The values of normal cough represent the mean of arbitrary units and (±) SEM in mild inflammation represent the maximal limit of normal values; in severe inflammation represent threshold of pathological values. (Reproduced from Ref. [20] with ermission from Publisher).

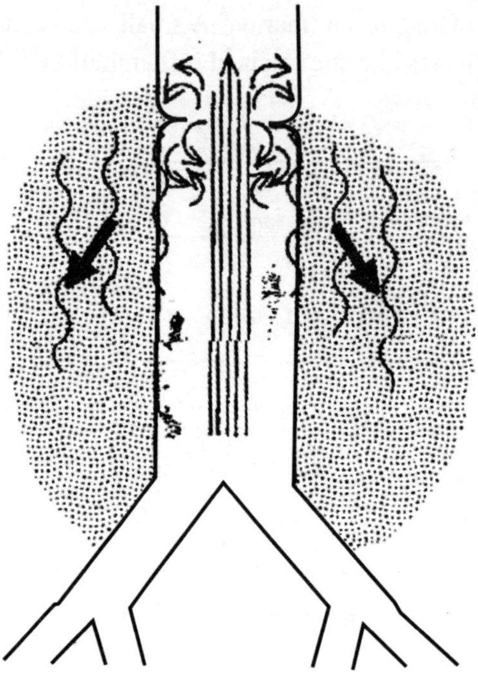

Fig. 2.4 Schematic representation of the creation of the second cough sound. When the vocal cords approach each other at the end of the expulsive phase of cough, the air stream between them causes their vibration as well as that of other laryngeal structures, thus creating sound. In pathological condition, this sound is modified by the presence of other sounds that originate from the presence of mucus and the partial obstruction of the laryngeal lumen.

2.4.3 Interpretation of the Second Cough Sound

The second cough sound has unambiguously a laryngeal origin. When the vocal cords approach each other at the end of the expulsive phase of cough, the air stream between them causes their vibration as well as that of other laryngeal structures and creates a sound (Fig. 2.4). The pitch of the vibration is determined mainly by the degree of the stretch of vocal cords, by their approximation to one another and by the mass of their edges.

Therefore, in laryngeal inflammation and other pathological processes in the laryngeal area, the intensity of the second sound, its duration and character change noticeably. Leith[8,45] reported that the second cough sound is generated in the larynx, but no further clarification was forthcoming.

The origin of the second sound has been affirmed from clinical findings. This does not appear in patients after laryngectomy or chordectomy or in paralysis of the vocal cords. In mild paralysis, with decreased movement of the vocal cords after repeated coughing, the second sound may reappear. The second cough sound is also absent in patients suffering from persistent cough of

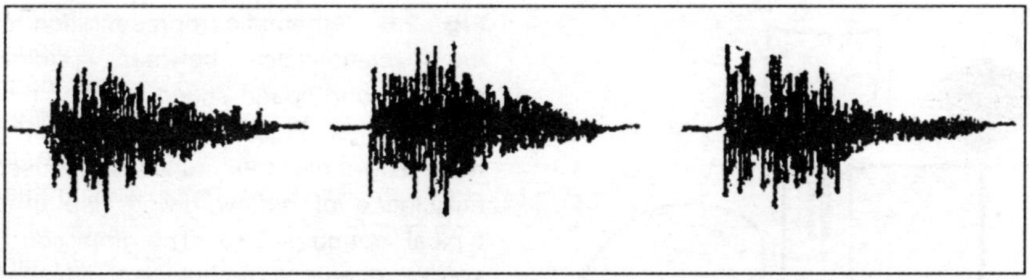

Fig. 2.5 Tussiphonograms of cough of psychogenic origin, taken from three girls (recorded on a multiscriptor). The similarity of monosounds is striking.

psychogenic origin; and this sound in them, is either hollow or bovine (Fig. 2.5). Thus, we can summarise, that the first cough sound represents a pathological situation in the airways that is located near the area of tracheal bifurcation and the second sound gives information about the laryngeal bifurcation itself. An intermediate cough sound, that is, one between two distinct cough sounds, or the absence of the second one, points to pathological processes in the trachea or in tissues affiliated to the trachea (Fig. 2.6).

2.4.4 Cough Sound Changes in Disease

The timbre of spontaneous as well as voluntary cough changes with disease. During the course of mild inflammation of the airways, the first and second cough sound becomes split into two, three, or one more, but without changes in intensity or duration (0.45 s). If the changes occur during the first sound with inflammation, the disease is likely to be below the level of the bifurcation of the trachea (Fig. 2.3). If changes are seen with reference to the second sound, the laryngeal area is likely to be involved (Fig. 2.4). In severe inflammation, the cough record represents a large and long monosound. The sound intensity increases by 50 to 400 per cent and its duration increases by 50 to 100 per cent[20] (Fig. 2.3).

In patients with bronchial obstruction and copious sputum output, the record shows multiple flow spikes and long cough sequences. Thus, it can be seen that differentiating between a record of a normal cough or that during pathological conditions is simple and allows not only identification of the healthy and ill subjects but also a distinction between acute and chronic respiratory diseases. It is important to keep in mind that subjects do not influence the cough sound pattern

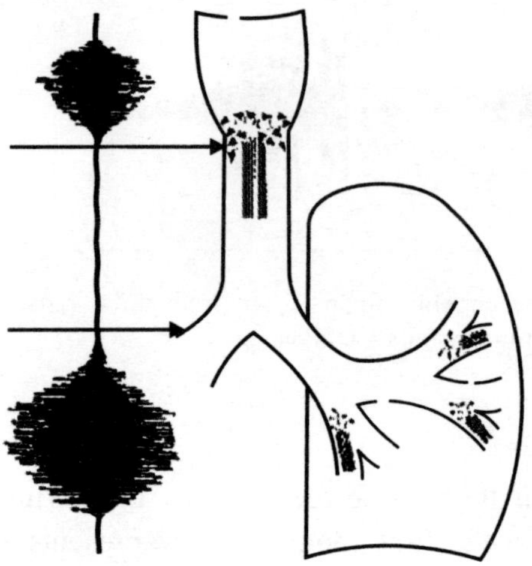

Fig. 2.6 Schematic representation of the relationship between airflow changes and cough sound creation (i.e. summary of Figs 2.2 and 2.4). The narrowing of the airways causes turbulence of airflow giving rise to a typical cough sound. The first cough sound reveals a pathological situation below the level of the tracheal bifurcation; the second sound gives information about the laryngeal area and the intermediate part reveals processes in the trachea and its surrounding areas. Tussiphonogram records correspond to the area of the airways from which the sound is supposed to arise. (Reproduced from Ref. [20] with permission from Publisher).

or its duration although they may alter the cough sound intensity if required by the investigator.[20]

2.4.4.1 *Objective Evaluation of the Cough Sound Pattern*

For carrying out an objective evaluation of the cough sound pattern, a histographic analysis is required (Fig. 2.7). The histogram represents the frequency of single efforts of the time–amplitude wave according to their amplitude level. The connection of the tops of individual bars yields a hyperbola in physiological cough. In pathological condition of the airway, the middle high efforts of the amplitude wave are augmented, whereas the low efforts are decreased and the hyperbola therefore plateaus off and tends to create a straight line. Thus, the pathological pattern is easily distinguishable.

2.4.5 Other Indications of Cough Sound and its Recording

Since alterations in cough sound pattern may be present at a time when other clinical findings are not explicit enough to determine an exact diagnosis in those instances such tussiphonographic findings may be utilised to detect the presence

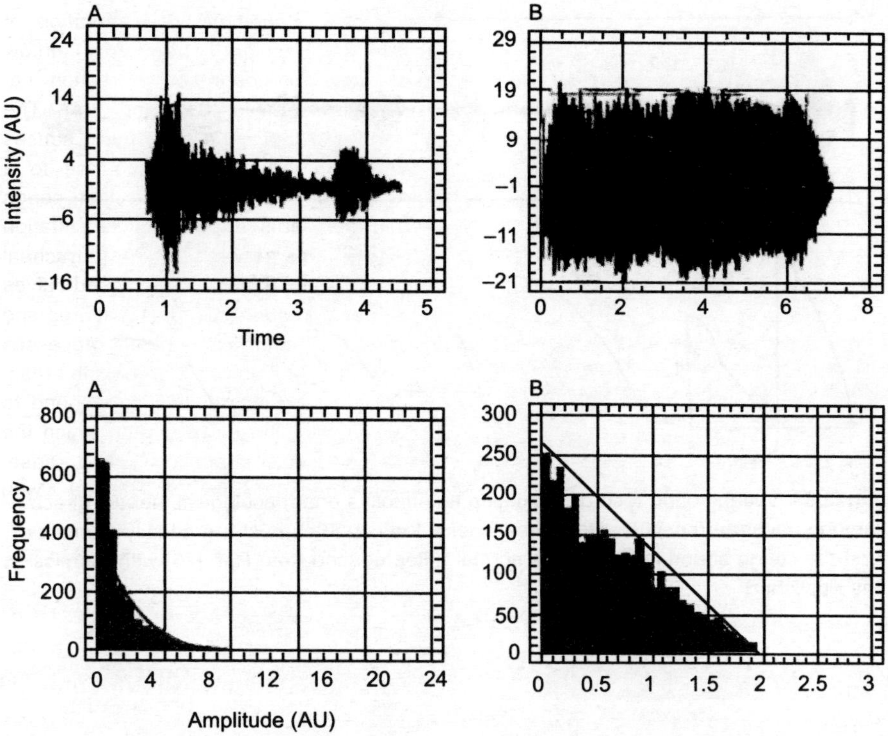

Fig. 2.7 The objective evaluation of cough sound pattern. **Upper graphs:** cough sound record in a healthy subject (A, upper graph). Cough sound record in a patient with chronic bronchitis (B, upper graph). **Lower graphs:** histographic expression of samples of sound amplitude (arbitrary unit—AU) according to their frequency of occurrence. The connection of the tops of bars gives a hyperbola, that is, normal pattern (A, lower graph) or a straight line (B, lower graph), indicating a pathological pattern. (Reproduced from Ref. [20] with permission from the Publisher).

of inflammation, if any. The advantage of a timely diagnosis is important for effective treatment of chronic respiratory diseases in order to prevent a worsening of the state. The tussiphonogram is useful not only for screening of respiratory diseases and for assessing their severity but most importantly, for clinical determination of the effectiveness of treatment (Figs 2.8 and 2.9).

Since it would be useful to know whether tussiphonography is capable of detecting minor pathological changes in the airway and lungs, we related the indices of voluntary cough sound to that of pulmonary function test results in a

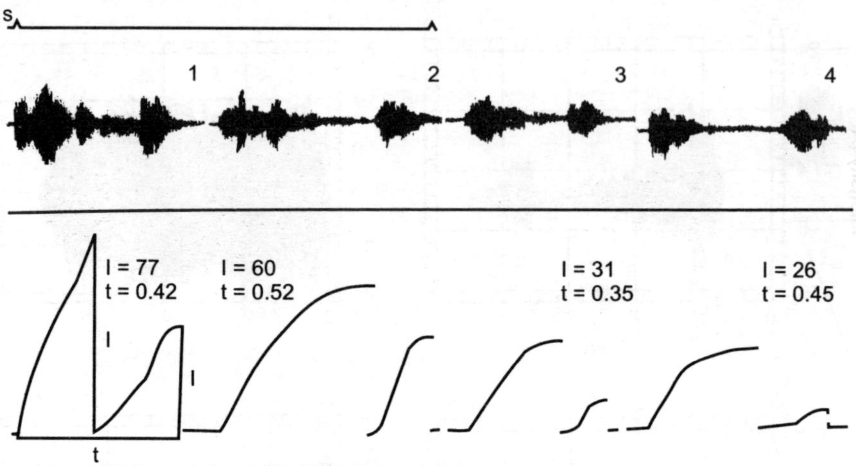

Fig. 2.8 Cough sound records indicating an effective pharmacological therapy of acute-laryngo-tracheo-bronchitis. After three weeks, the cough character gradually normalised, and the cough sound intensity was normal. (Reproduced from Ref. [76] with permission the Publisher)

group of asthmatics before and after treating them with pulsatile electromagnetic therapy. It may be pointed that this therapy influences the pulmonary function minimally.

After magnetotherapy in 18 patients, the expiratory forced lung capacity increased by 7.3 per cent and peak inspiratory flow increased by 31.7 per cent; the averaged voluntary cough sound intensity decreased by 37.8 per cent; the sound duration shortened by 11 per cent and the sound pattern showed a tendency towards normalisation. The improvement in the above mentioned cough indices was absent in 17 patients who were also treated with magneto-therapy, but at the same time suffered from respiratory viral infection, and in 22 patients who were treated only with climatotherapy and antiasthmatics. Changes of flow–volume loops in patients were not in close relation to the other indices that were observed.

The correlation analysis showed a functional connection in relative differences of cough sound indices and some pulmonary function tests. The results confirmed the usefulness of tussiphonography in indicating even mild pathological changes in the respiratory tract.[49]

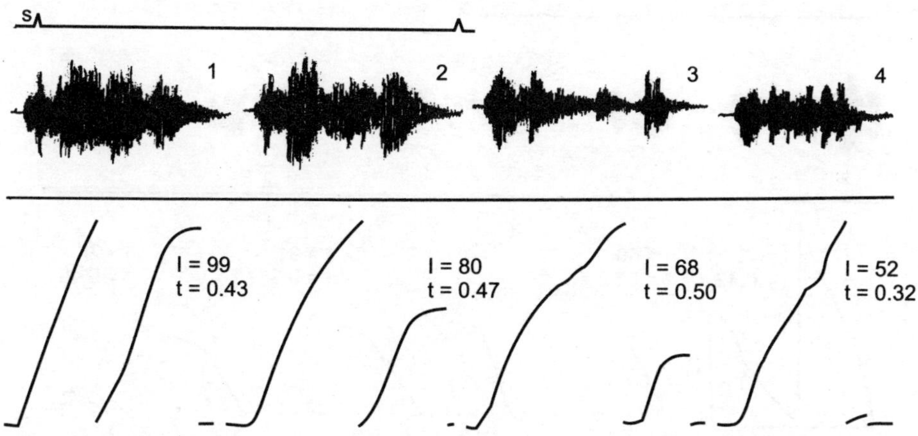

Fig. 2.9 Cough sound records indicating a less effective pharmacological therapy (over four weeks; 1–4) of a patient suffering from viral inflammation of the airways. Records from top to bottom are; 1 s time marks, acoustic pressure, integral of the acoustic intensity pressure (I = AU). The record of the last cough. 4 shows a decrease in the intensity but not a significant decrease in the occurrence of cough efforts. (Reproduced from Ref. [76] with permission from Publisher)

Since sound records taken repeatedly, essentially represent an unchanged pattern in healthy persons, these patterns then can be standardised for normals. We undertook to observe healthy subjects during a 24-hour long examination, and found that when certain short-term changes did appear, they could be explained as being due to the production of mucus in response to variations in temperature, humidity, pollution (cigarette smoke), in the environment (Fig. 2.10).

Earlier, studies on cough sound recordings were made mostly at night since cough frequency is relatively constant during sleep. It was thus possible to make meaningful observations on the effect of antitussive drugs on its intensity and duration.[50,51] A further advantage was based on the fact that while asleep, the subject's responses cannot be influenced by extraneous factors, his own emotions or by the noise of a busy clinic.[52] Another reason being, that significant cough attacks in asthmatics, occurred mostly at night. However, at present, these problems can be overcome by using modern methods of isolating the subject.

Some investigators find a microphone unsuitable for recording cough sounds.[36,53–56] Others are unable to discriminate between speech and background

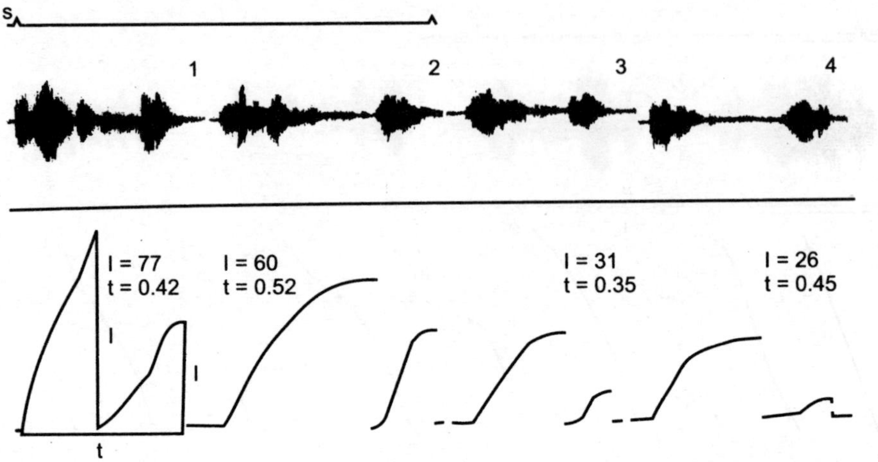

Fig. 2.10 Cough records obtained repeatedly in healthy volunteers present an unchanged pattern during a 24-hour long examination. Records from top to bottom are, 1 s time marks, acoustic cough pressure, integral of acoustic pressure intensity (I), time of cough duration (t). (Reproduced from Ref. [76] with permission from Publisher)

noise or are unable to decide on the appropriate recording distance from the microphone or be able to eliminate the noise of switching the recorder on or off.

For provoking a cough experimentally, citric acid aerosol is used. It is interesting to note that the voluntary cough sound does not differ greatly from that caused by citric acid[57] (Fig. 2.11).

Gramophone records have been found suitable to analyse and screen respiratory diseases from the sound of common cough. These were published by Schmidt and Voigt* and by Hirschberg and Szende.** According to their criteria, the cough sound records of patients who suffered from some respiratory disease or another could be correctly identified as arising from a pathological state (Fig. 2.12).

The suitability of tussiphonography for clinical diagnosis is based on its ability to differentiate it from records of other sounds such as noisy breathing, a

* Schmidt and Voigt
** Hirschberg and Szende

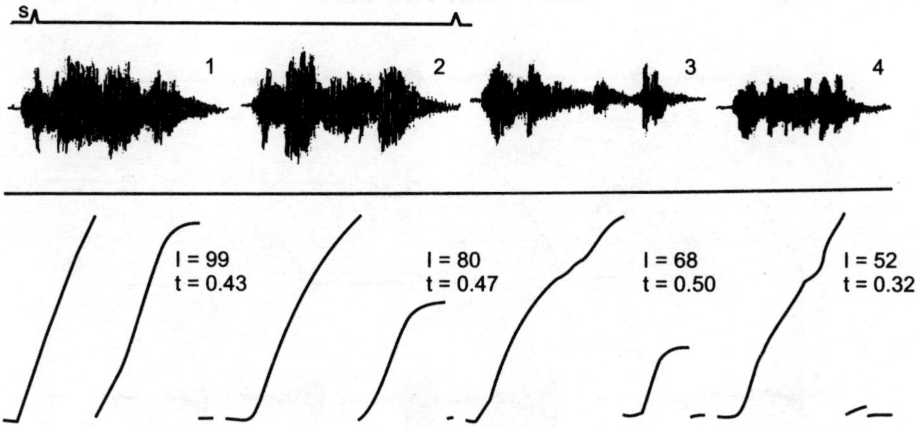

Fig. 2.11 Comparison of voluntary cough with that elicited by citric acid in a healthy volunteer (HV) and in a patient with bronchitis (BR).

dog's barking, a cry or the cackling stridor of newborns (taken from Hirschberg´s and Szende´s collection of 'sounds'). The records distinctly reflect the quantitative and qualitative differences of the evaluated sound samples. This reconfirms that the usual method of common cough sound recording is suitable even for evaluating the influence of sound phenomena related to the respiratory organs.

The currently held belief is that, a persistent and irritant cough represents airway hyper-reactivity. We, therefore, examined the cough sound record to see how the changes could be symbolised. Investigations were made on 74 patients with bronchial hyper-reactivity (56 females, 19 males; mean age 46 years) who were hospitalised in the Martin Faculty Hospital (Slovakia). Bronchial hyper-reactivity was determined on the basis of a clinical check-up and routine pulmonary function tests (with stress on FEV_1 and MEF_{25-75}) and a bronchoprovocation test (acetylcholine, PC_{20}). The values were compared with cough sound values in 60 volunteers who were free from any respiratory disease. The voluntary cough sounds of both these groups were recorded with the help of a microphone (Sony, optimal frequency response 50–16,000 Hz) on a tape

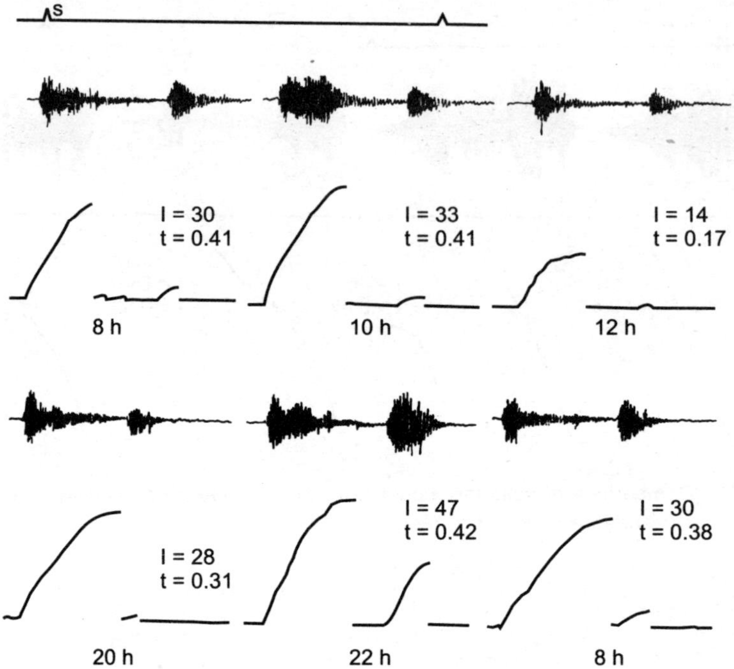

Fig. 2.12 Gramophone record of cough sounds: **A,** in tracheobronchitis (1); chronic bronchitis (2); and bronchial asthma (3); (From Schmidt and Voigt); **B,** tracheolaryngitis (1); chronic bronchitis (2); and bronchial asthma (3) (From Hirschberg and Szende). Records from top to bottom in each trace are, cough sound; integral of acoustic pressure intensity (I); *t*, time of cough duration in seconds.

recorder (Sony TC 133 Japan, optimal frequency response 20–10,000 Hz) and analysed by a computer (Hardware, PC AT 38+ADVANTECH A/D card PLC 812 PG, using a software for routine data acquisition). No changes that could suggest airway hyper-reactivity were found; but in all cases, the records reflected the typical changes of chronic airway inflammation. Figure 2.13 depicts the typical sounds of dry cough taken from healthy volunteers (A) and from patients who showed hyper-reactivity of the airways (B). The latter record shows an increase in the frequency with a close connection between the first and second sounds.

Figure 2.14 compares spectrograms from a healthy volunteer (first traces) and a patient with airway hyper-reactivity (second traces).

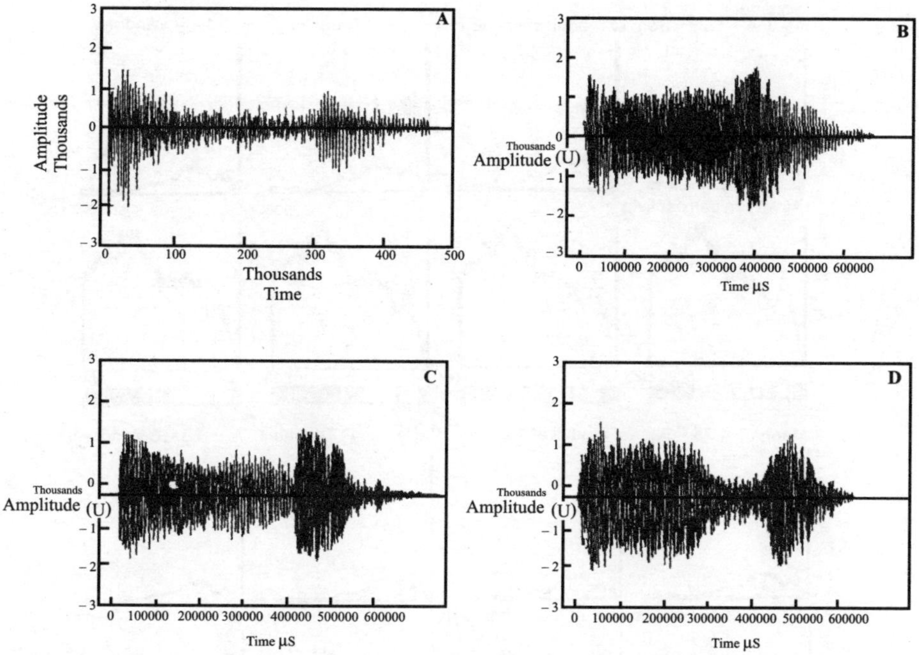

Fig. 2.13 Comparison of cough sound records: **A,** from a healthy volunteer; **B–D,** with cough sound records from three patients suffering from hyper-reactivity of airways. It may be noted that their records reveal chronic inflammation of the bronchi.

Thorpe and his collaborators[59] found that only one third of asthmatic patients have the second cough sound as compared to non-asthmatic subjects. Thus, the absence of the second sound can be considered as a sign of asthma. However, in our observations there was no connection between the presence of asthma and the absence of the second sound. In our view, to consider the presence of the second sound as a sign of asthma without a clinical examination is incorrect. The cough sound may, however, be a combination of one or two sounds which is a consequence of the glottis mechanism. Moreover, vibrations of lung tissue can also contribute to cough sound creation; this was demonstrated in cats in experimentally induced lung oedema.

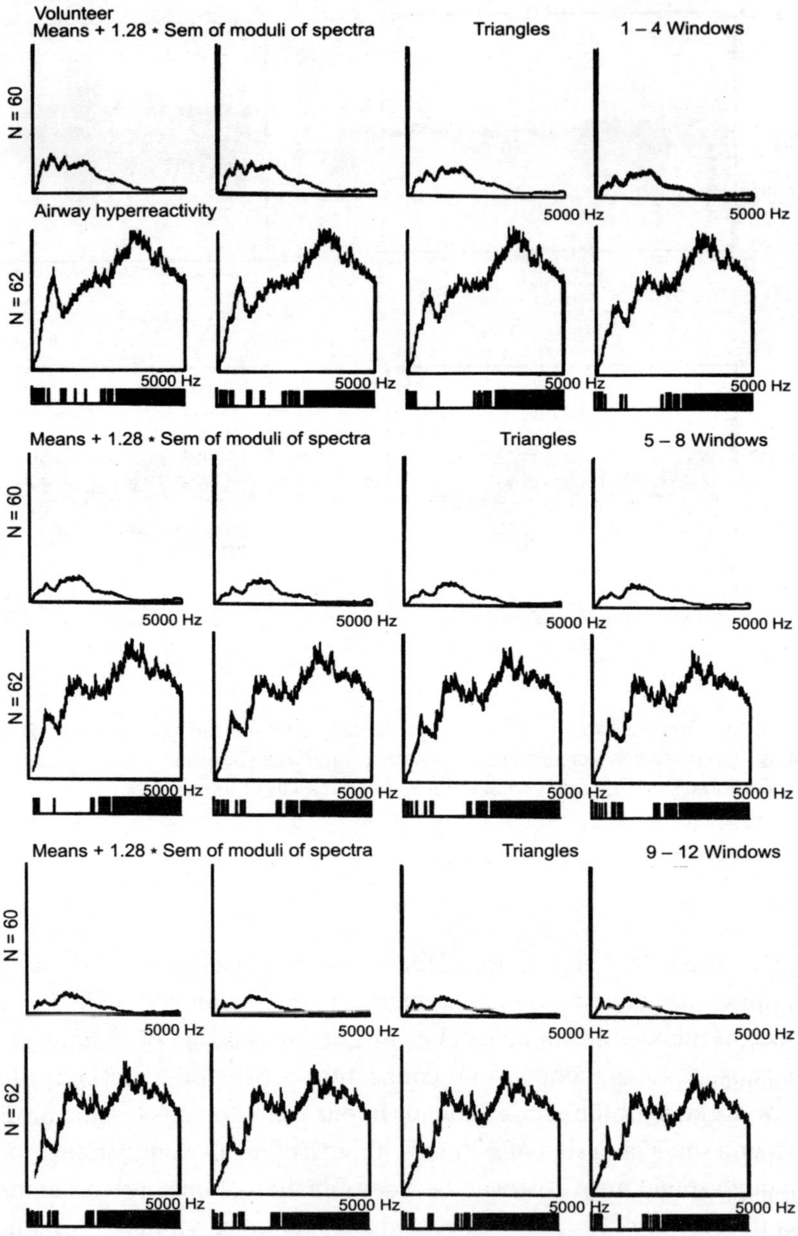

Fig. 2.14 Comparison of cough sound spectra from a healthy volunteer with that of 12 consecutive windows from a patient with airway hyper-reactivity. Sampling rate 12.500 Hz, time shift between windows 10.24 ms, bars indicate statistical significance ($p < 0.05$).

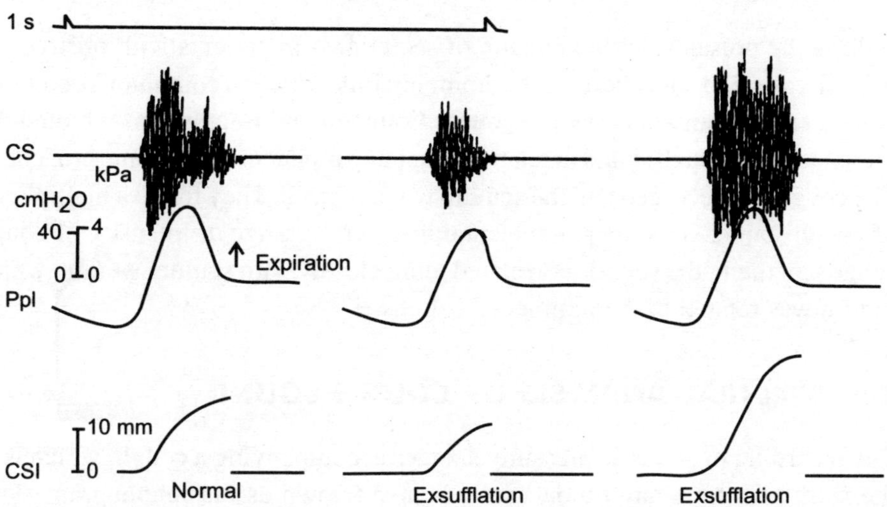

Fig. 2.15 Effect of exsufflations and insufflations of pig gastric mucin in cat airways and their comparison with normal situation. Records: time, 1 second time marks; CS, cough sound; Ppl, pleural pressure; CSI, integration cough sound intensity. (Reproduced from Ref. [11] with permission from Publisher)

2.4.6 Role of Mucus in Cough Sound Creation

With regard to the creation of pathological cough sounds, empirical evidence suggests that the main factor responsible for its production is the presence of mucus in the airways. It is well known in clinical practice that administration of mucolytics can lower or increase the intensity of the cough. This has been confirmed experimentally in response to administering natural, undiluted egg albumin or pig gastric mucin into the airways of anaesthetised cats. It produced obvious changes in the character of the cough sound and significantly increased its intensity and effort. Thereafter, the removal of the egg albumin or pig gastric mucin produced the opposite effects that is, a decrease in the sound (–41%) and intensity of effort (–52%) of the cough, simultaneously with changes in the character of cough sounds (Fig. 2.15). In cats, no clear-cut patterns of cough sounds, as in humans, have been described. Apart from this, it was interesting to note that unlike humans, the cough sound was often present not only during the expiratory phase but also during the inspiratory phase.[11]

Other authors emphasise the importance of mucus production for the cough sound creation, too.[59–61] Clinically, the quality of sounds produced by coughing reflects the presence and expulsion of secretions. In patients with obstructive lung disease, expectoration more commonly follows when continuous coughing is seen rather than after a single cough. Loundon and Baughman[60] studied the presence of the cough sound in relation to sputum production in chronic bronchitis. The cough was recorded and the sputum was collected. They found a multiplicity of cough sounds in some patients; and in others, a range of intensity of cough sounds. In them, the sounds correlated more closely with sputum weight, which in turn was related to the number of coughs.

2.5 SPECTRAL ANALYSIS OF COUGH SOUND

The recording of acoustic pressure changes accompanying a cough, which is in the form of a time-amplitude wave, is also known as tussiphonogram. This allows one to characterise the cough sound, intensity and duration. Furthermore, it also helps to predict whether the course of cough will be acute or chronic and to identify the damaged part of the respiratory tract from which the cough originates. The cough sound has another important property. It is the sound timbre, which can be quite distinct among coughs of different nosological units and typical for some of them. For example, a brassy or bitonal sound is so characteristic that it may suffice in itself for the diagnosis of lymphoid gland tuberculosis and bronchial compression.[38] A 'barking' type of cough is typical in subglottis stenosis. The deep, hollow and ringing cough sounds also come from the trachea. A metallic sound is due to congenital rigid stenosis of trachea. 'Whooping' is typical of pertussis infection.[38] The evaluation of various types of cough sound timbre serves spectral frequency analysis.

The cough sound timbre is determined by the fundamental frequency just as for the other sounds, which may be regarded as reflexely generated perturbations of respiratory functions, for example, sneezes, hiccoughs, and sighs. The fundamental frequency and its harmonics and overtones are produced by the narrowed parts in airways and by periodic vibrations of the vocal cords as a consequence of mechanical interaction between expired air and the vocal cords. The value of the fundamental frequency is defined by taking into consideration the ranges found by various authors, that is, from 300 to 700 Hz under normal conditions.[7,38,39,62,63]

Debreczeni et al[64] stated that the averaged spectra of the first voluntary sounds in healthy subjects shows two peaks at about 350 and 650 Hz. These peaks are nearly the same in the case of cough sounds recorded with or without

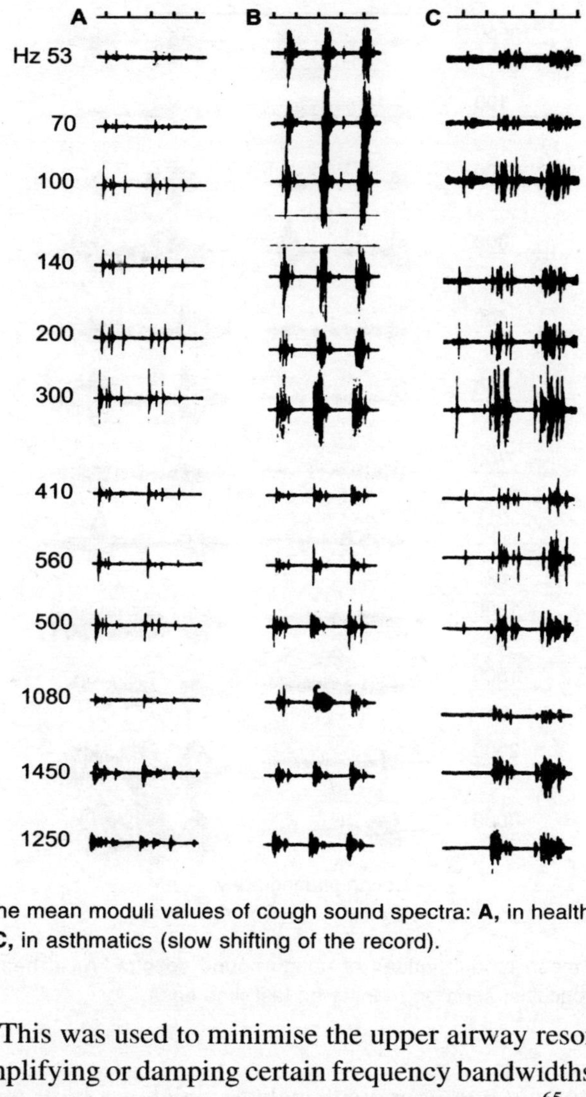

Fig. 2.16 The mean moduli values of cough sound spectra: **A,** in healthy subjects; **B,** in bronchitics; **C,** in asthmatics (slow shifting of the record).

a noise clip. This was used to minimise the upper airway resonator functions, that is, for amplifying or damping certain frequency bandwidths, which emerge in (resonating) cavities of the upper airways and the chest.[65] The fundamental frequencies and the overtones may deviate from normal in the case of pathological sound production.[38]

When the airflow is blocked, for example, an obstacle in some part of the respiratory tract produces a sound called 'noise'. Noise production may be independent from the sound producing function of larynx as in the case of respiratory noises, coughing, hoarseness, and pressed sounds.[38] Normally, any pathologically produced sounds may contain noises, quasi periodic vibrations

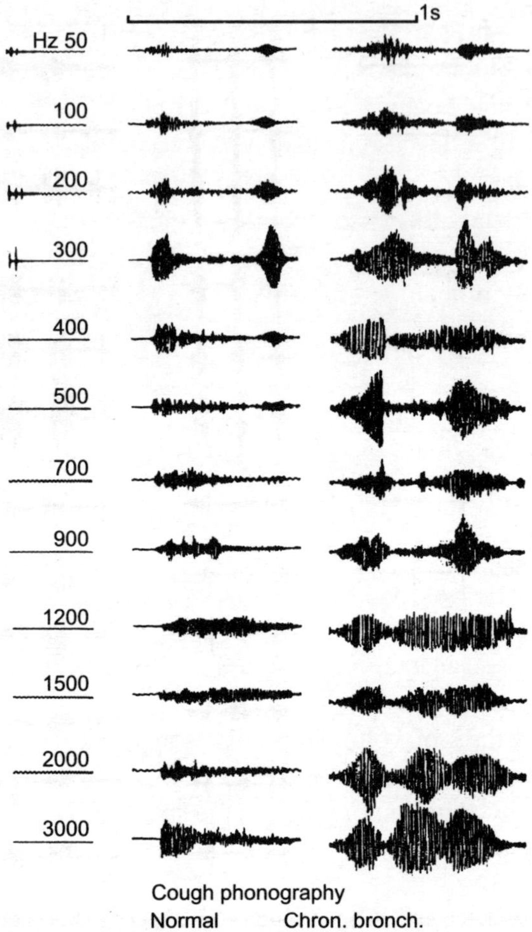

Fig. 2.17 The mean moduli values of cough sound spectra: **A,** in healthy subjects; **B,** those with bronchitis; seen on running on fast time base.

created by the tongue, uvula and soft palate, which are built up of voiceless bursts. The noise produced by turbulent flow of air at some constricted place of the tract, that is, when stenosis causes an increase in pressure and air can only escape by causing audible friction, then this noise resembling aspiration, is produced, or when in the airways there is transient stenosis followed by a moment of total obstruction and subsequent dilatation, the blocked air escapes causing a typical turbulent burst. This may also appear as typical coughing. Acoustically, this noise can be described as an increase in intensity of the noise bands followed by a decrease, precisely reflecting the concurrent mechanism of breathing.[38,39] The noise production may be independent of the quality of sound. However, normally any pathologically produced sound may contain noise, which is created by turbulent airflow in narrowed parts of the airway and its frequency can reach 20 kHz.[38,39]

One way to study the cough sound timbre is to assess the intensity band at several levels. We found that the frequencies 200, 300 and 500 Hz were the most expressive in healthy subjects (Fig. 2.16A); whereas in the cough of bronchitics, the width of all bands was increased and the frequencies 50–300 Hz were accentuated (Fig. 2.16B). In patients suffering from bronchial asthma, the changes had a similar character, but the registered frequencies were stronger at all levels of frequencies (Fig. 2.16C).

The differences between phonographic records of normal and pathological conditions can be seen clearly if run on a fast time base (Fig. 2.17).

The spectrogram of the voluntary cough in healthy volunteers was found to be relatively unchanged over 30 days of observation that it was seen for; there were only a few sporadic instances of a decrease in frequency intensity at 100, 140, and 200 Hz, and an increase in the intensity of frequency at 1,080 and 1,450 Hz.[66]

The mean values of voluntary cough sound spectra do not significantly change in bands from 40 to 1,450 Hz after administration of 30 mg codeine sulphate in healthy subjects for 2 hours; the spectrogram of control cough also remains unchanged.[66]

Olia et al[67] studied the FEV_1 values and cough spectrograms in 275 healthy non-smokers belonging to a similar age group. The subjects coughed towards a microphone at a distance of 70 cm. Cough was recorded using a personal computer with an A/D converter (sampling rate 10 kHz, 8-bit resolution) and divided into: a first part with the frequencies presenting rapid variations of energy, a second part with relatively stable frequencies (continuous bands, CB) and a third, which was an inconstant part. After digitisation, they analysed by FFT the first and second coughs of each bout. Analysing the intermediate continuous band (between lowest and highest continuous bands) and their percentage distribution with a step of 500 Hz, they found significant differences in males and females from 1001 to 1500 Hz (34% vs. 27.1%), 1501 to 2000 Hz (8.2 % vs. 18.5 %) and 2001 to 2500 Hz (27.5% vs. 15.6 %), in spite of there being the same number of continuous bands in males as well as in females (p = ns). The differences in percentage distribution are probably a consequence of anatomical

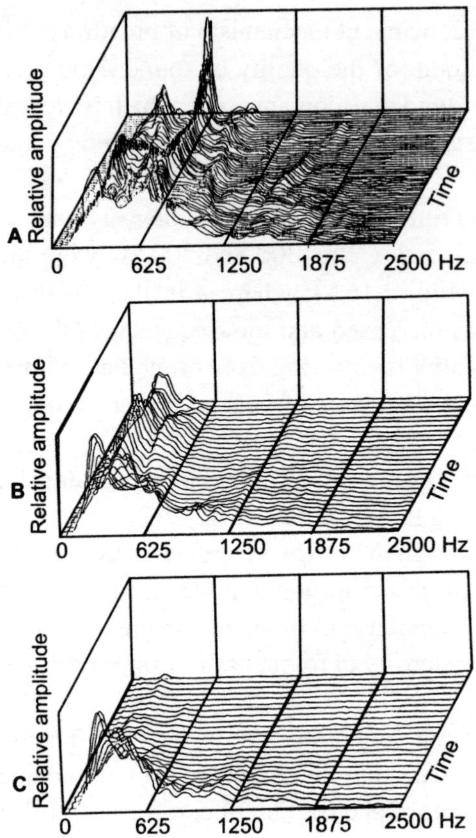

Fig. 2.18 The mean moduli (terminus techniques = from modulation = changes of basic oscillations of high-frequency of wave) values of cough sound spectra: **A,** in bronchitis (duration of 56 win. 102.40 ms, lengths of signal 576.0 ms, sampling frequency 11, 000 Hz); **B,** in healthy volunteers with double cough sound (duration of 29 win. 102.40 ms, time shift 12.80 ms, length of signal 460.80 ms); **C,** with mono cough sound (duration of 25 win. 102.40 ms, time shift 12.80 ms, length of signal 409.0 ms).

differences of the geometry of airways involved in the production and presence of cough.

Olia et al,[68] with further help of FFT analysis, performed a preliminary study investigating some acoustic parameters of spontaneous or voluntary cough. They studied patients with chronic lung disease. Ten to twenty coughs from each patient were recorded on tape and subsequently digitised in a personal computer with 8-bit resolution at a sampling rate of 20 kHz. These sounds were subjected to spectral analysis through short-time FFT on a sliding window of 256 samples (12.8 ms) with 50 per cent overlap between subsequent windows giving a time resolution of 6.4 ms. For each cough, they studied the morphology of time expanded waveform and spectrogram, duration, maximum frequency, frequency spectrum changes over time and acoustic energy distribution at various frequencies.

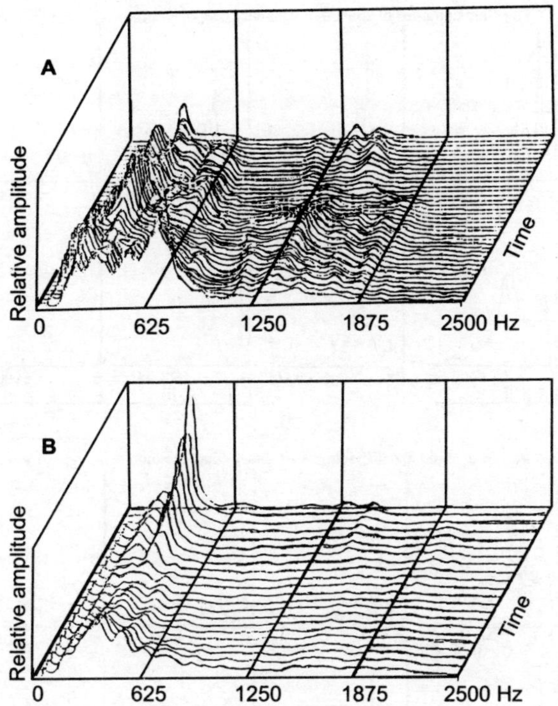

Fig. 2.19 Comparison of the mean moduli values of cough sound spectra: **A,** in adult asthmatics; **B,** with those of asthmatic children.

The cough sounds presented a marked heterogeneity either when heard casually or graphically or when plotted in terms of time or frequency. However, in most cases, it was possible to identify on the spectrogram, a first explosive phase characterised by a rapid transient increase in acoustic energy and also by rapid changes in energy content at various frequencies, which were followed by a second part where acoustic energy changed more slowly and the frequency distribution remained relatively stable. The explosive part was significantly shorter (95 ± 4 ms) than the constant part (302 ± 14 ms), and had a significantly lower peak (876 ± 55 vs. 1079 ± 63 Hz) and median (1546 ± 3 vs. 1763 ± 68 Hz) frequencies. Olia and his collaborators[68] infer from these results that inter- and intra-heterogeneity of the characteristics of cough sound may create a severe obstacle in the development of a reliable method of cough detection based on acoustic parameters.

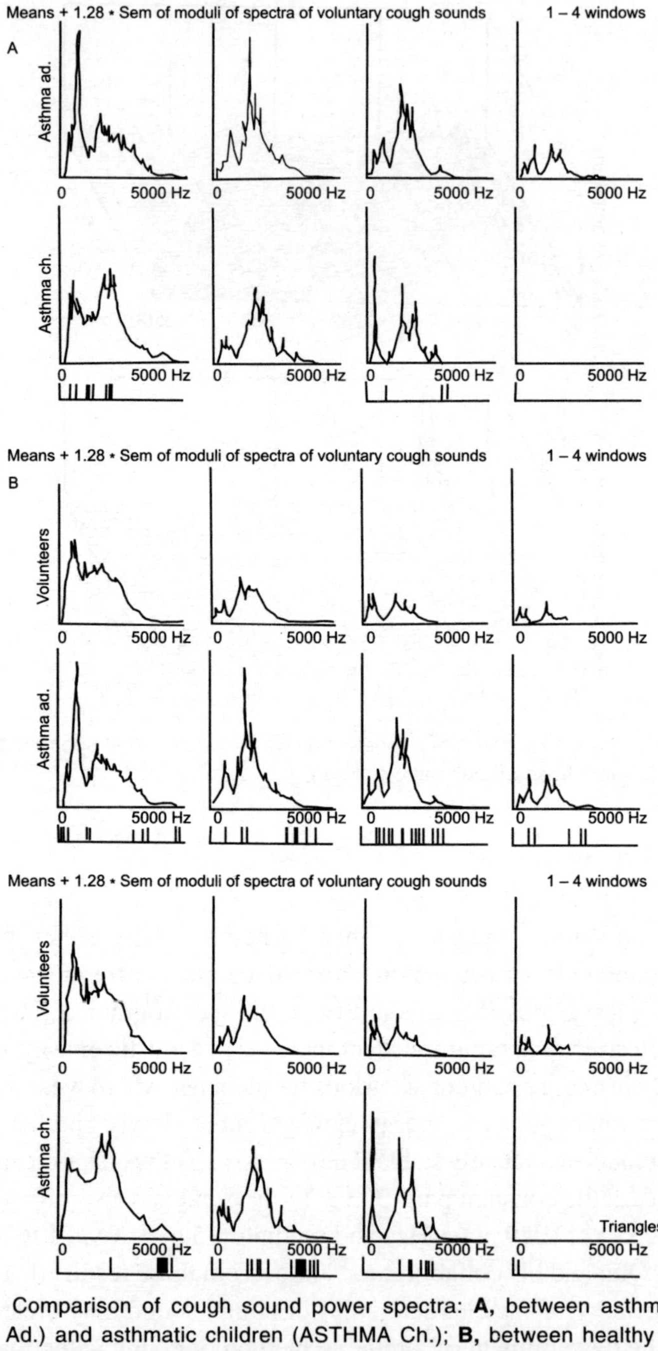

Fig. 2.20 Comparison of cough sound power spectra: **A,** between asthmatic adults (ASTHMA Ad.) and asthmatic children (ASTHMA Ch.); **B,** between healthy volunteers (VOLUNTEERS) and asthmatic adults (ASTHMA Ad.); **C,** between healthy volunteers (VOLUNTEERS) and asthmatic children (ASTHMATIC Ch.).

Distribution of acoustic frequencies of cough in COPD patients after bronchodilators therapy showed a wider and more homogeneous percentage distribution of continuous bands on the spectrogram.[69] Piirila and Sovijarvi[70] saw that the spectrograms of the sound of spontaneous cough of asthmatics were characterised by duration of a prolonged wheezing sound and by lower frequency than those of patients with chronic bronchitis and tracheobronchial collapse syndrome. For comparison, we present the mean modular spectra of cough sounds of patients suffering from chronic bronchitis (males and females) (Fig. 2.18A) in relation to differences in cough sound spectra of healthy volunteers (mean values of the double sound and the monosound.).

2.6 ANALYSIS OF COUGH SOUND FREQUENCY IN ADULTS AND CHILDREN WITH BRONCHIAL ASTHMA

The timbre of cough sound may be typical and characteristic in some diseases of the airways and lungs. The sound timbre is determined by its frequency, the distribution of which varies in different pathological conditions. If it is properly identified, it could be of value for diagnosis. The only problem is that cough sound frequency considerably varies between subjects and within coughs from the same subject. In spite of this conclusion, we were curious about the characteristic patterns of cough sound in those who suffered from bronchial asthma.

Bronchial asthma in adults and children used to be diagnosed on the basis of clinical criteria.[71–73] The patients examined were stable clinically and on a given regimen of medication and were selected from a group of 200 asthmatics with approximately similar levels of disease and therapy (corticoids and individually specific bronchodilators). Voluntary cough was recorded on tape and digitalised in a personal computer with 8-bit resolution at a sampling rate of 10 Hz. The sounds were subjected to spectral analysis through FFT on an overlapping window of 256 samples (12.8 ms). The method was basically identical to those published.[41,44,74,75] Experiments were conducted to evaluate the energy spent in coughing by integrating the power spectrum in the frequency domain from 50 to 2500 Hz. The frequency distribution was compared between asthmatics and healthy volunteers (without signs of chest infection). The results showed that the intensity of frequencies increased in 3 to 4 waves over a frequency span ranging from 100 to 900 Hz (elevation of amplitude) (Fig. 2.19A). The intensity of frequencies decreased afterwards. They appeared again between 1000 and

2000 Hz in further spectra, but with lower amplitudes of frequencies, the sound signal was about 64 per cent longer in adult asthmatics than in asthmatic children. The range of frequencies was larger in asthmatic children versus asthmatic adults; asthmatic adults versus healthy volunteers and asthmatic children versus healthy volunteers.

The spectrogram in children had a smoother course during the first part of spectrum and a smaller elevation of amplitude than before, during the last part of spectrum (Fig. 2.19B). That means the spectrum in children resembled the spectrum in adults. The visual similarity was also statistically confirmed. The power spectra compared among asthmatics showed only sporadic statistical differences, only about 1 per cent (Fig. 2.20A). On the other hand, comparison of power spectra of adult asthmatics with those of healthy volunteers showed pronounced, statistically significant increases of about 40 per cent (Fig. 2.20B). The differences between percentages are also statistically significant. The power spectra also increased when comparing asthmatic children with healthy volunteers, that of asthmatic children being in the third window (Fig. 2.20C).

Despite all our efforts, we did not find many characteristic changes in the sound spectrum, which could be utilised for establishing differential diagnosis.

2.7 THE SENSITIVITY OF TUSSIPHONOGRAPHY FOR ASSESSING THE EFFECTIVENESS OF TREATMENT

Our previous studies have demonstrated that the tussiphonogram is suitable not only for the detection of pathological conditions in the respiratory tract but also for the assessment of the effectiveness of treatment. We were curious about the possibility of detecting the small pathological changes in the airways and lungs by tussiphonography. Therefore, the changes of voluntary cough sound indices were compared with pulmonary function tests in selected group of asthmatics before and after a pulsatile electromagnetic therapy in which the effect of therapy on pulmonary function tests was minimal. After magnetotherapy in patients, expiratory forced lung capacity was increased by 7.3 per cent and peak expiratory flow by 31.7 per cent; on an average the voluntary cough sound intensity decreased by 37.9 per cent, the sound duration shortened by 11 per cent and the sound pattern showed a tendency to normalisation. However, these cough indices did not improve with magnetotherapy in those patients who suffered from respiratory viral infections also or those treated only with climatotherapy or antiasthmatic drugs. Changes of flow volume loops in these patients did not bear as close a relationship as did other indices. The correlation analysis showed a functional connection in relative differences of cough sound indices and some pulmonary function tests. The results confirmed the suitability of tussiphonography as an indicator of even mild pathological changes in respiratory tract.[76]

2.8 CONCLUSION

In spite of various findings in spectral analysis, no specific indices that could diagnose asthma or other nosological units have yet been found. Such an indication could be of great clinical interest and merits for further investigation.

REFERENCES

1. Sant' Ambrogio G. An airway defensive reflex. In: Andrews P, Widdicombe J, editors. Pathology of the gut and airways. London, Chapel Hill: Portland Press, 1993;pp89–96.
2. Widdicombe JG. Symposium in the cough reflex-Summary. Bulletin Europėen de Physiopathologie Respiratoire 1987;23(Suppl 10):73–4.
3. Korpas J, Tomori Z. Cough and other respiratory reflexes. Basel, Munchen, Paris, New York, Sydney: Karger; 1979;p356.
4. Widdicombe JG. Physiology of cough. In: Braga PC, Allegra L, editors. Cough. New York: Raven Press; 1989;pp2–25.
5. Widdicombe JG, Chung F. Cough: pharmacology and therapy. Pulmonary Pharmacology and Therapeutics 2002;15:185–6.
6. Leith DE, Butler JP, Sneddon SL, Brain JD. Cough. In: Macklem PT, Head J, editors. Handbook of Physiology, Vol.3, the Respiratory System. Part 1. Bethesda: American Physiological Society; 1986;p.316–36.
7. Braga PC, Allegra L. Cough. New York: Raven Press, 1989;p244.
8. Leith DE. Cough. In: Proctor DF, Reid IM, editors. Respiratory Defence Mechanisms. Part 2. New York: Dekker, 1977; pp585–92.
9. Korpas J, Sadlonova J, Salát D, Masarova E. The origin of the cough sounds. Bulletin Europėen de Physiopathologie Respiratoire 1987;23(Suppl. 10):47–50.
10. Piirila P. Acoustic properties of cough and crackling lung sounds in patients with pulmonary diseases. Dissertation Medical. Faculty of the University of Helsinky. Chest 1989;96:46–53.
11. Korpas J, Widdicombe JG, Vrabec M. Influence of simulated mucus on cough sounds in cats. Respiratory Medicine 1993;87:49–54.
12. Korpas J, Widdicombe JG, Vrabec M, Kudlicka J. Effect of experimental lung oedema on cough sound creation. Respiratory Medicine 1993;87:55–59.
13. Piirila P, Sovojarvi ARA. Objective assessment of cough. European Respiratory Journal 1995;8:1949–56.
14. Morice AH. The epidemiology of chronic cough. In: Korpas J, Widdicombe JG, editors. Cough: recent advances in understanding. European Respiratory Review 2002;12(85):222–5.

15. Mazzone SB, Canning BJ. Plasticity of the cough reflex. In: Korpas J, Widdicombe JG, editors. Cough: recent advances in understanding. European Respiratory Review 2002;12(85):136–242.
16. Ashurst L, Smith JA, Jack S, Woodcock AA, Earis JE. Subjective recognition of coughs sounds by respiratory professionals. European Respiratory Journal 2003;172.
17. Bullar JF. Experiments to determine the origin of the respiratory sounds.
18. Martini P, Mueller H. Studien ueber das Bronchialatmen. Deutche Archive fur Klinikal Medicine 1923;143:159–71.
19. Cabot RC, Dodge HF. Frequency characteristics of heart and lung sounds. Journal of the American Medical Association 1925;84:1793–5.
20. Korpas J, Sadlonova J, Vrabec M. Analysis of cough sound: an overview. Pulmonary Pharmacology 1996;9:261–8.
21. Korpas J, Tomori Z. Cough. Karger Gazette 1980;40:6–7.
22. Kohts O. Experimentale Untersuchungen uber den Husten. Virchows Archive fur Pathologischen Anatomie 1984;60:191–216.
23. Hogyes E. Kiserletek a kohogesrol. Orvosi Hetilap 1875;19:148–50.
24. Coryllos PN. Action of the diaphragm in cough: experimental and clinical study in the human. American Journal of the Medical Sciences 1937;194:523–35.
25. Hoglund NJ, Michaelson M. A method for determining the cough threshold with some preliminary experiments on the effect of codeine. Acta Physiologica Scandinavica 1950;21:168–73.
26. Ross B, Gramiak R, Rahn H. Physical dynamics of cough mechanism. Journal of Applied Physiology 1955;8:264–8.
27. Bickermann HA, Itkin SE. The effect of a new bronchodilator aerosol on airflow dynamics of the maximal voluntary cough of patients with bronchial asthma and pulmonary emphysema. Journal of Chronic Diseases 1958;8:629–36.
28. Calesnic B, Christensen JA, Munch JC. Antitussive action of proporyphene in citric acid induced cough response. The American Journal of Medical Sciences 1961;242:560–4.
29. Schmidt-Voigt J. Husten ALS Leitsymptom bei inneren Erkrankungen. Munchen: Lehman Verlag; 1962; p111.
30. Leiner GC, Abramowitz S, Small MJ, Stenby J. Cough peak flow rate. American Review of Respiratory Diseases 1967;96:666–77.
31. Langlands J. The dynamic of cough in health and chronic bronchitis. Thorax 1967;22:88–95.
32. Friebel H. Experimenteller Husten. In: Eichler O, Farah A, Herken H, Welch AD, editors. Handbuch der experimentellen Pharmakologie. Vol.XVI/2. Berlin, Heidelberg, New York: Springer Verlag 1969;p19–76.
33. Nemerovskij LI. Pulmofonografija. Moskva: Medicina 1981;p158.
34. Yanagihara N, Leden H, Werner-Kukuk E. The physical parameters of cough. The Larynx in a normal single cough. Acta otolaryngologica 1966;61:495–509.
35. Braga PC, Allegra L. Clinical methods for the study of cough. In: Braga PC, Allegra L, editors. Cough. New York: Raven Press 1989;p73–93.
36. Renovanz H, Rench H. Tussometrie. Munchen Diesenhofen: Dusti Verlag 1979;p102.
37. Kelemen SA, Cseri T. Die Phonetik des willkurlichen Hustens. Atemwege und Lungen Krankheiten 1981;7(4):222–5.
38. Hirschberg J, Szende T. Pathological cry, stridor and cough in infants. Budapest: Akademiai Kiado, 1982;p156.

39. Korpas J, Sadlonova-Korpasova J. Cough registration in men. Folia Medica Martiniana 1984;10(1):167–93.
40. Korpas J, Sadlonova J, Salat D, Debreczeni LA. Tussiphonography: A new tool for diagnosis of airway inflammation. Proceedings of Ist High Tatras International Health Symposium. In: Salat D et al, editors. Health and quality of life in changing Europe in year 2000. New York, Bratislava, Tatranska Polianka; Symposium International, 1992;252–7.
41. Subburaj S,Hirtum AV, Quanten, Berkmans D. An algorithm to automatically identify coughs sounds from clinical recordings. European Respiratory Journal 2003;172.
42. Kelemen SA. Cseri T. The phonetics of voluntary cough. Acta Physiologica Academiae Scientiarum Hungaricae 1980;10:595–608.
43. Mussel MJ. The need for standards in recording and analysing respiratory sound. Medical and Biological Engineering and Comparation 1992;30:129–39.
44. Subburaj S, Pervez L, Rajagopalan TG. Methods of recording and analysing cough sounds. Pulmonary Physiology 1996;9:269–79.
45. Leith DE, Butter JP, Sneedom SL, Brain JD. Cough. In: Handbook of Physiology. Sect III. The Respiratory System. Bethesda, MD: American Physiological Society, 1986;pp.315–36.
46. Salat D, Saratoga V, Korpasova-Sadlonova J, Palecek D. Changes in cough sound of voluntary cough in acetylcholine induced obstruction of the airways. Bratislavske lekarske Listy 1986;85:466–71.
47. Leden H, Isshiki N. An analysis of cough at the level of larynx. Acta oto-laryngologica 1965;81:616–25.
48. Korpas J, Sadlonova J, Salat D, Masarova E. The origin of cough sound. Clinical Respirology Physiology 1987;23(10):40–50.
49. Korpas J, Salat D, Sadlonova J, Vrabec M, Kudlicka J. The sensitivity of tussiphonography for assessing the effectiveness of treatment. Bratislavské lekárske Listy 2000;101(2):71–7.
50. Wohlrabe H. Tussometrie mit integration und kehlkopfmikrofon. In: Renovanz H, Rensch H. editors. Tussometrie. Munchen Diesenhoffen: Dusti Verlag, 1979;p.67–74.
51. Gravenstein JS, Beecher HK. Ein beitrag zur auswertung hustendampfender substanzen am menchen. Arzneimittel Forshung; 1955;364–7.
52. Ruhle KH, Matthys H. Fergleich zweier antitussiva mittels. Tussometrie. In: Renovanz HD, Rensch H. editors, Tussometrie. Munchen, Dresdenhoffen: Dusti Verlag; 1979;p.102.
53. Franta M. Stationare Hustenuberwachung mit Kehlkopfmikrophon und verfahren zur ambulanten Hustenuberwachung. In: Renovanz HD, Rensch H. editors, Tussometrie. Munchen, Diesenhoffen: Dusti Verlag; 1979;p.102.
54. Wieser O. Erfahrungen mit zwei tussometrie anlagen. In: Renovanz HD, Rensch H, editors. Tussometrie. Munchen Diesenhoffen: Dusti Verlag; 1979;p.102.
55. Renovanz HD. Methoden der Tussometrie. In: Renovanz HD, Rensch H. editors. Tussometrie. Munchen Diesenhoffen: Dusti Verlag; 1979;p.102.
56. Weist FR. Beitrag uber den Einsatz einer Hustenuberachungsanlage in der Klinik in der Theorie zur Praxis. In: Renovanz HD, Rensch H, editors. Tussimetrie. Munchen Diesenhofen: Dusti Verlag, 1979.
57. Korpas J, Vrabec M, Sadlonova J. Comparison of chemically induced cough sounds. In: Salat et al, editors. Proceedings of 3rd High Tatras International. Health Symposium. Tatranska Polianka; Symposium International, 1994;pp147–51.
58. Korpas J, Kelemen AS. Tussiphonographic analysis of coughs sound recordings performed by Schmidt-Voigt and Hirschberg and Szende. Acta Physiologica Hungarica 1987;70:167–70.

59. Thorpe CW, Toop LJ, Dawson KP. Towards a quantitative description of asthmatic cough sounds. European Respiratory Journal 1962;5:685–92.
60. Loundon RG, Baughman RP. Sounds of cough associated with sputum production in chronic bronchitis. European Respirology 1993;6(17):415.
61. Forster WM. Mucus secretion and mucus clearance in cough. In: Chung KF, Widdicombe JG, Boushey HA, editors Cough: causes, mechanisms and therapy London, San Francisko: Blackwell; 2003;pp.207–16.
62. Debreczeni LA, Korpas J, Vertes Ch. Sadlonova J, Radich K, Laszlo A. Role of spectral analysis of the voluntary cough sounds in screening. Proceedings of 1st High Tatras International Health Symposium. Editors Salat D, Badalik L, Krcmery V, editors. New York, Bratislava, Tatranska Polianka; Symposium International, 1992;256–71.
63. Debreczeni LA., Korpas J, Salat D, Korpasova-Sadlonova J, Vertes Ch, Masarova E, Kavcova E. Spectra of the voluntary first cough sounds. Acta Physiologica Hungarica 1990;75:117–31.
64. Debreczeni LA, Korpas J, Salat D. Spectral analysis of cough sound recorded with and without a nose clip. Clinical Respirology Physiology 1987;23 (10):57–61.
65. Otis AB. Two functions of breathing, respiration and sound production. In: Lenfant C, editor. Lung Biology in Health and Disease. Vol. 25. New York: Marcel Dekker; 1988;519–34
66. Korpas J, Nosalova G. Dalsie poznatky o tusifonografii. Ceskoslovenskáfy-siologie 1981;30:3–4.
67. Olia PM, Sestini P, Vagliasindi M. Acoustic parameters of voluntary cough. In healthy non-smoking subjects. Respirology 2000; 5:271–5.
68. Olia PM, Sestini P, Rossi M, Triscari F, Vagliasindi M. Acoustic parameters of cough in chronic lung diseases. European Respiratory Journal 1993;6(17):P0209.
69. Olia PM, Sestini P, Vagliasindi M. Distribution of acoustic frequencies of cough in COPD patients before and after bronchodilator therapy. Eur Respir J 2000;16(31):p671.
70. Piirila P, Sovijarvi ARA. Differences in acoustic and dynamic characteristics of spontaneous cough in pulmonary diseases. Chest 1984;96:46–53.
71. International Consensus Report on Diagnosis and Treatment of Asthma. National Heart, Lung and Blood Instistute, National Institutes of Health, Bethesda Maryland 20892. European Respiratory Journal 1992;5:601–41.
72. Siafakas NM. ERS Consensus Statement: optimal assessment and management of chronic obstructive pulmonary disease. European Respiratory Review 1996;6(39):270–5.
73. Lenfant C. Global initiative for asthma. National Heart, Lung and Blood Institute, London, 1998;p28.
74. Earis JE, Cheetham BMG. Current methods used for computerized respiratory sounds. European Respiratory Review 2000;77:586–70.
75. Olia PM, Sestini P, Vagliasindi M. Distribution of acoustic frequencies of cough in healthy subjects. European Respiratory Journal 2000;16 (31):3905.
76. Sadlonova J, Korpas J, Salat D, Vrabee M. Possibilities to observe pathological conditions of the airways on the basis of tussifonography. Proceedings—Ist High Tatras International Health Symposium—Health and quality of life in changing Europe in the year 2000;258–65.

3 Expiration Reflex

J Korpas

3.1 INTRODUCTION

Expiration reflex is an airway defensive response characterised by a brief, intense expiratory effort, which is coordinated with adduction and abduction of the vocal folds. This reflex is different from cough, in that there is no preceding inspiratory effort or typical cough sounds. It is possible to elicit it by mechanical or chemical stimulation of the vocal folds of both humans and laboratory animals.[1–4,52] The role of expiration reflex is to prevent the penetration of foreign materials into the lower airways and to remove mucus and debris from the subglottic area.

Like the cough reflex, the expiration reflex, too, can be divided into three phases.[5] The first comprehensive phase is characterised by a simultaneous increase in abdominal and expiratory intercostal muscle activity and the contraction of laryngeal adductor muscles associated with narrowing of the glottis. This coordinated muscle activity results in an increase in intrathoracic pressure. The second, or expulsive, phase is marked by decreased glottal resistance due to relaxation of the adductor and contraction of the abductor muscles along with continued activity in the expiratory pump muscles. In the third phase, that is, constrictive, the expiratory pump muscle activity is decreased and the laryngeal adductor activity and the laryngeal resistance is increased.[4]

The sensory receptors responsible for the expiration reflex are located deep in the mucosa of the vocal fold margins, and belong to the group of rapidly adapting receptors. They are relatively few in number and this can explain

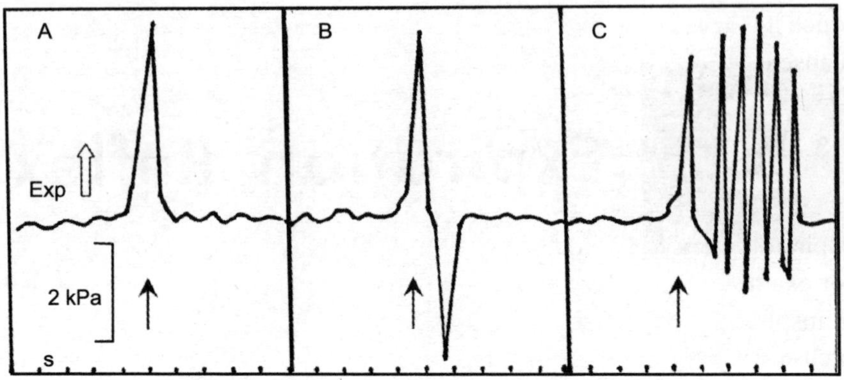

Fig. 3.1 A fit of coughing or a single expiratory effort with or without an initial inspiratory effort seen in an anaesthetised cat: **A,** a typical expiration reflex; **B,** expiration reflex followed by an inspiratory effort; **C,** spontaneous coughing.

their stability in pathological conditions of the laryngeal area.[1,6,7] In laboratory animals, laryngeal afferent fibres travel in the superior laryngeal nerve and project to various subnuclei of the caudal nucleus and of the tractus solitarius.[8,9] In humans, the afferents run mainly in the recurrent laryngeal nerve.[10] Baeky et al[10] have described the connections, through which the nucleus tractus solitarius second-order neurons distribute afferent information to the medullary respiratory network.

3.2 DISCOVERY OF THE EXPIRATION REFLEX

Nearly 30 years ago, we observed that in anaesthetised cats, the insertion of a nylon fibre through a tiny opening in the trachea and stimulation of the laryngeal mucosa by it evoked either a fit of coughing or a single expiratory effort with or without an initial inspiratory effort (Fig. 3.1). The later response was unexpected, as according to Bucher and Jacot,[11] the initial inspiration is a physiological requirement of the cough effort and without this, cough cannot be expected to occur. However, our investigation yielded that an intense stimulation can elicit expiratory efforts, and that the preceding inspiratory effort is not necessary[1,3] and that this airway defence reflex was hitherto unknown. We, therefore, defined this as a mechanical stimulation of laryngeal mucosa by which it is possible to elicit an expiratory effort even when the inspiratory effort is absent.[12]

3.3 INDEPENDENT EXPIRATORY EFFORTS DESCRIBED IN LITERATURE

Expiratory efforts without a preceding inspiration have also been described. For example, Stehaelin[13] found that almost every cough effort is preceded by an inspiration. In anaesthetised dogs, when the cough stimulus is sufficiently intense, a subsequent expiratory effort is not necessary for eliciting an expiration reflex.[13] In anaesthetised dogs, Kandarazki[14] recorded independent expiratory efforts between cough attacks after applying pressure, on the larynx from the outside (with fingers) or by electrical stimulation of the superior laryngeal nerve in dogs. He did not consider this as an independent reflex and he did not specify why it was so. Expiratory efforts were visible only from records. Widdicombe[15] recorded single expirations from mechanical stimulation of the trachea of cat. Pressmann and Kelemen[16] also observed a similar phenomenon after stimulation of the proximal and the superior laryngeal nerve in cats. Korpas and Tomori[17] described spontaneous 'expiratory gasping' in cats during hypothermia. Kuhn and Friebel[18] found that a pronounced inspiration is not essential for giving rise to the cough 'expiratory efforts'. Trendelenburg[19] described independent expiratory efforts in humans after exposure to sulphur dioxide (SO_2). Kade and Bucher[20,21] observed single expiratory efforts after mechanical stimulation of the laryngeal fossa in pigeons. They considered these phenomena as a specific expiratory activity, but not cough. We do not find any similarity between these phenomena and the expiration reflex except that both consist of expiratory efforts.

3.4 EXPIRATION REFLEX IN CATS

Independent expiratory efforts have also been observed in conscious cats. The strength of expiratory efforts recorded through intrapleural pressure changes equalled the strength of bronchial cough. In conscious cats, the intensity of independent expiratory efforts was ten times higher than that in anaesthetised cats. On the other hand, the incidence of expiratory phenomena followed by subsequent cough attacks were six times more frequent in anaesthetised animals than in conscious ones. Therefore, we have been focusing on these reflexes, which we do not consider as typical cough. We undertook to locate the receptive fields from which these independent expiratory efforts appear to originate, by stimulating the mucosa of vocal folds, larynx and epiglottal area of anaesthetised cats. The most effective site for evoking expiratory efforts was found to be the medial margin of the vocal folds. This finding indicates that there is a high concentration of sensory receptors in this area, which could be responsible for eliciting this reflex. Stimulation of the vocal folds was always effective when a small loop of nylon fibre was used. This produced a double expiratory effort, possibly because it would have stimulated two closely situated receptor sites, or produced two stimulations with a short refractory phase.[22,23]

We observed that an independent expiratory effort was sometimes followed by a deep inspiration (Fig 3.1B). At other times, it was followed by a cough attack (Fig 3.1C). These variations were, however, independent of the intensity of stimulation.

The stimulus is most effective when applied to the medial margin of the vocal folds in experimental animals and least effective when applied to the laryngeal part, that is, distal to the vocal folds and the epiglottal area. We did not observe any independent expiratory efforts as described by Tomori and Stránsky[22] in spite of repeated stimulations of the nasal and pharyngeal mucosa. In addition to seeing it in cats, independent expiratory efforts can also be elicited in other laboratory animals such as mice, rat rabbits, guinea, pigs, ferrets, and dogs.[1,2,24,37,50,52]

3.5 DIFFERENTIATION OF EXPIRATION REFLEX FROM COUGH REFLEX

Although Widdicombe[25] considers the expiration reflex as a 'fragment of cough, but it has to be pointed that apart from differences in the physiological properties of the two reflexes, the function of cough is more complicated and amongst others, it is to keep the airways and lungs clear of mucus and debris.

Repeated administration of 10 mg of codeine per kg body weight to anaesthetised cats, inhibited cough that seemed to arise from the tracheobronchial region, but it did not affect independent respiratory (expiratory) efforts that were still present. This was seen in both conscious cats and in those in whom anaesthesia (thiopental) had been increased. In the latter case, cough diminished but mechanical stimulation still evoked independent expiratory efforts.[26] This observation confirms that the cough reflex and expiration reflex are not identical.

3.6 ROLE OF EXPIRATION REFLEX

The role of the 'expiration reflex' which is a vigorous expiratory effort elicited mechanically or chemically from the vocal folds,[26] is to prevent invasion of foreign bodies into the airways and to expel phlegm and debris from the subglottal area, thus ensuring continuous airflow. It can be considered as belonging to a class of defensive airway reflexes, which have as yet not been described.[22,23,25]

3.7 OTHER PROPERTIES OF EXPIRATION REFLEX

Expiratory efforts resembling the expiratory reflex can also be seen after stimulating different parts of the airways, but a uniformly similar response is not always produced from these sites. In other words, the site from which it originates changes, as does its intensity when it actually appears. They can, thus, not be regarded as being the same as an expiration reflex.[1] Identifying the essential differences between cough and expiratory reflexes was not possible until pneumotachographic studies became available. These showed that in the latter case, the expiratory airflow and air volume increased, but before a significant change could occur in them, their values fell to that of normal respiration.[1,22]

Expiratory reflex can be elicited not only by mechanical stimulation of the vocal folds but also by electrical stimulation of the superior laryngeal nerve.[27–30] Chemical stimulation can also be effective and this can be seen after administration of intranasal xylene vapours in anaesthetised rabbits.[31] In dogs, it was possible to see the expiratory reflex after squirting water into the larynx or by a small balloon positioned in the rostral tracheal segment.[32,33]

It may be noted that the expiration reflex may be elicited independently of the phase of respiratory cycle,[22,23,34,35] although, it is best seen in late inspiration or early expiration as confirmed by Holmer et al.[29] Moreover, it is superimposed on the respiratory generator and 'cough centre', where it interrupts inspiratory or expiratory airflow. When it appears along with cough, it never merges into it but always precedes it[1,3,32] (Fig. 3.2).

Ontogenetic studies have revealed that the reflex appears in the first few days after birth in cats, when sneezing and coughing from tracheobronchial tree are still absent.[36] This was also seen in newborn rats (first day),[37] although the respiratory response from the bronchi (rats lack cough reflex) was present only after the 15th day.[1,37]

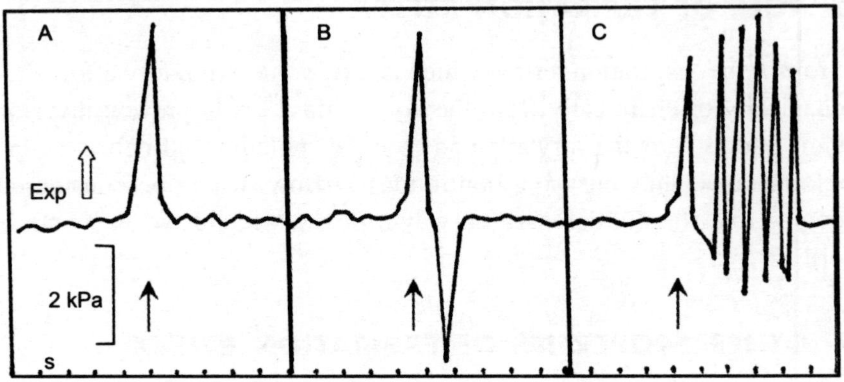

Fig. 3.2 Comparison of the expiration reflex (ER) with tracheobronchial cough (TBC) evoked by touching the vocal fold margin and the tracheobronchial mucosa of the bronchial bifurcation (mechanical stimulation), in an anaesthetised cat. The initial inspiratory effort is lacking in ER in contrast to TBC. V′, flow rates; P_{tp}, transpulmonary pressure.

Sullivan et al[32,33] provided further evidence about differences in cough and the expiration reflex. During the state of wakefulness, irritant laryngeal stimuli caused cough, expiration reflex, and tracheal smooth muscle contraction. During slow wave sleep or rapid eye movement sleep, these responses disappeared, except for the expiration reflex. Similarly, we found a different response during progressive isobaric hypoxia, when the expiration reflex markedly diminished during the early stages of hypoxia ($FO_2 = 0.11$), whereas laryngeal and bronchial cough were well present until more marked hypoxia ($FO_2 = 0.07$).[38]

3.8 EXPIRATION REFLEX IN HUMANS

In humans, this reflex has the typical features that are seen in animals. Unlike cough, it consists of a single expiratory effort without a preceding inspiration (Fig. 3.3). It has a typical barking-like sound, which is very distinct from the cough sound. It can be elicited clearly by touching the vocal folds with a nylon fibre, nylon fibre loop, or thin catheter or by spraying distilled water, after anaesthesia of the oral, pharyngeal and epiglottal mucosa or during laryngeoscopy.[39–43]

The effect of a vigorous expiratory effort after the vocal folds are touched either with a laryngoscope or with a droplet of local anaesthesia is very well

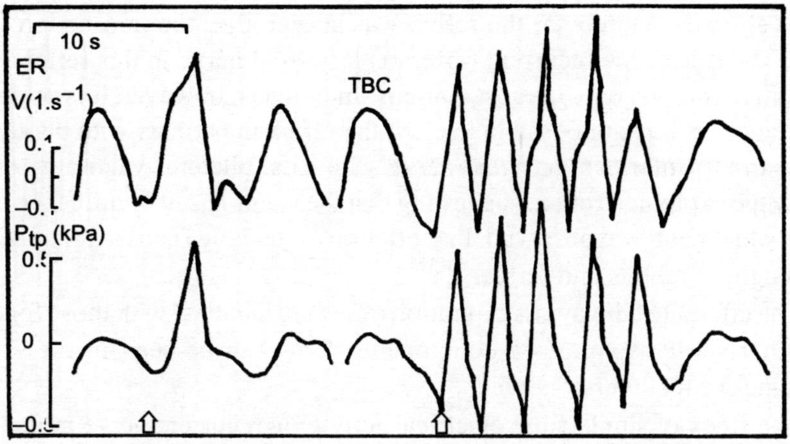

Fig. 3.3 Comparison of expiration reflex (ER) with cough reflex (CR) in a subject. The ER was elicited mechanically during laryngoscopy, after local anaesthesia and it was followed by a spontaneous cough.

known in laryngology and anaesthesiology,[39] but it is always regarded as a cough from the larynx.

3.9 REFLEX ARC OF EXPIRATION REFLEX

Many nerve endings have been seen in the mucosa of the vocal folds and the larynx using light microscopy. Unfortunately, these receptors have neither correlated with any reflex function[44–46] nor have there been any reports of detailed studies of this area using electron microscopy or immunofluorescent techniques. In an electron microscopic investigation of the epithelium of the vocal cord carried out by us,[6] we found no new nerve endings that were distinguishable from those, whose structure and function were already known. This has led us to conclude these also mediate the expiration reflex in animals and man (Fig. 3.3). However, we found some identifiable receptors in the supraglottal and subglottal areas, which possess the ability of rapid adaptation,[22] and those lying in the laryngeal mucosa and not in vocal folds, could be responsible for giving rise to the laryngeal cough.

The afferent pathway of the expiration reflex runs through the superior laryngeal nerve. This conclusion was arrived at, from single-fibre recordings as their frequency of discharge was seen to increase immediately on stimulating the vocal cords. Moreover, the reflex was absent after the transection of this nerve. The role of the recurrent (inferior) laryngeal nerve in this reflex is only an additive *(minor)* one, in most animals. In humans, however, it is of primary importance, as it is not possible to elicit the reflex in patients with paralysis of the recurrent (inferior) laryngeal nerve.[39] In cats, bilateral vagotomy did not modify the expiration reflex, suggesting that the vagus has little influence on it.[30] On the other hand, we observed that inflation of the lungs caused an increase in its strength in rabbits and ferrets.[31,51]

The efferent pathways of expiration reflex are identical with those for cough and other similar expiratory components. This can be seen in the efferent recordings of the lumbar nerves.[52]

The study of single-fibre electrical activity in recurrent nerve motoneuron showed that, if expiration reflex was elicited during inspiration, the activity in inspiratory motoneuron was interrupted in the compressive phase of the reflex, and the expiratory laryngeal motoneuron were activated. Conversely, if expiration reflex was elicited during expiration, bursting activity appeared in the expiratory laryngeal motoneuron during the compressive phase of reflex. No inspiratory activity was present during the expulsive phase following stimulation.[6]

A complete understanding of the central control of the expiration reflex is still a problem. A single centre does not coordinate the reflex, but rather by a network system in the brainstem. 'Multifunctional' population of medullar neurons in the Bötzinger complex supposedly produces its motor pattern. The rostral ventral respiratory group is also involved in the genesis of breathing and cough. However, in cats, other neurons may also play a vital role in production, shaping, and mediation of the motor pattern of the reflex; some may be localised in the rostral pons, lateral segmental field or the raphe medullar midline and other central structures.

3.10 EXPIRATION REFLEX IN PATHOLOGICAL CONDITIONS

The expiration reflex can be evoked in experimental inflammation of the vocal folds by spreading croton oil aerosol or turpentine oil aerosol into the larynx of cats. The reflex remains unchanged in croton oil inflammation; but in turpentine oil inflammation, its intensity decreases with time.[1,53] Since toxic or staphylococcal inflammation or experimental pleurisy does not alter the magnitude of the expiration reflex, one can also conclude that its elicitation does not bear any relationship to suppression of cough by inflammation.[54]

An inflammation of the laryngeal area produces a decrease in the intensity of the expiration reflex, but produces an increase in that of the laryngeal cough. This observation, therefore, allows us to assume that there are two kinds of simultaneously stimulated receptors having different sensitivities, to inflammation.[1,52–54]

The expiration reflex is the easier of the two to elicit, and the effect is more marked in some pathological conditions. Vocal folds infiltrated by tumour cells in humans respond weakly to stimulation of the affected site, and the resulting reflex is thus less pronounced. Moreover, it cannot be elicited on the affected side in recurrent laryngeal nerve paralysis and in functional dyskinesia,[39,52] and it is interesting to note that the expiration reflex under these conditions is replaced by an attack of coughing. Stimulation of the scar tissue in the larynx after vocal cordectomy does not produce the reflex but stimulation of the newly formed pseudovocal fold is effective after about 20 days.[1,39,52,53]

3.11 CONCLUSION

From the above-mentioned conditions, one can conclude that the expiration reflex is biologically significant as it can reappear not long after the recurrent laryngeal nerve is affected.

REFERENCES

1. Korpas J, Tomori Z. The expiration reflex. In: Herzog H, editor. Cough and Other Respiratory Reflexes. Basel, Munchen, Paris, London, New York, Sydney; S. Karger, 1979;pp189–217.
2. Korpas J, Tomori Z, Kaselaine Respiracne Reflexy (In Slovak) Bratislava: Veda 1975;p236.
3. Korpas J. Differentiation of the expiration and cough reflex. Physiologia Bohemoslovaca 1972;21:677–80.
4. Poliacek I, Stránsky A, Jakuš J, Barániová H, Tomori Z, Halásová E. Activity of the laryngeal abduction and adductor muscles during cough, expiration and aspiration reflexes in cats. Respiration Physiology 2003;52:746–62.
5. Korpas J. Aspects of airway defence mechanisms. Pathophysiology 1996;3:81–6.
6. Stránsky A, Tomori Z. Changes in laryngeal motoneurone activity and in laryngeal calibre during expiration reflex. Physiologia Bohemoslovaca 1979;28:365–73.
7. Jeffery P, Korpas J, Widdicombe JG. Intraepithelial nerve fibres of the cat larynx and the expiration reflex. Journal of Physiology (London) 1978;275:35P–36P.
8. Kalia M, Mesulam M. Brainstem projections of sensory and motor components of the vagus complex in the cat: II. Laryngeal, tracheobronchial, pulmonary, cardiac and gastrointestinal branches. Journal of Comparative Neurology 1980;193:467–508.

9. Lucier GE, Egizii R, Dostrovsky JO. Projections of the internal branch of the superior laryngeal nerve of the cat. Brain Research Bulletin 1986;16:713–21.
10. Backey DM, Moric KF, Nuding SC, Segers LS, Lindssey BG, Shannon R. Ventolateral medullary respiration network particularly in expiration reflex in cats. Journal of Applied Physiology 2004;96:2057–72.
11. Bucher K, Jacot C. Zum mechanismus des Hustens. Helvetica Pharmacologica Acta 1951;9:454–62.
12. Ivanèo I, Korpas J. K otázke laryngeálneho a tracheálneho kaša (in Slovak). Bratislavské lekárske Listy 1954;34:1391–6.
13. Stehaelin R. Respirations Krankheiten. Jahreskunde ärztliche Forbildung 1914;5:32–43.
14. Kandarazki M. Ueber den Husten nebst einigen Bemerkungen ueber den Einfluss des Chloroforms auf die Atmung der Tiere. Pflugers Archiv fur die gesamte Physiologie 1881;26:470–9.
15. Widdicombe JG. Respiratory reflexes from the trachea and bronchi of the cat. Journal of Physiology (London) 1954;123:55–70.
16. Pressmann JI, Kelemen G. Physiology of the larynx. The Physiological Review 1955;35:506–54.
17. Korpas J, Tomori Z. Uber den Einfluss der Hypothermie auf den Husten und die Atmung. .Physiologia Bohemoslovaca 1975;4:487–93.
18. Kuhn HN, Friebel H. Zur Einordnung des Hustenstosses in den Atemthytmus. Medicina Experimental 1960;3:329–35.
19. Trendelenburg U. Uber die wirkung einiger Hustenmittel auf Hustenreizschwele und Atmung. Acta Physiologica Scandinavica 1950;21:174–86.
20. Kade F, Bucher K. Charakteristik der expiratorischer Anfälle bei der Traube. Helvetica Physiologica Acta 1967;25:241–8.
21. Bucher K. Respiratory changes following reflexogenic twitches. Agents Action 1979;3:61–5.
22. Tomori Z, Stránsky A. Electroneurographic and pneumotacho-graphic analysis of the expiration reflex. Physiologia Bohemoslovaca 1973;22:589–601.
23. Tomori Z, Stránsky A. Mechanisms of expiration reflex. Bulletin de Physio – pathologie Respiratoire 1973;9:1281.
24. Tomori Z, Lemáková S, Holéczyová A. Defensive reflexes of the respiratory tract in dogs. Physiologia Bohemoslovaca 1977;26:49–54.
25. Widdicombe JG. Laryngeal and tracheal reflexes. In: Widdicombe JG. editor. Respiratory Physiology. London, Baltimore: University Park Press; 1974;pp279–82.
26. Korpas J. Differentiation of the expiration and cough reflex. Physiologia Bohemoslovaca 1972;21:677–80.
27. Dyachenko YA. The participation of bulbar "respiratory" and "nonrespiratory" neurones in the development of the expiration reflex (in Russian). Neirofiziologija 1990;22:670–80.
28. Dyachenko YA, Preobrazhenskij NN. Responses of bulbospinal neurones during expiration reflex in cats (in Russian). Neirofiziologija 1991;29:88–98.
29. Holmer BH, Marek W, Scheid P. Der Einfluss laryngealer Afferenzen auf inspiratorische und expiratorische Nerven und Muskeln der Katze. Atemwege und Lungenkramkheiten 1986;12:327–32.
30. Nishino T, Honda Y. Time dependent responses of expiration reflex in cats. Journal of Applied Physiology 1986;61:430–35.

31. Hanacek J, Korpas J. Modification of the intensity of the expiration reflex during short-term inflation of the lungs in rabbits. Physiologia Bohemoslovaca 1982;31:159–74.
32. Sullivan CE, Murphy E, Kozar LF, Phillipson EA. Waking and respiratory responses to laryngeal stimmulation in sleeping dogs. Journal of Applied Physiology 1979;47:17–25.
33. Sullivan CE, Kozar LF, Murphy E, Philipson EA. Arousal, ventilatory and airway responses to Bronchopulmonary stimulation in sleeping dogs. Journal of Applied Physiology 1979;47:17–25.
34. Tomori Z, Lemáková S, Gromysz H, Strásky A. Electroneurographic and pneumotachographic analysis of the expiration reflex. Physiologia Bohemoslovaca 1977;26:49–54.
35. Jakuš J, Stránsky A, Poliacek L, Bárányi H, Bošeová L. Effects of medullary midline lesions on cough and other airway reflexes in anaesthetised cats. Physiological Research 1998;47:203–13.
36. Korpas J, Kalocsayová G. Mechanoreception of the cat respiratory tract on the first days of the postnatal life. Physiologia Bohemoslovaca 1973;22:365–73.
37. Korpas J, Tatár M. The expiration reflex during ontogenesis in the rat. Physiologia Bohemoslovaca 1975;24:257–61.
38. Tatár M, Korpas J, Polacek H, Záhradný V. Changes induced by sever hypoxia in respiratory defence reflexes in anaesthetized cats. Respiration 1986;49:114–21.
39. Korpas J, Mišík A, Kalocsayová G. The expiration reflex in man. Physiologia Bohemoslovaca 1975, 24:253–6.
40. Nishino T, Hiraga K, Hiyuguchi T, Honda Y. Respiratory reflex responses to stimulation of tracheal mucosa in enflurane anaesthetised humans. Journal of Applied Physiology 1989;65:1069–74.
41. Nishino T, Hiraga H, Honda Y. Inhibitory effects of CO_2 on airways defensive reflexes in enflurane anaesthetised humans. Journal of Applied Physiology 1989;66:2643–6.
42. Nishino T, Taigo T, Issuno S. Cough and other reflexes on irritation of airway mucosa in man. Pulmonary Pharmacology 1996;9:285–92.
43. Tagaito Y, Issono S, Nishino T. Upper airway reflex during a combination of proposal and fentanyl anaesthesia. Anaesthesiology 1998;88:1459–66.
44. Widdicombe JG. Neurophysiology of the cough reflex. European Respirology 1995;8:1193–1202.
45. Widdicombe JG. Afferent receptors in the airways and cough. Respiratory Physiology 1998;114:5–15.
46. During M, Andres KH. Structure and functional anatomy of visceroreceptors in mammalian respiratory system. In: Hankann W, Iggo A, editors. Progress in Brain Research. Amsterdam: Elsevier; 1988;p139–54.
47. Fillenz M, Widdicombe JG. Receptors of the lung and airways. In: Antrum H. Handbook of Sensory Physiology. Berlin: Springer Verlag; 1971;p.81–112.
48. Hayek H. Die menschliche Lunge. Berlin, Heidelberg, New York: Springer; 1970;p379.
49. Laitinen A. Ultrastructural organization of intraepithelial nerves in human airway tract. Thorax 1985;40:488–92.
50. Tucran J, Korpas J, Hanácek J. The effect of the short-term lung inflation upon expiration reflex intensity under normal and pathological conditions in ferrets. Physiologia Bohemoslovaca 1983;80:53–9.
51. Tomori Z, Stránsky A. Mechanisms of the expiration reflex. Bulletin de Pathophysiology Respiratoire 1973;9:1281.

52. Korpas J, Tomori Z. Cough and other respiratory reflexes. In: Herzog H, editor. Basel, Munchen, Paris-London, New York, Sydney: S. Karger, 1979;p368.
53. Korpas J, Bilcík P, Fraenkel E. Changes in coughing in cats with experimental and spontaneous inflammation of respiratory tract. Physiologia Bohemoslovaca 1965;14:488–94.

4 Cough from Airway Receptors

HANACEK J

4.1 INTRODUCTION

The main function of the respiratory system is to ascertain a sufficient supply of oxygen to meet the body's metabolic requirements and to eliminate carbon dioxide produced in the process. For this the patency of the airways has to be ensured. Many efficient mechanisms bring this about and these can be divided into two main subgroups—protective and defensive. The nature of their function classifies them to be either reflex or non-reflex in character.[1] The cough reflex is one of the most important defensive reflexes of the airway. It serves to protect the airways from the damaging effects of inhaled particulate matter, aeroallergens, pathogens, aspirate, and accumulated secretions.[2] Its manifestation is associated with a pathological process, predominantly localised in the airways and the lung parenchyma, but damage of tissue around the afferent endings of vagus nerve in other organs can also lead to the elicitation of cough. Thus, cough can be described as being exclusively mediated via the vagus nerve,[3] and it is generally accepted that primary afferent nerves regulating the cough reflex are of vagal origin. The specific vagal afferent nerve subtypes subserving a primary role in producing and controlling cough and the modulatory role of other vagal afferent nerves in cough reflexes, have been studied extensively.[4–6] Our knowledge of the bronchopulmonary afferent nerves involved in the induction of cough and its modulation has increased over the last few years,[2,4,7–9] and this has enabled us to clarify the results of some of our earlier experiments as well as to look at newer ways of understanding the complex phenomenon of cough in patients.

Stimulation of bronchopulmonary mucosal membrane usually leads to changes in the activity of autonomic afferents supplying the airways. It results in, for example, changes in the frequency and amplitude of breathing and giving rise to particular sensations, such as an urge to cough and dyspnoea.[9] These constitute an important part of the mechanism involved in maintaining physiological homeostasis and defending the gas exchange system and in addition are signs of lung pathology.

The various bronchopulmonary afferent nerves that have been described so far can be differentiated according to several criteria. Currently, the most frequently used scheme of classification is based on nerve fibre conduction velocity and fibre size, ganglion origin of cell body, nature of the stimulus to which they respond, rates of adaptation to maintain suprathreshold stimuli, and their neurochemistry.[9] Till recently, bronchopulmonary afferent nerves were considered to belong to one of the three general categories, namely slowly adapting pulmonary stretch receptors (SARs), rapidly adapting pulmonary stretch receptors (RARs), and C-fibres. This scheme of classification, however, does not consider all the mentioned nerve properties. On the other hand, it may also be assumed that all kinds of airway afferents play some role in the induction of the cough reflex or its modulation.

New data on possible interactions between afferent innervation of the airways and the production of cough and bronchospasm have emerged recently.[10,11] These pathways can participate significantly in regulating the intensity of the cough reflex. The principle underlying these interactions could be similar to that in the somatosensory system, e.g. in initiation of allodynia by the interaction of C-fibres and low threshold mechanoreceptors.[12] Further knowledge in this field would help us to understand better, the mechanisms involved in increasing or decreasing cough intensity.

Sensitivity to tussive stimuli is often increased in subjects with airway inflammatory disease.[13,14] It is well known that the threshold of airway afferent nerves to various stimuli can vary, as the nerve endings are known to get sensitised, especially during airway mucosal inflammation.[15,16] Not all mechanisms underlying an increase in excitability of airway nerve-endings at the sites of inflammation are known as yet, but constitute a subject, which is currently under intense investigation. One of the possible explanations for the increased excitability of these nerve endings could be an induction of neurokinin synthesis, which under normal conditions is not present in them.[17] This process, whereby a change occurs in the neuronal excitability, receptor expression, neurotransmitters chemistry and nerve structure is termed 'nerve plasticity'. These changes can lead to either an increase or a decrease in the overall responsiveness of the concerned afferent nerve endings.[18]

4.2 TYPES OF AIRWAY NERVE ENDINGS

Detailed data about the characteristics of the airway afferent nerves involved in the induction of cough and its modulation can be found in the following papers and reviews.[9,19,20] From these and other studies, it is well known that vagal afferent nerves are the primary pathways between bronchopulmonary system and the central nervous system (CNS). Inputs from the vagus nerve endings are processed and integrated at different levels of the CNS, and ultimately give rise to respiratory sensations and various reflexes whose inputs are coordinated in the brainstem and serve an important host-defence function.[9] Thus, the airway defense reflexes are mediated by afferents that are mainly of vagal origin.

4.2.1 Rapidly Adapting Pulmonary Stretch Receptors

This subgroup of vagal afferents belongs to low-threshold mechanosensitive bronchopulmonary A-fibres that respond as a burst of action potentials during the dynamic phase of inspiration and expiration, but cease to respond during the maintained static phase of lung inflation.[9] Hence, they are called the rapidly adapting pulmonary stretch receptor fibres (RARs). They are very sensitive to mechanical stimuli influencing the airways, for example, lung inflation and deflation, mechanical distortion of the airway wall due to airway spasm, mucosal oedema or mechanical probing.[21] Activation of RARs leads to increased inspiratory activity, increased rate of breathing, bronchospasm, vasodilatation, mucous secretion, and cough.[2,9,21] The 'cough fibres' as described by Widdicombe[22] are myelinated fibres that conduct action potentials in the A-delta range. Their properties are very similar to RARs mentioned above, so it is reasonable to think that 'cough receptors' belong to the RARs subgroup. Hunter and Undem[23] have shown in experiments carried out on guinea pigs that RARs are situated in the submucosal tissue, i.e. just beneath the epithelium. According to the observation of Riccio et al,[24] this type of nerve fibres arises from cell bodies situated in the nodose ganglia. Embryonically, neurons within the nodose ganglia are thought to be derived from the epibranchial placodes. Thus, based on the nature of their specific stimuli, their location within the airways and possibly their embryonic origin, the RARs represent quite a distinct subpopulation of airway afferents in guinea pig trachea and bronchi.[18]

The RARs project to distinct region within the nucleus tractus solitarius (NTS) of the brainstem[25] and are associated with different reflex outputs. The primary excitatory transmitter at synapses between central portion of RARs and second-order neurons in the NTS, is glutamate.[26]

4.2.2 Slowly Adapting Pulmonary Stretch Receptors

The basic features of airway slowly adapting pulmonary stretch receptor fibres (SARs), were first described by Adrian.[27] When the lungs are maintained in an inflated state, these nerve fibres respond with a continuous discharge. In general, the activity of SARs leads to inhibition of inspiration, and of parasympathetic activity and a consequent relaxation of airway smooth muscle.[28] SARs influence the timing and pattern of inspiratory and expiratory motor activity during eupnoea.[29] The activity of SARs is manifested by Hering-Breuer inflation reflex (HBIR). These receptors are believed to lie in the smooth muscles of the airway wall, especially the trachea and larger bronchi.[30] SARs appear not to affect inspiratory amplitude and inspiratory and expiratory phase timings during multiple cough episodes.[31] Evidence, however, appears to support the idea that they are necessary for expression of the cough motor pattern.[32,33] Although, Ezure and Tanaka[34] have found an inhibitory linkage from the SARs to the RARs at the level of the second-order neurons (P-cells and rapidly adapting receptor cells, respectively), this mechanism can be responsible for manifestation of HBIR. These authors also showed that not all the P-cells are inhibitory. Yet, the role of SARs in the induction of the cough reflex and its modulation is not well understood. It is known that HBIR is present in newborns and babies.[35,36] In adults, during non-REM sleep, HBIR is seen only when the inflating lung volume is greater than 1 L.[37] In contrast, Fernando and Saunders[38] have shown, that in man even a single deep inspiration influences the following few breaths. There is some evidence to support the idea that increased activity of SARs leads to an increased activity in expiratory motoneurons and expiratory muscles.[39]

4.2.3 C-fibre Endings

The vagal afferent C-fibres innervate the entire respiratory tract from the larynx to the lung parenchyma. They are thin and non-myelinated. Some of them are accessible to stimuli via the arterial circulation; others react to stimuli via the pulmonary circulation. Examples of the former subgroup are the bronchial C-fibres and of the latter, the pulmonary C-fibres.[40] The cell bodies of C-fibres which supply extra thoracic airways (in guinea pigs) are localised nearly exclusively, in the jugular ganglia, whereas the intrapulmonary C-fibre are derived from neurons in both the jugular and nodose ganglia.[24] Kummer and co-workers[41] showed that other properties of these two types of C-fibres are also likely to differ. This difference is presented by the synthesis of neurokinins and calcitonin-gene related peptide (CGRP) in the neurons of the jugular C-fibres, which the nodose ganglion neurons (whose fibres innervate intrapulmonary airways) do not exhibit. The C-fibre endings are relatively insensitive to mechanical stimuli (high-threshold mechanoreceptors) but are rather sensitive to potentially damaging stimuli such as inflammatory mediators, acids, changes in osmolarity, and chemicals such as capsaicin and bradykinin.[24,41] These types of nerve endings are also called 'nociceptors', although most of them that are present in the airways do not transmit pain signals to the CNS. Reflexes resulting from stimulation of C-fibres include inhibition of inspiration and expiration (apnoea), rapid shallow breathing, bronchoconstriction, bradycardia and increase in bronchial blood flow.[40] Stimulation of pulmonary C-fibres (which are identical to Paintal's juxtapulmonary capillary or J receptors) evoke the so-called J-reflex, which is characterised by a decreased muscle force[42] and some respiratory reflexes. The nociceptive C-fibres localised in the airways release neurokinins via axon reflexes, which lead to neurogenic inflammation; they also communicate with second-order neurons through release of neurokinins.

4.3 ROLE OF AIRWAY SENSORY NERVE ENDINGS IN INDUCTION OF COUGH AND ITS MODULATION

There is still no consensus about the role of the various airway nerve endings in the induction and modulation of cough.[43–47] Cough is generally thought to be initiated predominantly, via the stimulation of mucosal nerve endings that are located in the larynx and along the trachea and up to its bifurcation. This conclusion is based on the presence of a very rapid discharge in response to a mechanical stimulation of all of these structures.[48] There is evidence that other airway receptors may also participate in the cough reflex induction and its modulation.[5,24,47]

The influence of the various airway receptors on cough production is either stimulatory or inhibitory. Examples of stimulatory reflex inputs are viral, bacterial, and chemical inflammation of the mucosa of the lower airways.[15] A reflex inhibitory input occurs because of damage to the epithelium or by stimulation of those airway receptors that inhibit cough reflexely.[15,47] Much attention has been devoted to defining the role of RARs and C-fibres in cough induction and modulation, but it seems logical that for understanding the complex reflex of cough, it is necessary to know the effect of inputs from the main types of airway and lung receptors and from receptors localised in other parts of the body as well.

4.3.1 Reflex Input from Slowly Adapting Pulmonary Stretch Receptors to Cough

Arising from Bucher's pivotal studies,[49,50] it has been believed by some that the SARs are important in the control of the strength of the cough reflex. Since then, a few groups of researchers have tested this hypothesis,[32,33,45,46] but evidence obtained both supports it and refutes it. Thus, any role of SARs in the control of cough at all, is still not very clear. From a clinical point of view, the strength of the cough reflex is important. Cough of an appropriate intensity is able to clear out the mucus or foreign bodies from the airways, but if it is not strong enough, then cleaning of the airway will not be adequate. Such a situation may lead to airway obstruction, resulting in a limitation of the main functions of the lung.

The question arises whether SARs are important for the regulation of cough intensity and other airway defensive reflexes, or not. The answer to this question was sought primarily in animal experiments[32,33] and later on in clinical studies in man.[45,46] The methods by which one can obtain relevant answers are both by exclusively blocking as well as stimulating the airway SARs. The main drawback of both the methods is that neither can select these fibres exclusively. Therefore, the results obtained by using either method, would be open to debate.

4.3.1.1 Influence of Blocking SARs on Cough Reflex Strength

Bucher[50] suggested that stimulation of airway SARs can increase the intensity of cough and that their block ought to be able to reduce it. A possibility to test the hypothesis arose when a method for the selective blockade of SARs was

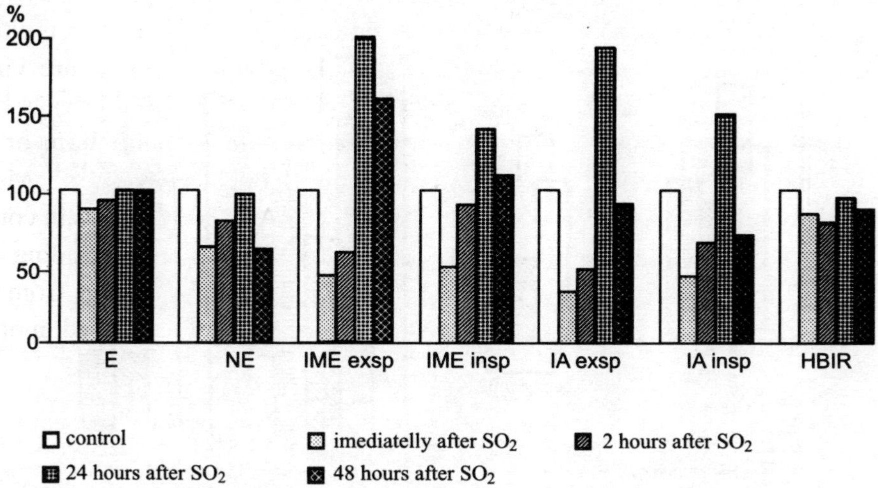

Fig. 4.1 Changes in cough reflex elicitability (E) and cough reflex strength [expressed as number of cough efforts (NE); maximal expiratory cough effort (IME_{exp}); maximal inspiratory cough effort (IME_{insp}); sum of all expiratory efforts in one cough bout (IA_{exp}); sum of all inspiratory efforts in one cough bout (IA_{insp}); Hering-Breuer inflation reflex strength (HBIR)] in rabbits before, immediately after 10–15 minutes of inhalation of sulphur dioxide (SO_2, 200–300 ppm), and at intervals during recovery. Values are expressed in % scale. Control values are taken as 100%. (Reproduced from Ref. [53] with permission from Publisher).

developed.[51] One such method that worked in rabbits was inhalation of a high concentration of sulphur dioxide (200 ppm) which blocked the SARs and from which they recovered soon after the gas inhalation was over. The blockade of airway SARs in rabbits in this manner resulted in a profound inhibition of cough induced by stimulation of airway mucous membrane by chemical or mechanical irritants.[32] The inhibition of 'cough reflex elicitability' (CRE) was manifest as the percentage of trials successful in eliciting cough by two thirds of its control value, when provoked by blowing ammonia (2 ml of 1×10^{-3} molecular concentration) into the larynx (separated from the lower airways). The parameters of cough reflex strength (CRS) were decreased to about 40 to 55% of their control values. The important finding was that only expiratory parameters that denote intensity of cough were inhibited by blocking the SARs; the inspiratory cough efforts were not significantly influenced (Figs 4.1 and 4.2). An even more pronounced inhibitory effect of the blockade of SARs was seen on cough induced by mechanical and chemical stimulation of tracheo-

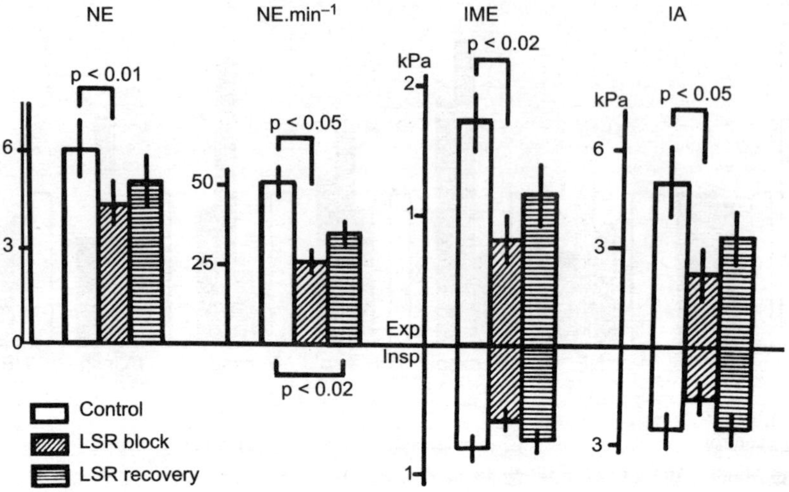

Fig. 4.2 Influence of blocking slowly adapting pulmonary stretch receptor fibres (SARs) by sulphur dioxide (SO_2) on cough reflex strength in anaesthetised rabbits. Cough was induced by stimulation of larynx (LSR) with ammonia. Control before LSRs block—during SARs block; LSR recovery—SARs recovery from block; NE.min^{-1}, number of cough efforts per minute; other abbreviations are as in Figure 4.1 (Reproduced from Ref. [32] with permission from Publisher).

bronchial mucosa.[32] Blowing ammonia gas into the lower airways caused an immediate cough in each of the stimulation before SARs blockade, but only in one out of 13 stimulations when the SARs were blocked. Therefore, the reduction of CRE was even more marked than when the cough was induced from the larynx. Mechanical stimulation (soft catheter) of the tracheobronchial tree always caused coughing before SARs were blocked, but immediately after SARs block, this was seen only in 25% of the attempts. Additionally, the intensity of the cough episodes was far weaker than those seen in the control situation. Similar results were noted by Sant' Ambrogio et al.[33] They found that mechanically induced cough from laryngeal mucosa of rabbits is profoundly inhibited by SARs block and that such a blockade results in the failure to elicit cough by mechanical stimulation of trachea and carina.

However, these observations do not still resolve the dilemma of being able to attribute the cough reflex inhibition seen in experiments using SO_2 for blockade of SARs, exclusively to the latter. On the other hand, it is rational to suppose that airway RARs and C-fibres, too can be influenced by the presence of SO_2.

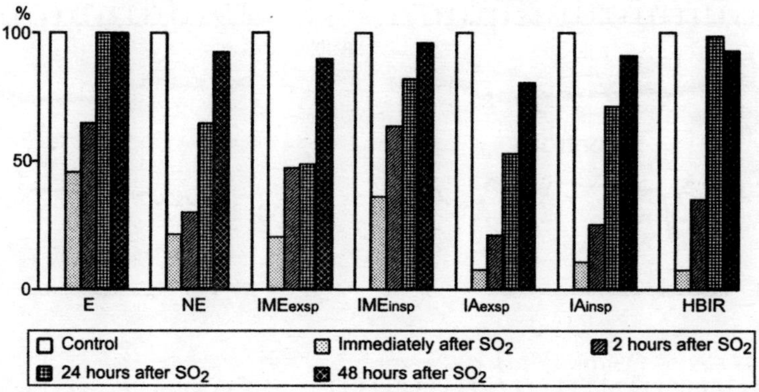

Fig. 4.3A Changes in cough reflex elicitability (E), cough reflex strength (expressed by the same parameters as in Figure 4.1) and Hering-Breuer inflation reflex (HBIR) duration in cats before, immediately after 10–15 minutes of inhalation of sulphur dioxide (SO_2) (of the same concentration as in rabbits), and after intervals during recovery (intervals are the same as in Figure 4.1). Cough was induced by mechanical stimulation of the interior of trachea and bronchi. Values are expressed in % scale. Control values are taken as 100%. (Reproduced from Ref. [53] with permission from Publisher).

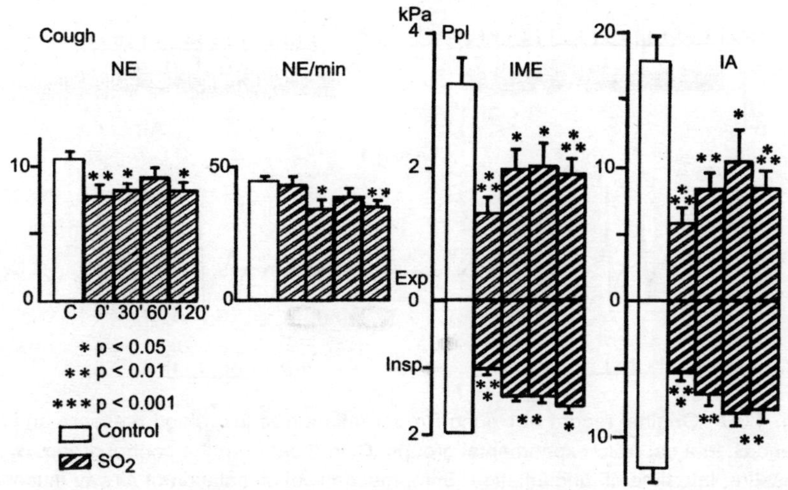

Fig. 4.3B Changes of cough reflex strength in anaesthetised cats before, immediately after and up to 2 hours after sulphur dioxide (SO_2) inhalation. Exp, expiration; Insp, inspiration; NE.min^{-1}, number of cough efforts per minute; other abbreviations as in Figure 4.1. (Reproduced from Ref. [53] with permission from Publisher).

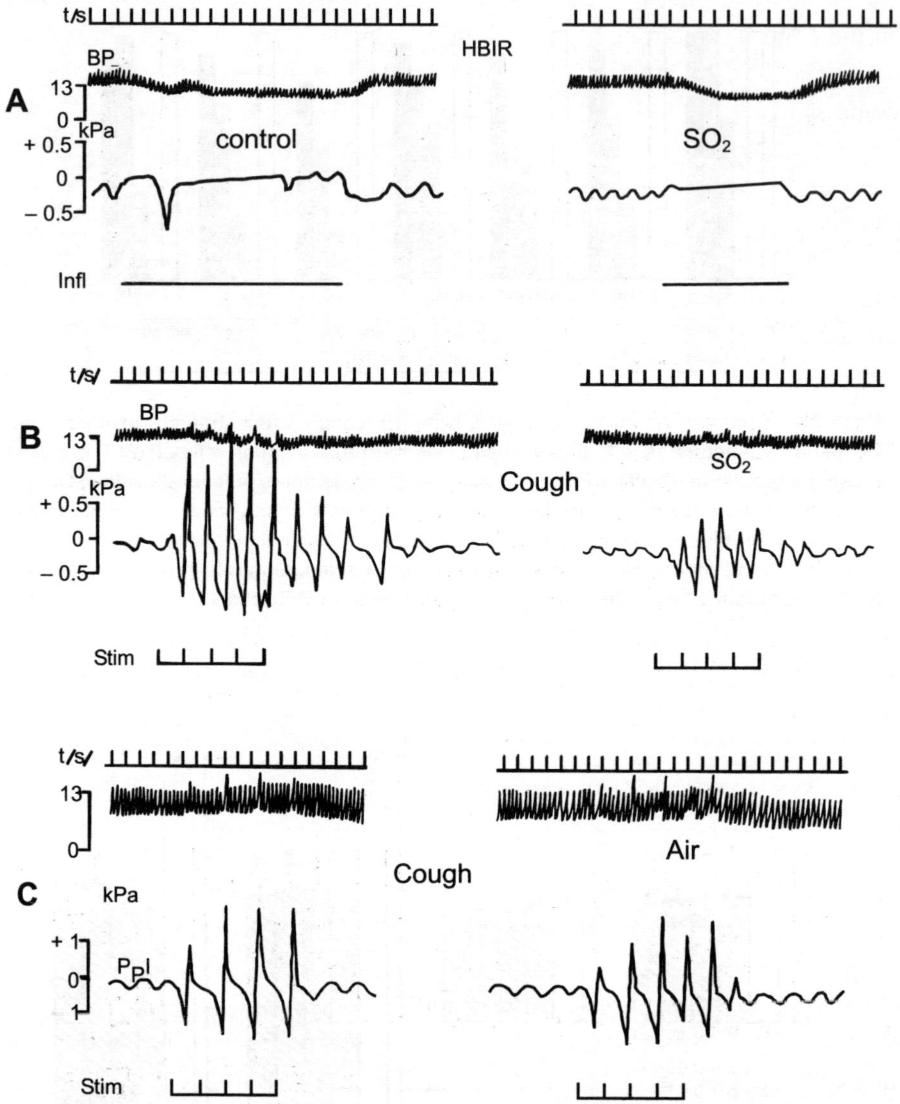

Fig. 4.3C Original record of Hering-Breuer inflation reflex, blood pressure and cough: **A** and **B,** in a cat from experimental groups; **C,** in a cat from the control group. BP, blood pressure; Infl, time of lung inflation; Stim, mechanical stimulation of airway mucosa; Ppl, intrapleural pressure. (Reproduced from Ref. [53] with permission from Publisher).

On the contrary, the results of Sant' Ambrogio and coworkers[33] have shown that tracheal RARs are not significantly influenced by SO_2 breathing. Thus, it seems plausible to think that inhibition of cough seen in experiments on rabbits can be ascribed mainly to the block of SARs. The possibility that inhibitory effect of SO_2 inhalation on cough are due to stimulation of lung C-fibres, is evident from the findings of Tatar and coworkers.[52] They were able to abolish the cough reflex during the 20–30 seconds of apnoea induced by C-fibre stimulation. In our studies[32] and in some of those carried out by Sant' Ambrogio and coworkers,[33] evidence of a notable stimulation of lung C-fibres, such as reflex apnoea, followed by rapid shallow breathing was not available. Thus, it is doubtful that these receptors could have exerted an inhibitory influence in our experiments that we have described above. Further evidence for the notion, that inhibition of the cough reflex in experiments with SO_2 is not due to blockade of RARs was provided by Sant' Ambrogio and coworkers.[33] They found that in dogs, SO_2 breathing did not abolish either the Hering-Breuer inflation reflex (HBIR) or the production of mechanically induced cough from the trachea. Unfortunately, they did not evaluate the quantitative parameters of cough, so they were not able to show whether there was any change in the cough strength after SO_2 breathing. In our experiments on cats,[53] we found that SO_2 breathing does not influence the HBIR and CRE, as it does in dogs. However, with SO_2 breathing, CRS decreased immediately and remained so for 2 hours after which it was increased for up to 48 hours (Figs 4.3A to C).

From this, one can conclude that the activity of airway SARs is important for cough generation. Afferent inputs from them permit the cough to develop and are important for the production of tracheobronchial cough and they facilitate the production of laryngeal cough. This stimulatory effect of SARs on cough represents a different action from the well-known inspiratory inhibitory effect of these afferents on breathing.[54,55] The inhibition of the CRS found in our experiment with cats[53] cannot be ascribed to decreased activity of SARs, but rather partly to the inhibition of airway RARs, a change in the resting membrane potential of these nerve endings or probably due to stimulation of C-fibres that inhibit cough[52] by a direct central influence.

Some data that supports the role of airway SARs in the control of cough in man were provided by Higenbottam's group.[56] They reported that the cough response to stimulation of laryngeal mucosa by distilled water in patients with heart-lung transplants (with lungs denervated below the level of the tracheal anastomosis), was strikingly lower compared to that in normal controls.

However, under these conditions, inputs from all types of lung vagal afferents are also excluded, yet these authors believe that the observed inhibition of cough was due to the absence of inputs from the SARs. Lavorini et al[85] presented another indirect evidence that supports a facilitatory role of SARs on the cough reflex. These authors have shown that voluntary and reflex cough, in laryngectomised patients was significantly less than subjects with intact larynx. One cannot overlook the fact that this observed difference could also be ascribed to the absence of the compressive phase of cough due to the missing larynx. Absence of this phase results in a decrease of airway pressure and can become the reason for a decreased output of airway SARs. Thus, a decreased cough response seen in heart-lung transplant patients and in laryngectomised patients is similar to what was observed in our studies[32] on rabbits and that by Sant' Ambrogio's group when SARs in the lower airways of their experimental animals were blocked and cough was provoked by stimulation of the laryngeal mucosa.[33] Therefore, it seems reasonable to think that the activity of airway SARs plays an important role not only in the inspiratory off-switch, but in cough development as well.

4.3.1.2 Influence of Stimulation of SARs on Cough and Expiration Reflexes

Another approach that could help answer the question whether airway SARs are involved in the induction of cough and its modulation, is to stimulate the SARs and study their influence. Since the natural stimulus for this type of receptors is an increased pressure inside the airways, the result of such stimulation would be an increased activity of SARs leading to an inhibition of inspiration (Hering-Breuer inflation reflex). Javorka and coworkers[57] found that in anaesthetised cats a continuous positive airway pressure (0.24–0.98 kPa) led to a weakening of inspiratory and expiratory components of the defence reflexes such as mechanically-induced sneezing, tracheobronchial cough and aspiration reflex. Tatar and Nagyova,[58] who used short-lasting inflation pressures (0.5–1.5 kPa) to stimulate airway SARs in anaesthetised cats found no significant effect on the strength of sneezing and cough reflexes, but they observed that frequency of sneezing and cough efforts tended to increase.

On the other hand, Romaniuk et al[46] obtained results that clearly oppose the notion that stimulation of airway SARs enhance cough. They showed that

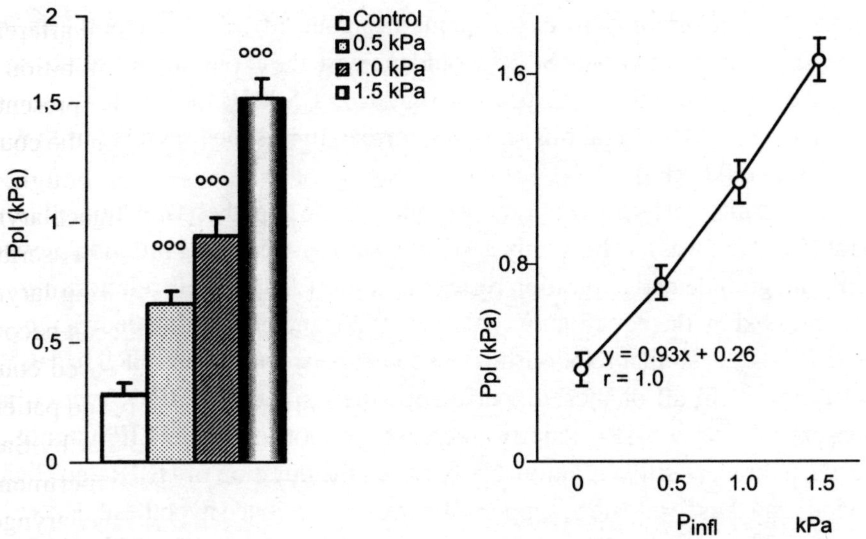

Fig. 4.4 In anaesthetised rabbits an almost linear relationship between: **A,** lung inflation pressure magnitude; **B,** expiration reflex strength. P_{pl}, intrapleural pressure; P_{infl}, lung inflation pressure; ooo, p<0.001 between each step of inflation pressure and control value. (Reproduced from Ref. [65] with permission from Publisher).

in dogs, an increased vagal stimulation resulting from airway occlusion at the end of inspiration and maintained throughout the subsequent expiration, did not affect expiratory muscle activity during cough. In contrast to the above, in a clinical study carried out in anaesthetised humans, Nishino et al[45] showed that lung inflation with continuous positive airway pressure (1 kPa) did not exert any influence on the types, latencies and duration of reflex responses to mechanical irritation of the trachea, but the intensity of expiration reflex and cough reflex were augmented. They attributed the augmentation of the reflexes rather to the mechanical properties of the chest wall and respiratory muscles than to increased activity of airway SARs.

In experiments on rabbits,[32] the blockade of airway SARs was seen to lead predominantly, to attenuation of expiratory components of the cough reflex. These observations gave rise to the hypothesis that the stimulation of airway SARs could influence the reflex event, composed only of a single expiratory effort. The only known airway defence reflex, of this type, is the expiration reflex,[59] which can be easily induced by mechanical stimulation of the medial margin of the vocal folds. It is characterised by a single expiratory effort without a preceding inspiration. In experiments designed to test the hypothesis that increasing activity of airway SARs would increase the expiration reflex strength, we used lung inflation pressures of 0.5, 1.0, 1.5 kPa, of 5 s duration, for stimulation of SARs in rabbits, cats and ferrets (in rats the pressures used were 0.2, 0.4, and 0.6 kPa).

The results were surprisingly consistent with the hypothesis mentioned above. In rabbits, there was an almost linear relationship between lung inflation pressure (LIP), magnitude and expiration reflex strength (ERS).[60] This relationship can be expressed by the equation: $y = 0.93\,x + 0.26$, and correlation coefficient $r =$ 1.0 (Fig. 4.4). A similar relationship was found between LIP and ERS in cats[61,62] and ferrets.[63] In all of these experiments, the duration of HBIR (which is a measure of airway SARs activity) increases proportionally to LIP magnitude. Hence, a direct positive relationship between the duration of HBIR and ERS is obvious and thus in our view, supports the above-mentioned hypothesis. However, in rats the data obtained does not quite do so. In these animals, LIP of 0.2 kPa leads to a significant increase of ERS compared to that in the controls. However, increasing LIP further does not augment the ERS[64] in spite of the duration of HBIR having increased in response to an increasing LIP.

4.3.1.3 Influence of Blocking Airway SARs on ERS

The airway receptors play an important role in the direct dependence of LIP magnitude on the ERS and are supported by observations made in rabbits after inhibition or after total elimination of vagal inputs from the lower airways.[61,62,65] When the lower airways were anaesthetised by spraying a local anaesthetic (Xylocaine, Astra), then the direct positive relationship between LIP and ERS was almost totally abolished (Fig. 4.5A). That anaesthesia was deep enough was ascertained by cough and HBIR being not inducible by the standard method of stimulation of the lower airways. After a partial recovery from airway anaesthesia (about 15–20 min later), the HBIR recovered somewhat and the dependence between LIP magnitude and ERS too, revived partially. One hour after instillation of the anaesthetics into the airways, a full recovery of HBIR and a normal relationship between LIP and ERS was re-established, but cough inducible from the tracheobronchial tree remained still absent.

Further evidence, which supports the view that enhancement of ERS by lung inflation is mediated by vagus nerves, was obtained from experiments carried out in cats.[62] The slope of direct dependence between LIP and ERS

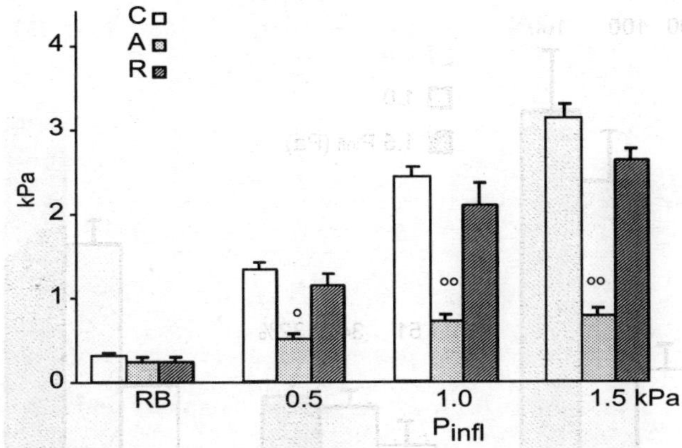

Fig. 4.5A Relationship between lung inflation pressure and expiration reflex strength in rabbits before, during, and after airway anaesthesia (with xylocaine). RB, breathing at rest; C, control values; A, during airway anaesthesia; R, recovery from airway anaesthesia; o, $p<0.05$; oo, $p<0.01$; ooo, $p<0.001$; other abbreviations as in Figure 4.4. (Reproduced from Ref. [65] with permission from Publisher).

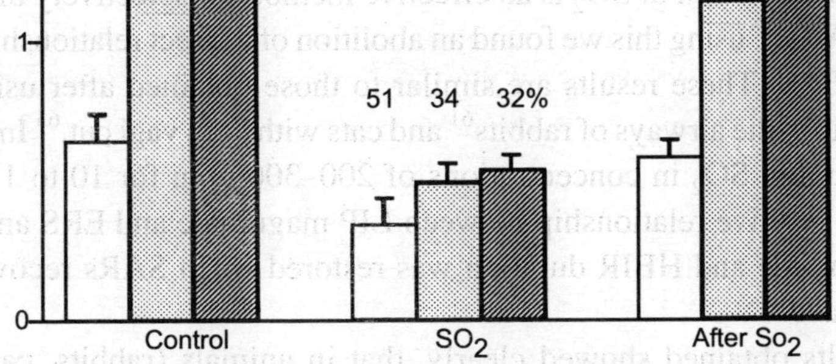

Fig. 4.5B Relationship between lung inflation pressure and expiration reflex strength in anaesthetised cats with both vagi intact (C), right vagus cut (RVC), and both vagi cut (BVC); o, $p<0.05$; oo, $p<0.01$; ooo, $p<0.001$; other abbreviations are as in Figure 4.4.

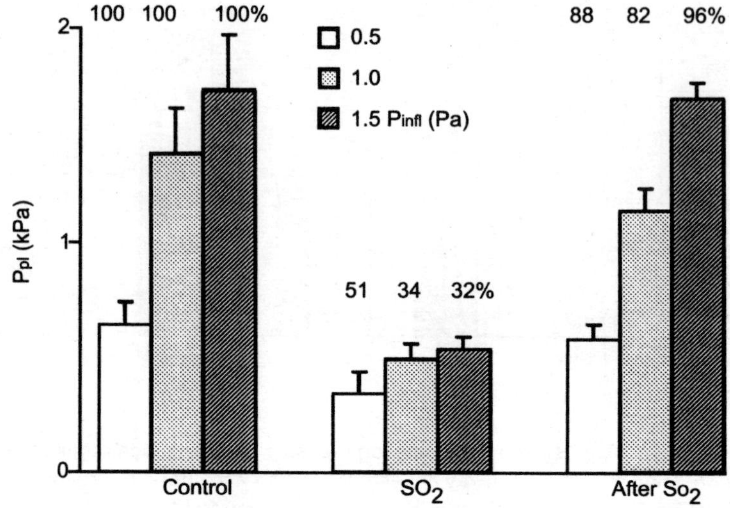

Fig. 4.5C Relationship between lung inflation pressure and expiration reflex strength (ERS) in anaesthetised rabbits before and during SARs block by inhalation of sulphur dioxide (SO_2), and during recovery period. Control, before SO_2 inhalation; SO_2, immediately after inhalation of SO_2; After SO_2, recovery period from SO_2 block. Values above columns denote ERS expressed as % of control values. (Reproduced from Ref. [65] with permission from Publisher).

was halved after the vagus on one side was cut and was almost totally abolished when both vagi were cut. The ERS at rest (i.e. no increased lung inflation), when either one or both vagi were cut, decreased significantly compared to the control values that were obtained (Fig. 4.5B).

Since inhalation of SO_2 is an effective method for selectively blocking the airway SARs,[51] using this we found an abolition of a direct relationship between LIP and ERS. These results are similar to those obtained after using a local anaesthetic in the airways of rabbits[61] and cats with both vagi cut.[63] Immediately after breathing SO_2 in concentrations of 200–300 ppm for 10 to 15 minutes, the direct positive relationship between LIP magnitude and ERS and between LIP magnitude and HBIR duration was restored when SARs recovered from the blockade.

Results obtained showed clearly, that in animals (rabbits, cats, ferrets) stimulation of SARs leads to increasing the expiratory effort, which is manifest as an enhancement of ERS. Furthermore, the blockade of airway SARs prevents the enhancement of ERS. These phenomena can only be partly attributed to the biomechanical properties of the chest wall, since when both the vagi are cut, only an insignificant increase in the ERS but a progressive increase in the LIP can be seen[61] (Fig. 4.5B). If the chest wall properties are important factors in the enhancement of ERS by increasing LIP, as supposed by Nishino et al[45] then this dependence should be present when both vagi are cut, but it is not so.

Accordingly, it is likely that the increased activity of airway SARs is responsible for the direct dependence between ERS and the magnitude of LIP. This conclusion is based on the fact that breathing of SO_2 leads to blockade of SARs and leaves RARs activity, largely unchanged[51] (Fig. 4.5C). Moreover, an increased LIP leads to only a short lasting burst of RAR activity only at the beginning of lung inflation.[66] Thus, they cannot be involved in the enhancement of ERS that is seen in our experiment, as we had induced expiratory reflexes only 3 to 4 seconds after inflating the lungs.[60] An increased activity of RARs by induction of pneumothorax was shown in studies carried out by Sellick and Widdicombe.[67] However, in our experiments on ferrets, the evidence obtained shows that pneumothorax induced by introducing 20 or 40 ml of air into the right pleural cavity, does not influence the direct dependence between LIP magnitude and ERS.[63] This is further evidence that RARs are not involved in the above-mentioned dependence.

The likelihood of bronchial or lung C-fibres influencing the direct dependence of LIP on ERS is very small. First, the C-fibres are rather insensitive to increased airway/intrapulmonary pressure as they belong to a group of high-threshold mechanoreceptors; and secondly, if they are stimulated, say by capsaicin, the result is an inhibition of inspiratory and expiratory components of the cough reflex rather than stimulation.[52]

Thus, we can conclude that experiments devoted to answering the question whether the stimulation of airway SARs can increase the strength of the various airway defence reflexes, gave different answers for cough, sneezing and expiration reflex. In cough and sneezing, there is no positive relationship between SARs activity and cough reflex strength, but in expiration reflex the stimulation of SARs exerts clear stimulatory influence on the strength of this reflex.

How can this difference be explained? The pathways from SARs to respiratory neurons in the brainstem are still largely unknown.[34] The second-order relay neurons of the SARs are distributed in the NTS and are called pump neurons or P-cells. These types of cells send axons to various respiration-related areas of the medulla and the pons, but their exact target neurons have not yet been determined. There is a widespread axonal projection of P-cells, i.e. those to the commissural subnuclei of the NTS on both sides. In these areas, the second-order relay neurons from the airways (RAR cells) are concentrated. Ezure and Tanaka[34] have shown that stimulation of airway SARs leads to increased activity of P-cells and that their activity in turn inhibits the RAR cells in rats. The inhibition of RAR cells by P-cells during lung inflation functions as a mechanism by which activation of RARs-related pathways in the brainstem are inhibited. This could explain the neuronal mechanisms underlying the Hering-Breuer inflation reflex,[34] but not the one responsible for increasing ERS, that is seen in our experiments.

Ezure and Tanaka[34] do not think that all P-cells are inhibitory. There is some evidence that also suggests that there exists an excitatory connection between P-cells to certain types of respiratory neurons in the brainstem,[29,69] but a lack of knowledge about the network in which P-cells are involved, prevents a complete understanding of SARs-evoked respiratory reflexes.[70]

It is logical to assume that an enhancement of ERS during lung inflation can occur only by an increased activity of expiratory muscles. Studies published by Cohen,[71] Bianchi and Barillot[72] and von Euler[73] have shown that stimulation of airway SARs facilitates the expiratory neurons in medulla oblongata as well as of the expiratory muscles. Another insight regarding the relation between LIP and ERS has been provided by the observation[74,75] that lung inflation excites expiratory premotor neurons characteristically present in the caudal ventral respiratory group (cVRG) of medulla by pressures less than 4 cmH_2O,[78] and inhibits them at pressures that are at higher levels. In our experiments, we used LIP in the range of 5 to 15 cmH_2O. Thus, we should have expected to see this group of expiratory neurons to have been inhibited. One explanation of this discrepancy that is offered could be explained by the observation of Bolser and Davenport[76] that cVRG premotor expiratory neurons undergo a post-inhibitory rebound when inflation is removed (as also shown by Bajic et al.).[75] However, it does not quite explain the direct relationship between LIP magnitude and ERS, which we saw in our experiments;[60–63] it was seen during lung inflation but not at the end of it. Another notion presented by Bolser and Davenport[77] derived from existing data which appears acceptable enough, is that SARs input has an excitatory effect both on tracheobronchial cough[32,33] as well as on the amplitude of the ERS and that these effects are presumably mediated through the action of pump cells. We suppose that the predicted connections from P-cells to brainstem expiratory neurons and expiratory muscles[29,69] are mainly involved in increasing ERS when LIP is increased, but they could be only partly involved in the regulation of expiratory efforts of cough. Bolser and

Davenport[54] in accordance with the model of the central regulatory systems for cough present this hypothesis. The model of a plausible regulatory system could be a combination of the original one proposed by Shannon and coworkers[82,83] and actual experimental data obtained by Bolser's group.[31,83] According to this, the pulmonary vagal afferent information is primarily processed by second-order interneurons located close to and in various subnuclei of the NTS. These interneurons include pump cells, mediating SARs information;[77] second-order RARs relay neurons,[78] laryngeal second-order neurons,[79] and relay neurons mediating pulmonary C-fibre reflexes.[80] All these groups of neurons are probably involved in production of, and/or modulation of cough under different conditions. The underlying idea of this model is the suggestion that separate gating mechanisms regulate afferent input to the burst-timer of laryngeal and tracheobronchial cough. The authors of this model developed the hypothesis that separate regulatory elements control laryngeal and tracheobronchial cough. This means that there is a separate gating mechanism for laryngeal and tracheobronchial cough. By using this model, it is possible to explain why there are differences in the influence of SARs stimulation, on cough and expiration reflex. Although results obtained by Ezure and Tanaka[34] show that stimulation of SARs inhibit RARs-relay neurons, there is yet no evidence for an excitatory connection from P-cells to motoneurones driving the expiratory muscles, in animal, other than the rat. Jordan[84,85] had also presumed such a mechanism;[84,85] but unfortunately, there is no data that supports this idea.

4.3.2 Reflex Inputs from Rapidly Adapting Stretch Receptors and C-fibres to Cough

Pathological processes, symptoms and signs such as bronchoconstriction, increased ventilation, apnoea, tachypnoea, increased mucus secretion, unpleasant chest sensations and cough in the airways and lungs are expected to arise by stimulation of bronchopulmonary afferent nerves.[68] It is rational to suppose that these reflexes do not occur as a result of stimulation of separate kinds of airway afferent nerve endings, but rather that they are the consequence of some integrative input from some or all of them. While considering the mechanism of cough induction under pathological conditions, one has to take into account that more than one type of afferent nerve endings will be involved in this event. It is generally believed that a subgroup of airway RARs functions as the primary 'cough receptors'. Evidence for the participation of C-fibre afferents in eliciting cough reflex is controversial yet, as Tatar et al[47] showed that stimulation of airway and pulmonary C-fibres inhibits cough induced by mechanical stimulation of airway mucosa. When lung C-fibres are stimulated by an (intravenous) i.v. bolus of phenylbiguanide (PBG), cough induced by mechanical stimulation of larynx was completely abolished during the apnoeic phase and its strength, significantly reduced during the phase of rapid shallow breathing. It is well known that an i.v. injection of PBG provides a strong stimulus to pulmonary C-fibres, that generates a notable inhibitory effect on breathing, and which is typically seen as a long-lasting apnoea in anaesthetised animals[40] as well as in man.[86-88] Lee and coworkers[88] suggested that such an intense input may have altered the gating mechanism of the central neural circuit mediating the cough reflex or induced a short-term memory affecting the neuronal synaptic transmission. So it seems that cough inhibition by pulmonary C-fibre stimulation takes place at the central level of cough control.

According to another view, stimulation of C-fibre afferents by inhalation of capsaicin or of citric acid aerosol can consistently and reproducibly provoke cough in a dose-dependent manner in both animals and humans, and it is plausible to assume that tussive responses are elicited by indirect effects of C-fibre stimulation such as bronchoconstriction and hypersecretion of mucus, and by other mechanisms.[88] Amongst these could be pathways involved in induction of cough by C-fibre stimulation and as described by Joad and coworkers[92] and Barnes.[93] The authors have shown that stimulation of C-fibres in airways can lead to the release of substance P and subsequent activation of RARs via the synthesis and release of nitric oxide; that could lead to an increase in the interstitial fluid volume in airway mucous membrane. According to Barnes,[93] activation of airway C-fibres, particularly by capsaicin, evokes an axon reflex-dependent peripheral release of neuropeptides—substance P, neurokinin A and calcitonin-gene-related peptide. Based on these data, Widdicombe[94] and Sekizawa et al[95] put forward another hypothesis, which explains the induction of cough by both RARs and C-fibre stimulation. They suppose that chemical stimuli that induce cough may do so at first, by a direct action on RARs, and then by stimulating bronchial C-fibres which will then release tachykinins, which in turn stimulate RARs that lie close to postcapillary venules. The neurokinins would cause extravasation of plasma with an increase in interstitial fluid volume and opening of the paracellular pathways between epithelial cells, thus exciting RARs near the blood vessel and the epithelium. The strength and pattern of the cough response will depend on the relative direct excitation of the RARs and C-fibres (the former exciting and the latter inhibiting cough reflexely) and on the degree to which local release of tachykinins enhances the excitation of the RARs. Thus, local and central nervous integration would affect the ultimate cough response.

The neuropeptide-evoked RARs activation is unlikely to have a direct action on the afferent nerve endings, but it could possibly have one on the epithelial cells of the airways, which in turn could indirectly activate RARs.[96,97] Nevertheless, it seems undisputable that bronchopulmonary C-fibre afferents are involved, either directly or indirectly, in eliciting the cough reflex.[40,89–91]

Despite clear evidence that C-fibre stimulants readily evoke cough, it is not clear whether axon reflexes or any other type of peripheral interaction between C-fibres and RARs play a role in the defensive responses in the airways of humans or that of other species other than the guinea pigs.[2] This uncertainty is based on observations in dogs and cats that the effect of administering bradykinin and capsaicin into the airways can be abolished completely either by atropine or by vagotomy.[40,98,99] Fuller and co-workers[100] reported similar findings in humans. Morphological studies support the view that in humans, axon reflex does not play an important role in reactions induced by C-fibre stimulation.[101] However, the absence of the airway axon reflex in humans and other species is contrary to data showing that the C-fibre stimulants are very effective in provoking cough. From this, one can conclude that other mechanisms may also be potentially involved in C-fibres and coughing. Mazzone et al[2] supposed that peripheral interactions between C-fibres and RARs could occur independently of the axon reflex. This notion is based on the supposition that activation of C-fibres evokes CNS-dependent parasympathetic reflex-induced alteration in airway and vascular tone and induces mucus secretion.[40,99,100,102,103] These effects are mediated in a large part by acetylcholine released from airway parasympathetic nerves and may be sufficient to activate RARs in the airway mucous membrane that can result in coughing.

4.3.2.1 Central Processing of Input from Airway Rapidly Adapting Stretch Receptors and C-fibres

During the last few years, some new information on processing of inputs from afferent airway nerve fibres, responsible for cough induction and modulation, in the CNS had emerged.[54,81–82,104–106,108] These findings provide new knowledge to develop a model of the cough network. It is based on current knowledge about neurogenesis of cough[107] and the main ideas underlying the proposed model are:

1. a single network of neurons appears to mediate both cough and breathing,
2. the same network can produce such different actions as breathing and cough—also known as 'reconfiguration'. This can involve dynamic alteration of the excitability of key elements or recruitment of previously silent ones,
3. the excitability of this network during cough is additionally controlled by a 'gating mechanism' similar to that known from spinal cord pain regulation,
4. the gating mechanism of cough is a functional entity of unknown anatomical location, and
5. that it could represent single or multiple groups of interneurons interposed between NTS cough receptors relay neurons and the cough network; candidate populations of neurons may exist in raphe nuclei,[109] pons,[110] interposed with the nucleus of the cerebellum,[111] reticular formation,[112] and/or tegmental field.[107]

4.3.2.2 Changes of Cough Reflex due to Airway and Lung Inflammation

Cough is a common manifestation of acute and chronic inflammation of airway mucosa. The pathophysiological mechanisms that give rise to cough under such pathological processes are not well understood but are likely to result from one or all of the following causes:[112]

- irritation of nerve endings in airway mucosa by increased production of mucus,
- release of inflammatory mediators into the nerve endings environment,
- direct exposure of nerve endings to noxious substances present in the lumen of airway due to destruction of airway epithelium,
- enhanced effect of neuropeptides such as substance P, secondary to decrease of neutral endopeptidase on the epithelial cell surface,
- deformation of 'cough receptors' by accumulation of secretions and debris, and
- irritation of 'cough receptors' due to spasm of airway smooth muscles.

We suppose that destruction of the surfactant layer which (under normal condition covers the receptors on the surface of airways nerve endings), by inflammatory processes can be another reason for the sensitisation of airway 'cough receptors'. There are other factors which are involved in the development of chronic cough; for example, bronchial asthma, gastro-oesophageal reflux and chronic bronchitis, bronchiectasis.[113]

Hence, we can sum up our present knowledge on the mechanisms involved in cough manifestation during airway and lung pathological processes as being due to increased production of various tussigenic agonists in the airway wall, and due to increased sensitivity of cough reflex pathway.[18]

Cough intensity is very frequently increased in patients suffering from acute airway inflammation. This effect is ascribed to increased excitability of the nerve endings at the sites of airway inflammation. Unfortunately, we are largely ignorant about the mechanisms that underly increased nerve endings excitability under such conditions.

Recently, Kollarik and Undem[7] have shown that both the magnitude and rate of pH change are important variables in airway sensory nerve activation. These mechanisms may have relevance to changes of airway afferent nerve sensitivity that may occur in disorders in which airway pH decreases, such as airway inflammation. We have only some information on dynamics of nerve endings excitability during the progression and regression of airway inflammatory process. So we are not able to explain precisely why the cough intensity is so variable during airway and lung inflammation.

It is reasonable to assume that inflammatory or other types of pathological processes present in the airway mucosa can stimulate or inhibit the activity of airway 'cough receptors', which can result in increasing or decreasing of their excitability, and as a consequence result in the enhancement or inhibition (or disappearing) of the cough.

In our experiments performed on awake cats, in which experimental airway inflammation was induced by administering an aerosol of inflammatory agents, such as croton oil, turpentine oil, carrageenin or a suspension of *Staphylococcus aureus* (stabilised strain Wood 46, 1.5 ml, concentration 6×10^8 to ml^{-1}), the cough intensity was measured before the agent administration and during a 20-day period. The cough reflex was also induced by a mechanical (nylon fibre) or chemical (SO_2, 2 ml 10%) stimulation of the airway mucosa. The airway and lung inflammations were confirmed by respirophonography,[114] chest X-ray, white blood cells count and histological examination of samples taken from the airways and lungs. All these methods confirmed the presence of inflammatory processes with different intensities, in the respiratory system. The results of our experiments can be summarised as follows:

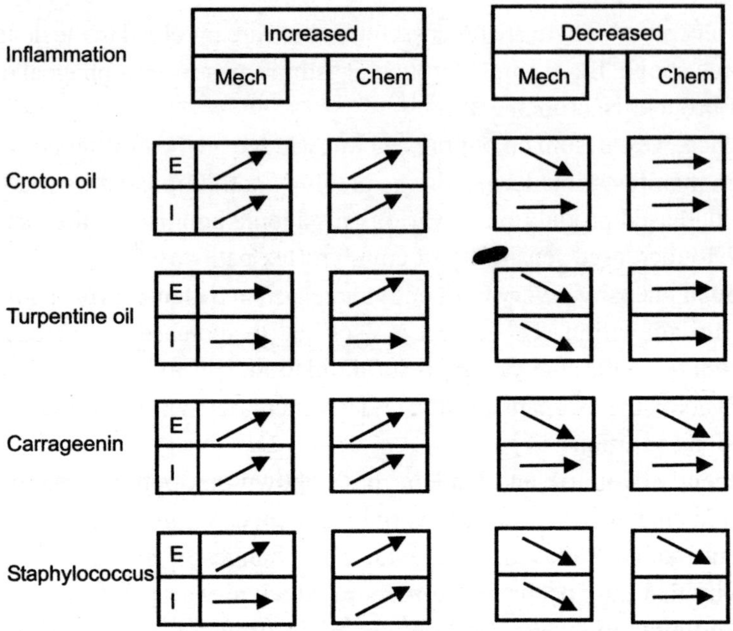

Fig. 4.6 Schematic representation of cough intensity changes during experimental inflammation of the airways and lungs of cats. Cough was provoked by mechanical (Mech) and chemical (Chem) means in awake animals, during airway or lung inflammation induced by aerosols of croton and turpentine oils, carrageenin and *Staphylococcus*. [= significant increase of the cough intensity; the change was significant compared to control values; = significant decrease of the change in cough intensity was significantly decreased compared to control values; = cough intensity unchanged compared to control values; (E) expiratory efforts of cough; (I) inspiratory efforts of cough.

1. Histological examination of airways and lungs has shown that the inflammatory agents that were used were successful in inducing inflammation in the airways and (in some cases) in the lung parenchyma. The intensity and character of the inflammation ranged from catarrhal to catarrhal-purulent. The inflammatory period can be divided into two phases. In the first phase, which lasted from the 2nd up to the 7th day after application of these agents, the signs of inflammation were present only in the airway mucosa. The second phase of inflammation occurred between 10 and 20 days. This phase was characterised by the inflammatory process proceeding into the airway mucosa although the inflammatory changes were also found in the

peribronchial and lung tissue. Erosions were seen in epithelial layer of airway mucosa; these were partly healed and covered over by metaplastic epithelium.

2. The intensity of cough induced by mechanical and chemical stimulation of airway mucosa in animals with airway or lung parenchymal inflammation changed significantly compared to that obtained before inflammation was induced.
3. During the entire period (20 days) that the cough intensity was monitored for, it was found that the phase of an increase in intensity of the cough (significantly higher) lasted for 2 to 4 days and that it was higher than in the pre-inflammatory period. During the same monitored period, another phase lasting for 2 to 5 days when the intensity of cough was significantly lowered compared to control value (Fig. 4.6) was also found.
4. Our results also show that there is a difference in the change in cough intensity when compared to that worked by mechanical or chemical means. In all types of inflammations, we were able to recognise when cough induced by SO_2 was enhanced; that evoked by mechanical stimuli during inflammation induced by all inflammatory agents (with the exception of turpentine oil), increased.
5. There is also a temporal difference in the enhancement of cough induced by mechanical or chemical stimuli during inflammation of the airways. The phase of enhanced cough provoked mechanically occurred earlier in inflammations induced by chemical agents (croton oil, carrageenin), i.e. about 4 to 5 days after agents were applied, as compared to that induced by *Staphylococcus* (5–7 days). We had also observed the enhancement of chemically induced cough earlier with inflammations induced by chemical agents (between 6 and 9 days) as compared to that induced by *Staphylococcus* (around 14th day after application).
6. Our experiments also showed a decreased intensity of cough induced by mechanical stimulation of airways in all types of inflammatory processes (Fig. 4.6). This decrease in cough intensity was present earlier (around 8–9 days) with inflammations induced by chemicals (croton and turpentine oils, carrageenin) than with inflammation induced by *Staphylococcus* (around 12th day).

We did not find a decrease in the chemically induced cough intensity during the entire episode of inflammation, induced by croton and turpentine oils, but observed a decrease in its intensity during inflammation induced by carrageenin and *Staphylococcus*. This decrease occurred very early on after *Staphylococcus* aerosol was introduced into the airways (around 4th day) and much later on during inflammation produced by carrageenin (around 11th day).

From these results, we can conclude that during experimentally induced airway inflammation in cats, there exists a phase when intensity of cough is increased but there is also a phase when cough is attenuated to as much as below the pre-inflammatory period. From the biological point of view, this is even more important than its enhancement. There are some data from clinical practice, which support our results. For example, Lemoine[115] had found a profound decrease in cough, in patients suffering from chronic bronchitis. Braestrup[116] had seen that cough disappeared in patients suffering from obliterating laryngotracheobronchitis.

The mechanisms that could be involved in the enhancement of cough seen in cats with inflammation of the respiratory tract have been listed at the beginning of this chapter. We suppose that more than one part of the cough reflex arc participates in the enhancement of cough under these conditions. First, the airway afferent nerve endings are sensitised and change their structure and function (plasticity of nerve fibres) due to inflammatory mediators,[117] which leads to an increased cough reflex sensitivity. Second, the inflammatory process in the airway can lead to enhancement of synaptic transmission at the level of second-order neurons in the brainstem that are involved in the mediation of the cough reflex. The enhancement of synaptic transmission can be not only due to an increased content of tachykinins in C-fibres but also in low-threshold mechanoreceptors.[118] Tachykinins are then transported to the central terminals of these afferents and then released into the synaptic cleft with second-order neurons. Such 'central sensitisation' can then supposedly lead to an enhancement of cough.

Even more difficult to explain is the underlying mechanism of attenuation of cough during airway and lung inflammation as seen in our experiments. We can only speculate that it could be due to destruction of the mucous membrane by inflammatory processes and secondary damage to airway afferents mediating cough. This is based on the observation of the time taken between morphological changes of airway mucosa and seeing decreased cough intensity.

Unfortunately, one cannot exclude other mechanisms that may be participating in this phenomenon too. One of them could be an inhibition of the central structures involved in integration of cough by an intensification of afferent inputs from airway nerve endings due to the presence of a high level of inflammatory mediators in the mucosa. Since strong activation of pulmonary J receptors due to pathological processes occurring in the lungs can activate the J reflex that inhibits the somatic muscles,[119] we can suppose that respiratory muscles too can be inhibited in a similar way and this could be the reason for the decrease in the intensity of cough.

An increase in the intensity of reflex cough in the presence of a diffuse inflammation of the airways was seen as expected, but the question that has to be answered is as to what kind of cough reflex changes, if any, would be seen when only local inflammation of airway is present. To answer this question, we used a slight modification of the method required for inducing local trachitis in cats.[120] A single silk stitch placed into the dorsal wall of cervical trachea was used for induction of trachitis.

Inflammation was restricted only to the trachea. No histological signs of inflammation were found in laryngopharyngeal and bronchial mucosa. With this, a significantly increased intensity of cough induced by mechanical stimulation of tracheal mucosa was found, with the maximum obtainable being seen between 15 and 17 days after insertion of the stitch. The cough induced from laryngo-pharynx and bronchi, however, remained unchanged. At about the 20th day after stitch insertion, the intensity of cough induced from trachea decreased to control level, but that obtained by stimulation of laryngo-pharynx and bronchi decreased significantly compared to pre-inflammatory period.

When the inflammatory process in the trachea was restricted to around 1 cm^2, by injecting 0.01 ml croton oil or turpentine oil diluted with olive oil in a ratio 1 : 20, into the tracheal mucosa (Hanacek, unpublished data), we also found an enhancement of cough induced by mechanical stimulation of trachea at or near the place of inflammation. Maximal cough intensity was present between 10 and 15 days after injection of chemical agents. During the entire duration when the cough was monitored, we did not see a decrease in its intensity below the control level, when induced from the trachea.

Interestingly, in local croton inflammation, but not in local turpentine inflammation, we observed a significant enhancement of cough induced from laryngopharyngeal mucosa. In both types of local tracheal inflammation, we had not seen enhancement of cough intensity when cough was induced by mechanical stimulation of bronchi. At the end of the observation period (between 17th and 19th days) the cough intensity induced from laryngopharyngeal and bronchial mucosa, in both types of inflammation, was significantly decreased below the control level. We can summarise the results obtained in experiments with local inflammation of trachea as follows:

1. Cough reflex intensity induced by mechanical stimulation of trachea is increased even when only local inflammation in the trachea is present.
2. In local trachitis induced by croton oil, the cough intensity provoked from laryngopharyngeal mucosa is enhanced, even though no histological evidence of inflammation was present at this place.
3. The unexpected result is that of a decrease in cough intensity induced from larygo-pharynx and bronchi in the absence of an inflammation in local trachitis produced by either method.

Other types of airway and lung pathology also influence the cough reflex intensity. In experiments carried out on anaesthetised rabbits,[121] we monitored cough intensity during the development of lung oedema induced by an i.v. injection of fatty acids. Cough was induced by blowing of NH_3 into the trachea by means of a syringe. We found attenuation of cough intensity-predominantly cough expiratory effort—from 5th to 60th minute after injection of fatty acids, with significant differences present during this time. Pulmonary oedema was confirmed by histological examination and by measurement of lung coefficient (ratio between lung weight expressed in grams and body weight expressed in kg).

Moderate but significant decrease in cough intensity induced by mechanical stimulation of laryngopharyngeal mucosa was also found in non-anaesthetised cats exposed for 14 days (10 h each day) to pure (100%) normobaric oxygen.[122]

Similar results were obtained in experiments carried out on awake guinea pigs,[123] where we found that animals with experimentally induced allergic airway inflammation and exposed to pure normobaric oxygen for 60 h had decreased the cough intensity induced by citric acid as when not exposed to oxygen at all.

What could be the main factors involved in enhancement and inhibition of cough intensity during the airway/lung damage which were present in our experiments? We suppose that primary factor is changed quality and quantity of afferent inputs from airways and lung parenchyma. The 'total activity' of airway and lung receptors during airway and lung pathology depends on at least on one of the following conditions:

1. *On the intensity and/or the phase of the inflammatory process*: In response to an increasing intensity of the inflammatory process, the activity of airway afferent nerve endings should increase too. There has to be some limit to the intensity of inflammation when the airway afferents could

be damaged or even destroyed and this could lead to decreasing the total activity of airway afferents to levels even lower than those seen during the pre-inflammatory period.

2. *On the type of chemical agents that induce pathological process in the airways and lung tissue:* Some of these may have a higher affinity for nerve tissue than to other types of tissues. This can lead to an intense damage of airway nerve endings and consequently, to decreasing the afferent output from the airways to the CNS. On the other hand, some other chemicals may lead to an overproduction of stimulants, which may result in increasing the output of airway afferents.
3. *On the size of inflammatory process in the airways and lungs*: With an increase in the size of the inflammatory reaction, more airway and lung afferents should be influenced, and consequently, the total activity of airway afferents could be profoundly increased.
4. *On the duration of inflammatory process*: It seems plausible to suppose that total activity of airway and lung afferents will be different in acute and in chronic airway inflammation because of different tissue characteristics and a different array of inflammatory mediators released.

Another level of the cough reflex arc at which it could be modulated, is the brainstem and other parts of CNS. We suppose that the gating mechanism controlling the parameters of cough and pain may function on similar principles. It is well known that the intensity of pain can be increased or decreased by functioning of a neuronal network at the dorsal horn of the spinal cord. It is possible that similar neuronal network can come into play at the level of NTS and the result could be an enhancement or inhibition of cough.

REFERENCES

1. Korpas J, Tomori Z. Cough and other respiratory reflexes. New York: S. Karger, 1979;356.
2. Mazzone SB, Canning JB, Widdicombe JG. Sensory pathways for the cough reflex. In: Chung F, Widdicombe JG, Boushey H, editors. Cough: Causes, Mechanisms and Therapy. 1st ed. Oxford: Blackwell Publishing, 2003;p161–71.
3. Irwin RS, Widdicombe JG. Cough. In: Murray JF, Nadel JA, editors. Textbook of Respiratory Medicine, 3rd ed. Philadelphia: Saunders, 2000;p553–66.
4. Widdicombe JG. Afferent receptors in the airways and cough. Respiration Physiology 1998;114(1):5–15.
5. Karlson JA. The role of capsaicin-sensitive C-fibre afferent nerves in the cough reflex Pulmonary Pharmacology 1996;9(5–6):315–21.

6. Sant' Ambrogio G, Sant' Ambrogio FB, Davies A. Airway receptors in cough. Bulletin Europèen de Physiopathologie Respiratoire 1984;20(1):43–47.
7. Kollarik M, Undem BJ. Mechanisms of acid-induced activation of airway afferent nerve fibres in guinea-pig. Journal of Physiology 2002;543(2):591–600.
8. Undem BJ, Carr MJ, Kollarik M. Physiology and plasticity of putative cough fibres in the guinea pig. Pulmonary Pharmacology 2002;15:193–8.
9. Carr MJ, Undem BJ. Bronchopulmonary afferent nerves. Respirology 2003;8:291–301.
10. Bolser DC, De Gennaro FC, O'Reilly RI, Hey JA. Central antitussive activity of the NK1 and NK2 tachykinin receptor antagonists, CP-99, 994 and SR 48968, in the guinea pig and cat. British Journal of Pharmacology 1997;121:165–70.
11. Mazzone SB, Canning BJ. Synergistic interactions between airway afferent nerve subtypes mediating reflex bronchospasm in guinea pigs. American Journal of Physiological Regulations: Integrative and Comparative Physiology 2002, 283:R86–98.
12. Ma QP, Woolf CJ. Involvement of neurokinin receptors in the induction but not the maintenance of mechanical allodynia in rat flexor motoneurones. Journal of Physiology 1995;486:769–77.
13. O'Connel F, Thomas VE, Studham JM, Pride NB, Fuller RW. Capsaicin cough sensitivity increases during upper respiratory tract infection. Respiratory Medicine 1996;90:279–286.
14. Pecova R, Frlickova Z, Pec J, Tatar M. Cough sensitivity in atopic dermatitis. Pulmonary Pharmacology and Therapeutics 2003;16:203–6.
15. Hanacek J. Changes of cough reflex intensity in unanaesthetized cats with experimental inflammation of airway and lung. Bratislavske Lekarske Listy 1986;85:444–50.
16. Pek W-Y, Boushey HA. Cough in lower airway infections. In: Chang F, Widdicombe JG, Boushey H, eds. Cough: Causes, Mechanisms and Therapy. 1st ed. Oxford: Blackwell Publishing, 2003;83–96.
17. Neumann S, Doubell TP, Lesie T, Wolf CJ. Inflammation pain hypersensitivity mediated by phenotypics switch in myelinated primary sensory neurons. Nature 1996;384:360–4.
18. Kollarik M, Undem JB. Plasticity of vagal afferent fibres mediating cough. In: Chung F, Widdicombe JG, Boushey H, editors. Cough: Causes, Mechanisms and Therapy. 1st ed. Oxford: Blackwell Publishing, 2003;p.181–92.
19. Paintal AS, Anand A, editors. Respiratory control mechanisms and sensations. Delhi: Vallabhbhai Patel Chest Institute, University of Delhi, 1998;245.
20. Chung F, Widdicombe JG, Boushey H, editors. Cough: Causes, Mechanisms and Therapy, Oxford: Blackwell Publishing, 2003;304.
21. Widdicombe JG. Neuroregulation of cough: implication for drug therapy. Current Opinion in Pharmacology 2002;2:256–63.
22. Widdicombe JG. Receptors in the trachea and bronchi of the cat. Journal of Physiology 1954;123:71–104.
23. Hunter DD, Undem BJ. Identification and substance P content of vagal afferent neurons innervating the epithelium of the guinea pig trachea. American Journal of Respiratory and Critical Care Medicine 1999;159(6):1943–8.
24. Riccio MM, Kummer V, Biglari B, Myers AC, Undem BJ. Interganglionic segregation of distinct vagal afferent fibre phenotypes in guinea-pig airways. Journal of Physiology 1996;496(2):521–30.

25. Davies RO, Kubin L. Projection of pulmonary rapidly adapting receptors to the medulla of the cat: an antidromic mapping study. Journal of Physiology 1986;373:63–86.
26. Haxhiu MA, Yamamoto B, Dreshaj IA, Bedol D, Ferguson DG. Involvement of glutamate in transmissions of afferent constrictive inputs from the airways to the nucleus tractus solitarius in ferrets. Journal of Autonomous Nervous System 2000;80:22–30.
27. Adrian ED. Afferent impulses in the vagus and their effect on respiration. Journal of Physiology 1933;79:332–58.
28. Mc Alexander MA, Myers AC, Undem BJ. Adaptation of guinea-pig vagal airway afferent neurons to mechanical stimulations. Journal of Physiology 1999;521:239–47.
29. Hayashi F, Cotes SK, Mc Crimmon DR. Respiratory neurons mediating the Breuer-Hering reflex prolongation of expiration in rat. Journal of Neuroscience 1996;16:6526–36.
30. Sant' Ambrogio G, Miserocchi G, Mortola J. Functional localization of pulmonary stretch receptors in the airways of the dog. Bulletin Européen de Physiopathologie Respiratoire 1974;9:1248–56.
31. Bolser DC, Davenport PW. Volume-timing relationships during cough and resistive loading in the cat. Journal of Applied Physiology 2000;89:785–90.
32. Hanacek J, Davies A, Widdicombe JG. Influence of lung stretch receptors on the cough reflex in rabbits. Respiration 1984;45:161–8.
33. Sant' Ambrogio G, Sant´Ambrogio FB, Davies A. Airway receptor in cough. Bulletin Européen de Physiopathologie Respiratoire 1984;20:43–7.
34. Ezure K, Tanaka I. Lung inflation inhibits rapidly adapting receptor relay neurons in the rat. Neuro Report 2000;11:1709–12.
35. Cross KW, Klaus M, Tooley WH, Weisser K. The response of the new-born baby to inflation of the lungs. Journal of Physiology 1960;151:551–65.
36. Rabbette PS, Fletcher ME, Dezatenx CA et al. Hering-Breuer reflex and respiratory system compliance in the first year of life: a longitudinal study. Journal of Applied Physiology 1994;76:650–6.
37. Hamilton RD, Winning AJ, Horner RL, Guz A. The effect of lung inflation on breathing in man during wakefulness and sleep. Respiration Physiology 1988;73:145–54.
38. Fernando SS, Saunders KB. Isocapnic and small hypercapnic single breath stimuli: evidence for an inhibitory inflation reflex in conscious man. The European Respiratory Journal 1994;7:869–74.
39. Bishop B, Bachofen H. Comparative influence of proprioceptors and chemoreceptors in the control of respiratory muscles. Acta Neurobiologiae Experimentalis 1973;33:381–30.
40. Coleridge JC, Coleridge HM. Afferent vagal C-fibre innervation of the lungs and airways and its functional significance. Reviews of Physiology, Biochemistry and Pharmacology 1984;99:1–110.
41. Fox A. Airway nerves: in vitro electrophysiology. Current Opinion in Pharmacology 2002;2(3):278–9.
42. Paintal AS. Sensations from J receptors. News in Physiological Science 1995;10:238–43.
43. Coleridge HM, Coleridge JCG. Pulmonary reflexes: Neural mechanisms of pulmonary defense. American Review of Physiology 1994;56:69–91.

44. Widdicombe JG. C-fibres, tachykinins and cough. In: Paintal AS, Anand A, editors. Respiratory Control Mechanisms and Sensations. Vallabhbhai Patel Chest Institute, University of Delhi, 1998;p66–81.
45. Nishino T, Sugimori K, Hiraga K, Honda Y. Influence of CPAP on reflex responses to tracheal irritation in anesthetized humans. Journal of Applied Physiology 1989;67:954–8.
46. Romaniuk JR, Kowalski KE, Dick TE. The role of pulmonary stretch receptors activation during cough in dog. Acta Neurobiologiae Experimentalis 1997;57:21–9.
47. Tatar M, Weber SE, Widdicombe JG. Lung C-fibre receptor activation and defensive reflexes in anaesthetized cats. Journal of Physiology 1988;402:411–20.
48. Widdicombe JG. Respiratory reflexes and defense. In: Brain J. D. et al., editors, Respiratory defense mechanisms, Part II. New York, Basel: Decker, 1977;pp593–630.
49. Bucher K, Jacot C. Zum mechanismus des hustens. Helvetica Physiologica Acta 1951;9:454–62.
50. BucherK. Tessalon, ein hustenstillender mittel von neuratigem wirkungsmechanizmus. Schweizarische Medizinische Wochenschrift 1956;86:94–6.
51. Davies A, Dixon M, Penman R, Widdicombe JG, Wise JCM. Effect of repeated exposure to high concentrations of sulphur dioxide on respiratory reflexes in rabbits. Bulletin Européen de Physiopathologie Respiratoire 1978;14:41–52.
52. Tatar M. Webber SE, Widdocombe JG. Lung C-fibre receptor activation and defensive reflexes in anaesthetized cats. Journal of Physiology 1988;402:411–20.
53. Hanacek J. Cough reflex changes in cats after sulphur dioxide breathing. In: editors. Salat D, Badalik L, Krcmery V. Day SB, Proceedings of 1st High Tatras International Health Symposium on Health and Quality of Life in Changing Europe in the year 2000, Postgraduate Medical School and School of Public Health. Bratislava, Czecho-Slovakia, 1992;pp272–9.
54. Bolser DC, Davenport PW. Functional organization of the central cough generation mechanism. Pulmonary Pharmacology and Therapeutics 2002;15:221–5.
55. Clark FJ, von Euler C. On the regulation of depth and rate of breathing. Journal of Physiology 1972;222:267–95.
56. Higenbottam T, Mackson M, Woolman P, Lowry R, Wallwork J. The cough response to ultrasonically nebulized distilled water in heart-lung transplantation patients. American Review of Respiratory Diseases 1989;140:58–61.
57. Javorka K, Michalik J, Caklos S, Bevilaqua J. Effect of increased intrapulmonary pressure on defense reflexes of the respiratory tract. Bratislavske Lekarske Listy 1982;77(5):612–20.
58. Tatar M, Nagyova B. Effects of lung inflation on airways defense reflexes. The European Respiratory Journal 1990;3:141.
59. Korpas J. Differentiation of the expiration and the cough reflex. Physiologia bohemoslovaca 1972;21:677–80.
60. Hanacek J, Korpas J. Modification of the intensity of the expiration reflex during short-term inflation of the lung in rabbits. Physiologia bohemoslovaca 1982;31:169–74.
61. Hanacek J. Relation between the airways receptors and the defensive reflexes of the respiratory tract. Folia Medica Martiniana 1984;10:45–65.

62. Hanacek J, Turcan J, Korpas J. The role of vagus nerve in mechanisms of expiratory reflex increase by lung inflation. Bulletin Européen de Physiopatholgie Respiratoire 1983;19:33–4.

63. Turcan J, Hanacek J, Korpas J. Influence of short-term lung inflation on the magnitude of expiratory reflex in the ferrets under normal condition and during experimental pneumothorax. Bratislavske Lekarske Listy 1983;79:705–11.

64. Turcan J, Hanacek J, Korpas J. Expiration reflex intensity in rats induced by the inflation of lungs. Physiologia bohemoslovaca 1981;30:465.

65. Hanacek J. Influence of sulphur dioxide breathing on defensive reflexes of the airways. Acta Physiologica Hungarica 1987;70(2–3):227–33.

66. Knowlton GC, Larrabee MG. Unitary analysis of pulmonary volume receptors. American Journal of Physiology 1946;147:100–14.

67. Sellick H, Widdicombe JG. The activity of lung irritant receptors during pneumothorax, hyperpnoea and pulmonary vascular congestion. Journal of Physiology 1969;203:359–81.

68. Widdicombe JG. Pathophysiology of lung reflexes. Bulletin Européen de Physiopathologie Respiratoire 1974;10:65–9.

69. Iscoe S. Control of abdominal muscles. Progress in Neurobiology 1998;56:433–506.

70. Miyazaki M, Tanaka I, Ezure K. Excitatory and inhibitory synaptic inputs shape the discharge pattern of pump neurons of the nucleus tractus solitarii in the rat. Experimental Brain Research 1999;129:191–200.

71. Cohen MI. Discharge pattern of brain-stem respiratory neurons during Hering-Breuer reflex evoked by lung inflation. Journal of Neurophysiology 1969;32:356–74.

72. Bianchi AL, Barillot JC. Activity of medullary respiratory neurons during reflexes from the lungs in cats. Respiration Physiology 1975;25:335–92.

73. von Euler C . The contribution of sensory inputs to the pattern generation of breathing. Canadian Journal of Physiology and Pharmacology 1981;59:700–6.

74. Cohen MI, Feldman JL, Sommer D. Caudal medullary expiratory neurons and intercostal nerve discharge in the cat: effects of lung inflation. Journal of Physiology 1985;368:147–78.

75. Bajic J, Zuperku EJ, Tonkovic-Capin M, Hopp FA. Expiratory bulbospinal neurons in dogs. I. Control of discharge pattern by pulmonary stretch receptors. American Journal of Physiology 1992;262:R1075–R1086.

76. Bolser DC, Davenport PW. Expiratory motor control during the cough reflex. European Respiratory Review 2004;85:243–8.

77. Berger AJ. Dorsal respiratory group neurons in the medulla of the cat: spinal projections, responses to lung inflation, and superior laryngeal nerve stimulation. Brain Research 1977;135:231–54.

78. Lipski J, Ezure K, Wong She RB. Identification of neurons receiving input from pulmonary rapidly adapting receptors in the cat. Journal of Physiology 1991;443:55–77.

79. Mifflin SW. Laryngeal afferent inputs to nucleus tractus solitarius. American Journal of Physiology 1993;265:R269–R276.

80. Bonham AC, Joad JP. Neurons in commisural nucleus tractus solitarii required for full expression of pulmonary C-fibre reflex in rat. Journal of Physiology 2001;441:95–112.

81. Shannon R, Baekey DM, Morris KF, Li Z, Lindsey BG. Functional connectivity among ventrolateral medullary respiratory neurons and responses during fictive cough in the cat. Journal of Physiology 2000;525:207–24.

82. Shannon R, Morris KF, Lindsey BG. Ventrolateral medullary respiratory network and a model of cough motor pattern generation. Journal of Applied Physiology 1998;84:2020–35.

83. Bolser DC, Hey JA, Chapman RW. Influence of central antitussive drugs on the cough motor pattern. Journal of Applied Physiology 1999;86:10017–1024.

84. Jordan D. Central nervous mechanisms in cough. Pulmorary Pharmacology 1996;9:389–92.

85. Lavorini F, Fontana GA, Cresci F, Polli G, Dallai S, Mutolo D, Panteleo T. Cough reflex in laryngectomized patients. The European Respiratory Journal 1994;7,25.

86. Leith DE. Cough. In: Brain JD, Proctor DF, Reid LF, editors. Respiratory defense mechanisms. New York-Basel, Dekker 1978;545–92.

87. Jain SK, Subramanian S, Julka DB, Guz A. Search for evidence of lung chemoreflexes in men: study of respiratory and circulatory effects of phenydiguanide and lobeline. Clinical Science 1972;42:163–77.

88. Lee L-Y, Kwong K, Lin YS, Qihai G. Hypersensitivity of bronchopulmonary C-fibres induced by airway mucosal inflammation: cellular mechanisms. Pulmonary Pharmacology and Therapeutics 2002;15:199–204.

89. Karlson JA, Fuller RW. Pharmacological regulation of the cough reflex—from experimental model to antitussive effect in men. Pulmonary Pharmacology and Therapeutics 1999;12:215–28.

90. Lalloo UG, Fox AJ, Belvisi MG, Chung KF, Barnes PJ. Capsazepine inhibits cough induced by capsaicin and citric acid but not by hypertonic saline in guinea pigs. Journal of Applied Physiology 1995;79:1082–7.

91. Winning AJ, Hamilton RD, Shea SA, Guz A. Respiratory and cardiovascular effects of central and peripheral intravenous injection of capsaicin in man: evidence for pulmonary chemosensitivity. Clinical Science 1986;71:519–26.

92. Joad JP, Kott KS, Bonham AC. Nitric oxide contributes to substance P-induced increases in lung rapidly adapting receptors activity in guinea pigs. The Journal of Physiology 1997;503:635–43.

93. Barnes PJ. Neurogenic inflammation in the airways. Respiration Physiology 2001;125:145–54.

94. Widdicombe JG. Sensory mechanisms of cough. Pulmonary Pharmacology 1996;9:383–8.

95. Sekizawa K, Jia YX, Ebihara T, Hirose Y, Hirayama Y, Sasakki H. Role of substance P in cough. Pulmonary Pharmacology 1996;9:323–8.

96. Sant' Ambrogio G, Widdicombe J. Reflexes from rapidly adapting receptors. Respiration Physiology 2001;125:33–45.

97. Bergren DR. Sensory receptor activation by mediators of defense reflexes in guinea-pig lungs. Respiration Physiology 1997;108:195–204.

98. Russell JA, Lai-Fook SJ. Reflex brnchoconstriction induced by capsaicin in dog. Journal of Applied Physiology 1979;47:961–7.

99. Ichinose M, Inoue H, Miura M, Yafuso N, Nogami H, Takishima T. Possible sensory receptors of nonadrenergic inhibitory nervous system. Journal of Applied Physiology 1987;63:423–929.

100. Fuller RW, Dixon CM, Barnes PJ. Bronchoconstrictor response to inhaled capsaicin in humans. Journal of Applied Physiology 1985;58:1080–4.

101. Lundberg JM, Hokfelt T, Martling CR, Saria A, Cuello C. Substance P-immunoreactive sensory nerves in the lower respiratory tract of various mammals including man. Cell and Tissue Research 1984;235:215–61.

102. Canning BJ, Reynolds SM, Mazzone SB. Multiple mechanisms of reflex bronchospasm in guinea pigs. Journal of Applied Physiology 2001;91(6):2642–53.

103. Lee L-Y, Pisarri TE. Afferent properties and reflex functions of bronchopulmonary C-fibers. Respiration Physiology 2001;125:47–65.

104. Mazzone SB, Geraghty DP. Respiratory actions of tachykinins in the nucleus of the solitary tract. Characterization of receptors using selective agonists and antagonists. British Journal of Pharmacology 2000;129:1121–31.

105. Jakus J, Stransky A, Poliacek I, Barani H, Boselova L. Effects of medullary midline lesions on cough and other airway reflexes in anaesthetized cats. Physiological Research 1998;47:203–13.

106. Jakus J, Stransky A, Poliacek I, Barani H, Boselova L. Kainic acid lesions to the lateral tegmental field of medulla: effect on cough, expiration and aspiration reflexes in anaesthetized cats. Physiological Research 2000;49:387–98.

107. Bolser DC, Davenport PW, Golder FJ, Baekey DM, Morris KF, Lindsey BG, Shannon R. Neurogenesis of cough. In: Chung F, Widdicombe JG, Boushey H, editors: Cough: Causes, Mechanisms and Therapy. 1st ed. Oxford: Blackwell Publishing, 2003;173–80.

108. Baekey DM, Morris KF, Nuding SC, Segers LS, Lindsey BG, Shannon R. Raphe neuron activity during fictive coughing. FASEB J 2002;16:628.

109. Baekey DM, Morris KF, Li Z, Nuding SC, Lindsey BG, Shannon R. Concurrent changes in pontine respiratory group neuron activity during fictive coughing. FASEB J 1999;13:A 824.

110. Xu F, Frazier DT, Zhang Z, Shannon R. Influence of the cerebellum on the cough motor pattern. Journal of Applied Physiology 1997;83:391–7.

111. Billig I. Foris JM, Enquist LW, Card JP, Yates BJ. Definition of neuronal circuitry controlling the activity of phrenic and abdominal neurons in the ferret using recombinant strains of pseudorabies virus. Journal of Neuroscience 2000;20:7446–54.

112. Pek W-Y, Boushey H. Cough in lower airway infections. In. Chung F, Widdidombe JG, Boushey H, eds. Cough: Causes, Mechanisms, and Therapy. 1st ed. Oxford: Blackwell Publishing, 2003;83–96.

113. Morice AH. The epidemiology of chronic cough. European Respiratory Review 2002;12(85):222–5.

114. Hanacek J, Korpas J. Vrabec M. Our experience with respirofonography. Ceskoslovenska Fysiologie 1976;25:343–6.

115. Lemoine JM. Tussigenic sensitivity of trachea and large bronchi in adults. Casopis Lekaru Ceskych 1968;107:763–5.

116. Braestrup PW. Acute obstructive laryngo-tracheobronchitis. Acta Pediatrica Scandinavica 1949;77:212–24.

117. Woolf CJ, Salter NW. Neuronal plasticity: increasing the gain in pain. Science 2000, 288:1765–1769.

118. Carr MJ, Hunter DD, Jacoby DB, Undem BJ. Expression of tachykinins in nonnociceptive vagal afferent neurons during respiratory viral infection in guinea pigs. American Journal of Respiratory and Critical Care Medicine 2002;165:1071–5.

119. Paintal AS. The mechanisms of excitation of type J receptors and the J-reflex. In: Porter R(ed). Breathing. Hering-Breuer Centenary Symposium. London, Churchill, 1970;59–71.

120. Hanacek J, Porubanova M, Korec L, Beseda O. Cough reflex changes in local tracheitis. Physiologia bohemoslovaca 1979;28(4):375–80.

121. Polacek H, Hanacek J, Ivan J, Gaman V, Tvrdik E. Plank L. Experimental cough induced by chemical stimulus in rabbits with pulmonary edema. Bratislavske Lekarske Listy 1985;83(1):53–62.

122. Brozmanova M, Hanacek J, Tatar M, Strapkova A, Szepe P. Functional and morphological changes of the respiratory organs in cats after long-term exposure to pure normobaric oxygen. Bratislavske Lekarske Listy 1996;97(5):251–9.

123. Brozmanova M, Hanacek J, Tatar M, Strapkova A, Szepe P. Effects of hyperoxia and allergic airway inflammation on cough reflex intensity in guinea pigs. Physiological Research 2002;51:529–36.

5 Influences on Cough

M TATAR

5.1 INTRODUCTION

Over the past 25 years, a great deal has been learnt about management of cough.[1] This information has been summarised in an evidence-based panel report written for cough specialists that includes diagnostic algorithms for chronic cough.[2] Studies have shown that in approximately 95 per cent of immunocompetent patients, chronic cough results from postnasal drip syndrome (PNDS), asthma, gastro-oeosophageal reflux disease (GERD), chronic bronchitis due to smoking or other irritants, bronchiectasis, eosinophilic bronchitis, or use of angiotensin-converting enzyme (ACE) inhibitor. In the remaining 5 per cent of cases, chronic cough is caused by a variety of other diseases, such as bronchogenic carcinoma, sarcoidosis, left ventricular failure, tuberculosis, and aspiration due to pharyngeal dysfunction.[2]

Most patients with postnasal drip-induced cough have symptoms or evidence of one or more of the following: postnasal drainage, throat clearing, nasal discharge, cobblestone appearance of the oropharyngeal mucosa, or mucus in the oropharynx. These upper respiratory tract symptoms may be absent in a small percentage of patients, yet that does not rule out the presence of a postnasal drip-induced cough.[3]

There is nothing distinctive about the clinical characteristics of cough associated with asthma,[4] and the clinical diagnosis of asthma is unreliable.[5] Since the methacholine challenge has a negative predictive value of 100 per cent[2] in the context of cough, so this test is extremely useful in ruling out asthma.

Diagnosing and successfully treating chronic cough due to GERD is a major challenge. Although GERD is amongst the three most common causes of chronic cough in all age groups, there is nothing about the character and timing of cough due to GERD that distinguishes it from other conditions;[4] moreover, it could be "silent" 75 per cent of the time.[6] GERD should always be considered a possible cause of cough when patients complain of typical and frequent gastrointestinal problems (e.g., heartburn and regurgitation) and especially when the chest radiograph is consistent with aspiration. GERD most likely causes chronic cough in patients with normal radiographs by a vagally mediated reflex mechanism. Cough in these diseases may become excessive and non-productive, and is potentially harmful to the airways and other organs.[2]

It is generally agreed that cough can be elicited from the larynx and the more proximal portion of the tracheobronchial tree.[7–12] Outside of the lower respiratory tract, cough could be elicited from the external auditory canals and eardrums.[13,14] The origin of cough is unique to structures that are innervated by the vagus nerves. There is clinical evidence that cough can be elicited, especially in pathological conditions, from many other organs such as the pharynx, nose and paranasal sinuses, pericardium, and gastrointestinal tract.[2] However, there is no conclusive evidence that afferent nerve endings localised in these organs can directly mediate the cough reflex. It is unlikely that cough arises from pharyngeal irritation, because cough has never been directly initiated from pharynx or other upper airway structures above the larynx.[15] Mazzone et al[12] proposed that afferent nerves innervating extrapulmonary viscera, play an integral role in regulating cough.

Although there are numerous studies on airways and pulmonary afferent nerve endings mediating the cough reflex, very few data are available regarding extrapulmonary mechanisms which may modulate cough intensity.[7,15] General anaesthesia, hypothermia and hyperthermia have a marked inhibitory effect on the pattern and strength of the cough reflex in cats.[7] For instance, in cats under pentobarbitone anaesthesia, the intensity of cough efforts and not their number per cough bout, decreases significantly as compared to what is seen when they are awake.[16] A significant decline in the intensity of chemically induced cough was present in conscious guinea pigs exposed to pure normobaric oxygen for 60 hours. Exposure of animals to 50 per cent oxygen for the same duration did not influence cough intensity.[17] It is well known that, in humans, an induced cough can be suppressed voluntarily, i.e. through the cortical pathways.[18]

An understanding of the neural extrapulmonary pathways involved in the regulation of the cough reflex may facilitate the study of new therapeutic strategies to modulate coughing for physiological reflex activity. Thus, it is important to discuss the influence of afferent inputs from the nasal mucosa, oesophageal mucosa, abdominal receptors, cardiac receptors and chemoreceptors on mechanically and chemically induced cough.

5.2 INFLUENCE OF NASAL RECEPTORS

Allergic diseases involving the nose and the sinuses are two important risk factors that can initiate an asthmatic attack[19] and nasal inflammation plays a significant role in the pathogenesis of asthma.[20–22] Reflex interactions between nasal stimulation and mechanically and chemically induced cough have not as yet been studied in experimental models.

The pathogenesis of chronic cough due to PNDS is not fully understood. The various mechanisms proposed for the appearance of cough in PNDS are: (i) stimulation of the hypopharynx by secretions from the nose and or the sinuses dripping on to it;[2] (ii) aspiration of inflammatory secretions from the nose and, or sinuses into the lower airways; (iii) reversible obstruction of extrathoracic airways;[23] and (iv) excessive drying of lower airways due to inadequate nasal airing.[24] All of these mechanisms incidentally, are able to give rise to a cough themselves.

Besides a direct activation of the cough reflex as mentioned in the foregoing account, it is also believed that the disease process that leads to a PNDS, also enhances coughing, albeit indirectly. Indeed, the cough reflex sensitivity (measured by the lowest dose of a tussigen that is effective in evoking a given intensity of cough) is substantially increased in patients with PNDS.[25,26]

Cough reflex hypersensitivity contributes to the pathogenesis of chronic cough; for instance, patients unlike healthy individuals may cough even in the presence of subthreshold levels of environmental stimuli. Interactions between the nasal passages and lower airways with regard to the cough reflex have not been studied systemically so far.[27,28] However, the effect of pathological changes in the nasal cavity on the cough reflex induced by the inhalation of tussive agents was studied in experimental allergic rhinitis in conscious guinea pigs.[29,30] Animals were challenged with ovalbumin intranasally and after the appearance of clinical symptoms of exudative rhinitis (sneezing, nasal rubbing, nasal discharge and nasal crackles), the cough response to gradually increasing concentrations

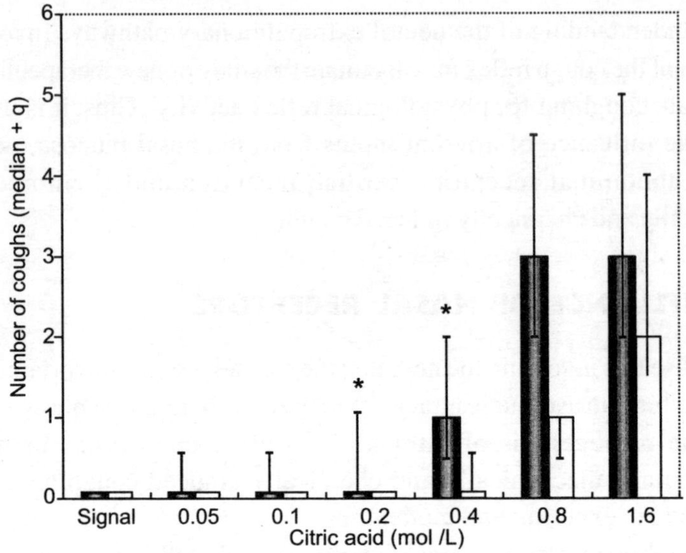

Fig. 5.1 The effect of inhalation of gradually increasing doses of citric acid aerosol on the number of coughs (median ± interquartile range) in awake guinea pigs with experimental allergic rhinitis (black columns) and in controls (white columns). * denotes p<0.05.

of citric acid was studied. For evaluation of cough, not only the parameters of expiratory airflow but also a spectral analysis of the cough sound was used. Use of this method made it possible to distinguish cough from sneezing.[31] The cough response in conscious guinea pigs with experimental allergic rhinitis was significantly increased during inhalation of lower concentrations of citric acid (Fig. 5.1). From these results, one can conclude that the sensitivity of the cough reflex was increased during ovalbumin-induced exudative rhinitis. Similar results were obtained when cough reflex sensitivity to capsaicin challenge was studied in pollen-sensitive patients with seasonal allergic rhinitis.[26] Their cough sensitivity to capsaicin was significantly increased not only in the 'pollen' season but also at other times.

So far, there is no clear experimental evidence as to the mechanism responsible for stimulation or sensitisation of laryngeal and tracheobronchial nerve endings that mediate cough reflex during rhinitis. Since nasal hypersecretion and a decreased nasal patency are frequent symptoms of experimental allergic rhinitis, and as guinea pigs are obligatory nasal breathers, it is possible that nasal mucus could move into the larynx and trachea in the form of a polydispersed aerosol. The intensity of citric acid-induced cough in conscious guinea pigs with bilateral resection of the superior laryngeal nerves was only slightly increased during experimental allergic rhinitis compared to control animals in whom the superior laryngeal nerves were resected, but who did not have any rhinitis.[32] This observation suggests that a decreased threshold of laryngeal mucosal nerve endings may play an important role in the phenomenon of increased sensitivity of the cough reflex during experimental allergic rhinitis in conscious guinea pigs. The small difference in the intensity of cough between control and rhinitic animals could be explained by the complementary role of tracheobronchial receptors.

Since symptoms of experimental allergic rhinitis last for 20 to 30 minutes after intranasal ovalbumin challenge in sensitised guinea pigs,[30,32] an important question that confronts us is, whether the changes in cough sensitivity are due to ovalbumin-induced rhinitis or due to sensitization to ovalbumin? When guinea pigs sensitised to ovalbumin were repeatedly challenged intranasally by ovalbumin and physiological saline in 4-day intervals, the intensity of citric acid-induced cough was significantly increased after ovalbumin challenge compared to that produced by intranasal saline.[33] Cough sensitivity was enhanced only when exudative inflammation of the nasal mucosa occurred after intranasal allergen challenge. When ovalbumin-sensitised animals were challenged intranasally with saline, the intensity of cough was not any different from that seen in control animals. Our observation regarding increased cough sensitivity in guinea pigs with experimental allergic rhinitis and in patients with pollen allergy suggests that a decreased threshold of nerve endings mediating cough could be an important pathomechanism in patients with seasonal allergic rhinitis. This hypothesis would be supported by the observation that the sensitivity of the cough reflex to a capsaicin challenge is decreased with successful treatment of the PNDS in patients with chronic dry cough.[25]

Another view that could be considered, is that the cough reflex hypersensitivity associated with PNDS results from increased sensory inputs from the upper airways. Several investigators in this field are sceptical about the cough reflex being elicited by the stimulation of nasal afferent nerve endings[10,15] The afferent inputs from the upper airways may interact with the neural pathways of the cough reflex to enhance cough.[34] The phenomenon of convergence and potentiation of disparate afferent pathways in the central nervous system (CNS) has been studied in the respiratory system and other visceral sensory systems.[35] The study of the role of afferent denervation of nasal mucosa on chemically-induced cough in conscious guinea pigs is limited by the methodological problems of blocking complicated innervation of the nasal mucosa. The injection of intraorbital anaesthetics has been used to block the ethmoidal nerves. This model was used to study the role of nasal afferent nerve endings in the regulation of breathing in anaesthetised guinea pigs.[36]

A bilateral intraocular injection of lidocaine was able to block the capsaicin-induced sneezing only in 30 per cent of conscious guinea pigs, therefore, we did not use this method in our studies which were specifically aimed at elucidating the role of nasal inputs, on the cough reflex.[37] The study was aimed to assess the effects of nasal administration of stimuli that are known to stimulate those sensory nerves that are known to affect the cough reflex. The intranasal administration of capsaicin enhanced the intensity of cough evoked by mechanical stimulation of tracheobronchial mucosa in anaesthetised cats as well as the intensity of cough evoked by mechanical stimulation of the larynx in anaesthetised guinea pigs and that intranasal capsaicin-enhanced citric acid-induced cough in conscious guinea pigs.[38] Capsaicin excites a subpopulation of afferent A d and C-fibres via the vanilloid receptor-1.

Sekizawa and Tsubone[39] reported that a substantial proportion (53%) of nerve endings in nasal mucosa are capsaicin sensitive. In addition to afferent signalling, activation of capsaicin-sensitive afferents evoke the local release of neuropeptides from nerve terminals. Neuropeptides, such as substance P (SP) and neurokinin A (NKA), exert powerful vasoactive and secretomotor effects leading to vasodilatation, plasma exudation and increased mucus secretions. Application of capsaicin to nasal mucosa can directly stimulate capsaicin-sensitive afferent nerve fibres, and it can also stimulate capsaicin-insensitive afferents indirectly via central and local reflex actions. Intranasal capsaicin-induced changes in the respiratory pattern consist of a transient increase in the respiratory rate and tidal volume, which return to baseline after approximately 30 seconds. Stimulatory effects of the application of intranasal capsaicin on breathing, were also observed in dogs.[40]

Since intranasally administered capsaicin was unlikely to reach more parts of the airways, we assume that the stimulatory effect on breathing was reflex in origin. Intranasal administration of capsaicin did not evoke cough in anaesthetised cats and guinea pigs. This observation is in agreement with the results reported in dogs[40] and extensive experimental evidence exists that shows that the origin of cough is unique to structures innervated by the vagus nerves.[15]

However, intranasal capsaicin enhanced the intensity of cough evoked by mechanical stimulation of tracheobroncheal mucosa in anaesthetised cats.[38] The number of coughs elicited by a certain level of mechanical stimulation, was increased immediately after administering capsaicin to the nasal mucosa. This effect was transient and reversed completely to the pre-challenge control levels, after 5 minutes. The average change in oesophageal pressure per cough was not affected. In anaesthetised guinea pigs, intranasal capsaicin significantly increased the intensity of the cough bout when cough was induced mechanically, from both laryngeal and tracheobronchial mucosa. The number of cough efforts was significantly increased for cough induced from the larynx, but not from the tracheo bronchial mucosa. The reason for this discrepancy is not known. It is possible that with more pronounced nasal stimuli, the difference would be statistically significant.A simple analysis of this study suggests that the central terminations of nasal sensory afferent neurons synapse directly on to the secondary sensory neurons of the cough pathway. This mechanism, termed as convergence, has been proposed in regulation of the bronchomotor tone.[35] Like vagal afferents, the trigeminal nerve afferents from the nose also project to the nucleus tractus solitarius offering a morphologic substrate for such interactions.[41] Convergence may also contribute to a heightened cough reflex sensitivity in another extrapulmonary disorder, i.e., GERD.[42]

Another possible interpretation of our results is that the intranasal stimulation affects cough by influencing the ventilatory drive. Application of intranasal capsaicin increased the ventilatory drive in anaesthetised cats and enhanced the mechanically induced cough. Thus, cough during nasal stimulation could be facilitated by interactions of afferent inputs from nasal mucosa with those of the brainstem neuronal network that integrates and coordinates cough with the respiratory cycle. In addition, increase of specific airway resistance following intranasal capsaicin has also been found.[38] Thus bronchoconstriction could also contribute to the modulation of the cough response during stimulation of the nasal mucosa.

Besides the sensitisation of the cough reflex centrally, it is possible that certain peripheral mechanisms could also sensitise it. These would include an influence on the innervation of the larynx and the more peripheral airways.[43] However, there is no clear experimental or clinical evidence available that could suggest as to the mechanisms that are responsible for either stimulation of or sensitization of laryngeal and tracheobronchial nerve endings mediating the cough reflex during rhinitis. A likely mechanism of the heightened cough reflex sensitivity that is seen, is microaspiration of nasal secretion into the lower airways due to laboured breathing through the nasal cavity, especially when their patency, due to inflammatory processes, is enormously decreased.[23]

Although inflammation is produced by different factors, but it results nevertheless in congestion of the nasal mucosa, and hypersecretion there from. Increased air velocity through the partially blocked nasal passages and nasal discharge could be a condition for aerosol production during laboured inspiration. Nasal discharge contains mediators released from inflammatory cells that could be breathed in, and which would modulate excitability of afferent mucosal nerve endings in the larynx as well as in the trachea.

The aim of the present study was also to test the assumption, that forced nasal breathing in rhinitic guinea pigs (that could enhance the creation of aerosol in the nasal cavity and probable microaspiration of nasal content into the lower airways) could increase the intensity of the mechanically induced cough. An increase in ventilation occurred by inhalation of carbon dioxide in anaesthetised guinea pigs with experimental allergic rhinitis. There was a significant enhancement of laryngeal cough in animals who were breathing through their nose in comparison to those who were breathing through a tracheostomy.[44] This conclusion supports the evidence obtained earlier, that cough reflex sensitivity due to allergic rhinitis was abolished by cutting off the superior laryngeal nerves in conscious guinea pigs.[32]

The intensity of the cough reflex with experimental allergic rhinitis was greater than usual, in both anaesthetised and conscious guinea pigs.[30,44]

5.3 INFLUENCE OF OESOPHAGEAL MUCOSA RECEPTORS

There are two proposed mechanisms for cough associated with GERD: (i) presence of acid in the distal oesophagus stimulating the mucosal afferent nerve endings and giving rise to this reflex, and (ii) microaspiration or macroaspiration of oesophageal contents into the larynx and the tracheobronchial tree. A number of studies have been carried out to examine potential mechanisms of reflex cough in patients suffering from gastro-oesophageal reflux.[45,46]

In summary, several observations point towards an oesophageal-tracheobronchial reflex mechanism of cough, induced by distal and non-proximal acid exposure or distal oesophagitis. However, the use of laryngoscopy and bronchoscopy, did not reveal any evidence of an acid-induced injury from aspiration, to be the cause.

GERD is a common cause of chronic cough[2] and though likely mechanisms have been discussed above, yet it is not quite clear as to which one of them actually mediates cough during gastro-oesophageal reflux. Ing et al[46] concluded that acid in the distal oesophagus precipitates cough, i.e. by an oesophageal-tracheobronchial reflex mechanism. This conclusion, however, is not supported by our findings.[47,48] Intra-oesophageal instillation of both HCl and capsaicin produced contractions of the oesophageal musculature and small fluctuations in the tidal volume in anaesthetised cats; these changes were more pronounced after the capsaicin challenge. In these instances, neither cough nor other respiratory reflexes (produced by forced expiration during a 5-minute stimulation of oesophageal mucosal nerve endings) were seen.

There was no significant difference in the intensity of mechanically-induced cough by instillation of intra-oesophageal physiological saline, HCl or capsaicin.[47] Neither was there any evidence of the presence of an oesophageal-tracheobronchial reflex mechanism, either for induction of or modulation of the intensity of citric acid-induced cough, in awake guinea-pigs undergoing an intra-oesophageal capsaicin challenge.[48]

In dogs, the oesophagus appears to have scant vagal innervation, but has a predominance of slowly adapting pulmonary stretch receptors (SARs) having a possible role in the mechanism of deglutition.

Moreover, the response to acidic solutions and other irritants, is poor. These receptors have properties that are different from those of vagal airway receptors; and furthermore, these do not suggest that in the presence of chemical irritants, they exert a noteworthy influence on the cough response.[49]

Our findings also suggest that the stimulation of vagal mucosal oesophageal nerve endings alone, is not trigger enough for cough. Patients with reflux oesophagitis have a decreased cough threshold, and this could be related to both laryngeal inflammation and acid flooding of the oesophagus.[50] This suggestion is supported by our recent study in patients with gastro-oeosophageal reflux disease.[51]

The acidification of distal oesophagus did not change the cough sensitivity in patients who did not complain of any respiratory symptoms. Cough sensitivity was significantly increased after Bernstein test (perfusion of distal oesophagus with 150 ml 0.1 N HCl during 15 minutes) in patients with reflux oesophagitis, who did complain of coughing.

We suggest that stimulation of afferent nerve endings in injured oesophageal mucosa can change cough sensitivity only in patients with evidence of some subclinical pathological changes in the airways.

5.4 INFLUENCE OF CARDIAC RECEPTORS

Stimulation of cardiac vagal receptors by chemicals such as veratrine, capsaicin, nicotine, or phenylbiguanide reduces phrenic nerve activity somewhat and gives rise to a reflex bradycardia.[52–54]

When the tracheobronchial mucosa was stimulated during an apnoea produced by intravenous veratrine, the intensity of mechanically induced cough was significantly decreased with two doses of veratrine (15 $mg.kg^{-1}$ and 30 $mg. kg^{-1}$) in anaesthetised cats.[55] The intensity of cough was attenuated with a significant decrease, seen both in the number of cough efforts and their intensity. When the mechanical stimulus was repeated during the resumption of breathing following apnoea (and hypotension), the main features of cough did not change significantly from control conditions. However, a decrease in both cough intensity and its duration was present during stimulation of the cardiac receptors by intracardial injections of 15 $mg.kg^{-1}$ veratrine which also produced the accompanying bradycardia, hypotension and a decrease in respiratory rate and tidal volume (Fig. 5.2). It may be noted that a large and an acute drop in blood pressure by itself, has no significant influence on cough.[56] As the pulmonary and left ventricular circulation time in the cat is about 3 to 4 seconds,[57] a cough produced by an intravenous injection of veratrine would have been produced not only by the stimulation of slowly adapting pulmonary receptors (SARs) but also by that of cardiac receptors. Thus, we can conclude that reflexes arising from the stimulation of cardiac receptors by veratrine, could also play a major role in the depression of cough that was seen. This argument is further supported by the evidence that the intensity of mechanically induced cough is not changed during lung inflation, by which the SARs would also have been stimulated.[58] A direct inhibitory effect of veratrine on cough receptors in the airways, however, is unlikely.

Thus, one can conclude that cardiac receptors are involved in similar cough downregulation effects which are produced during intense stimulation of either pulmonary or tracheobronchial C-fibres in anaesthetiased cats, suggesting an inhibitory effect on the cough reflex.[56,59] Such an intensive but transient inhibitory effect may have altered the gating mechanism of central neural pathways

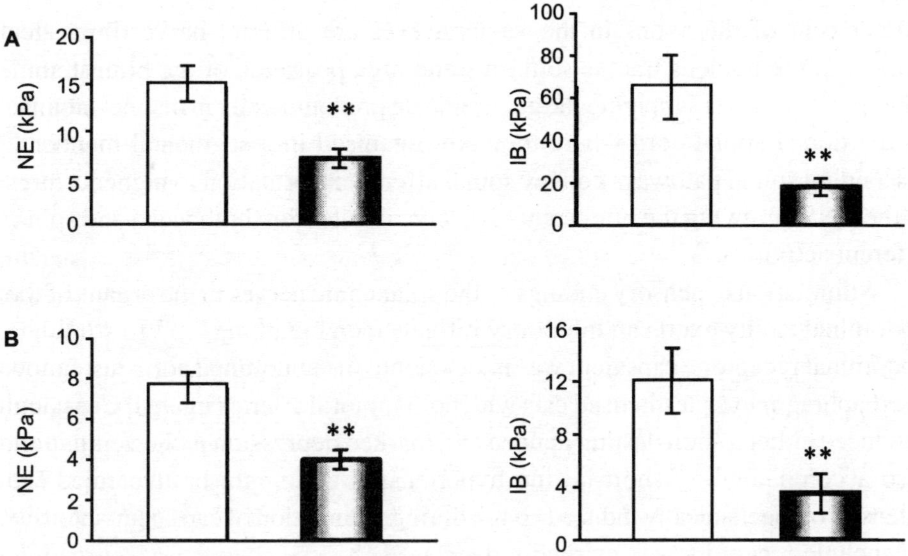

Fig. 5.2 Changes in the intensity parameters of mechanically induced cough: number of cough efforts (NE), and intensity of cough bout (IB) during control conditions (white columns), and during veratrine-induced inhibition of breathing (black columns) in anaesthetised cats. (A) – Intravenous injection of 15 mg.kg^{-1} veratrine. (B) – Intracardial injection of 15 mg.kg^{-1} veratrine through the catheter inserted into the left atrium. The chest wall was opened under artificial ventilation for the insertion of the catheter into the left atrium. It was subsequently closed and possible production of pneumothorax was permanently checked. Due to these thoracic interventions, the intensity of cough efforts was markedly decreased. **denotes p<0.01.

mediating the cough reflex.[60] Another possibility is that anaesthesia might upregulate inhibitory effects of C-fibres on cough.[61] A similar mechanism could occur in anaesthetised cats due to an intense stimulation of cardiac vagal receptors, which project to the nucleus tractus solitarius neurons.[54]

5.5 INFLUENCE OF SPLANCHNIC RECEPTORS

The vagal fibres as well as the spinal serosal afferents innervating the mucosa and muscle of the gastrointestinal tract, have also been shown to display capsaicin sensitivity.[62-64] Extrinsic gastrointestinal sensory neurons, which convey information from the gut to the brain, are vagal and spinal afferents, which originate from somata in the nodose and dorsal root ganglia.[65] Importantly, 80 to

90 per cent of the axons in the vagus nerves are afferent nerve fibres that project to the nucleus tractus solitarius and area postrema of the brainstem.[66] The spinal afferents supplying the gut terminate predominantly in distinct laminae of the dorsal spinal cord where they are organised in a segmental manner.[67] Ascending spinal pathways convey spinal afferent information to higher centres in the CNS, allowing the brainstem to receive inputs from both vagal and spinal afferent activities.[68]

Stimulation of sensory endings of the splanchnic nerves in the organs of the abdominal cavity exerts an inhibitory influence on breathing.[69,70] To stimulate abdominal receptors, capsaicin was injected into the abdominal aorta just below the diaphragm in anaesthetised cats with both femoral arteries ligated. Capsaicin produced either a short-lasting apnoea or a marked depression in the ventilation, also accompanied by short-lasting hypertension and slight bradycardia. The intensity of mechanically induced cough during stimulation of capsaicin-sensitive splanchnic receptors was markedly decreased.[71]

The intensity of cough was attenuated due to a significant decrease in both the parameters i.e. the number of cough efforts and the intensity of cough efforts. Cough elicited by long-lasting mechanical stimulation of tracheal mucosa in all the challenged animals was interrupted by an apnoea lasting 2 to 8 seconds after injecting capsaicin into the abdominal aorta (Fig. 5.3).

We conclude that the inhibition of cough is due to a depressive effect from the splanchnic receptor input into the central cough generator. This observation supports the view that several afferent inputs that inhibit ventilation centrally, are strong enough to attenuate the cough reflex. Downregulation of the cough reflex was also obtained when the interactions between mechanically induced cough and the stimulation of pulmonary C-fibre receptors,[56] cardiac receptors[55] and tracheobronchial C-fibre receptors[59] were studied.

5.6 INFLUENCE OF HYPOXIA AND HYPERCAPNIA

In the acute phase (15 minutes) of isobaric (inspiratory oxygen fraction (FIO_2) = 0.11), i.e. hypoxic hypoxia, the intensity of mechanically induced tracheobronchial cough was enhanced in conscious cats due to a significant increase in the intensity of cough efforts but without a change in the number of efforts.[72]

When airway mucosa was mechanically stimulated in anaesthetised cats in severe hypoxia ($FIO_2 = 0.07$) lasting 15 seconds, in which hyperventilation was

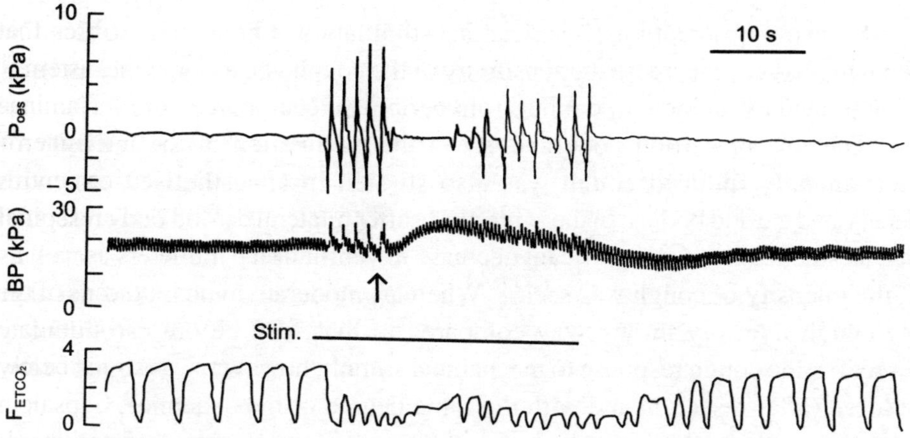

Fig. 5.3 Effect of splanchnic afferent nerve ending stimulation on the prolonged mechanically induced cough in anaesthetised cats. Changes in oesophageal pressure (POES), expiration upwards and blood pressure (BP) during continual mechanical stimulation of the tracheal mucosa with a FET CO_2 (and end tidal CO_2) nylon fibre (Stim.) and to an injection of 15 mg.kg^{-1} capsaicin into the abdominal aorta (-) in this duration.

due to an increased tidal volume, the intensity of tracheobronchial cough was also enhanced due to a significant increase in the intensity of cough efforts in comparison with the control cough induced under normoxic conditions (unpublished).

In the same animals, marked hyperventilation induced by an electrical stimulation of the sinus nerve was accompanied by enhancement of mechanically induced cough in comparison with the cough response under control condition.

Carotid and other peripheral chemoreceptors provide an important excitatory input to medullary respiratory neurons.[73] Afferents from peripheral chemoreceptors synapse in a region in close proximity to the nucleus tractus solitarius, in the brainstem.[74] The chemoreceptor projection site encompasses a midline area, which includes the commissural subnucleus of nucleus tractus solitarius. The chemosensitive neurons located in this site, fire tonically without any rhythmic relation to the phrenic nerve bursts, and are non-responsive to baroreceptor stimulation. These neurons may serve as a pre-central pattern generator for respiration. These chemosensitive neurons send projections to respiratory neurons.[75]

From our observations, it is clear that stimulation of breathing produced by acute hypoxia can increase the sensitivity of the cough generator, which in itself is facilitated by an increased input from peripheral chemoreceptors.

The role of carotid body activity in the modulation of the intensity of mechanically induced cough was also studied in anaesthetised cats with denervated carotid bodies. In the acute phase after bilateral carotid body resection in anaesthetised cats, a significant decrease in ventilation parameters as well as in the intensity of cough was seen.[76] Whereas, moderate hypoxia did not alter the cough intensity in any way compared to that seen before carotid body resection, the cough response to mechanical stimuli, however, was significantly reduced (after resection and with the same degree of hypoxaemia).

We suppose, therefore, that after the tonic afferent activity of peripheral chemoreceptors is removed, the ventilatory drive decreases and the sensitivity of cough generator to afferent discharges from nerve endings mediating the cough reflex, is acutely down regulated. This view has been put forward on the basis of the observation, that a marked depression in ventilation occurs during a mechanically-induced cough in the presence of pure oxygen whose intensity itself was markedly reduced.[77]

We conclude that the enhancement of cough during the initial phase of hypoxic hypoxia is due to an increased afferent input from the peripheral chemoreceptors. This is supported by a similarity in the response to electrical stimulation of the sinus nerve, during normoxia. The block of tonic carotid body activity either by carotid body resection or during pure oxygen inhalation led not only to hypoventilation but also to the inhibition of the intensity of cough.

The effect of more severe hypoxia on the intensity of cough, could be studied only in anaesthetised cats, because during severe hypoxia conscious cats become uncontrollably excited, and resist airway mechanical stimulation. During 7 minutes of severe hypoxic hypoxia ($FIO_2 = 0.7$), a significant decrease in the intensity of the cough reflex to mechanical stimulation was seen.[78] Compared to conscious cats, the hyperventilation seen in anaesthetised cats was due to an enormous increase in the respiratory rate, and not due to the tidal volume which was not different from control values.[72]

Mechanisms controlling the intensity of cough are less resistant to severe hypoxia than the mechanisms regulating ventilation. Despite increased afferent input from peripheral chemoreceptors, central local hypoxic depression is probably responsible for this effect. However, the effect of anaesthesia and the duration of tissue hypoxia in the brainstem cannot be excluded. Hypoxia can influence the central inspiratory drive by two mechanisms: (i) excitation of the respiratory neuronal net through increased activity of the peripheral chemoreceptors and (ii) direct central inhibitory effect on the neurons in the brainstem during severe hypoxia.[79,80]

A short-lasting increase in the peripheral chemoreceptor input into the medulla (either with a 15 seconds inhalation of hypoxic gas mixture or electric stimulation of the sinus nerve), induced hyperventilation and intensified the cough response. On the other hand, either short-lasting inhibition of the peripheral chemoreceptor activity (pure oxygen inhalation) or carotid body resection were accompanied by hypoventilation and inhibition of the cough response. However, during severe hypoxia with FIO_2 ranging from 0.21 to 0.06, minute ventilation increased while the intensity of cough decreased.

The intensity of mechanically induced cough was not affected during prolonged moderate isobaric hypoxic hypoxia ($FIO_2 = 0.11$) in healthy conscious cats.[81] Animals exhibited hyperventilation, due to marked increase of tidal volume, while the respiratory rate was not changed in comparison to control values. In the acute phase of hypoxic hypoxia, the intensity of cough was significantly increased in conscious cats.[72] The mechanisms responsible for the adaptation of the cough response to mechanical stimulation during prolonged hypoxia are unknown. The central hypoxic up regulation of cough response is presumably a short-term process.

The intensity of mechanically induced cough is modulated by hypercapnia; this was not significantly reduced in anaesthetised cats which were made to breathe 5 per cent carbon dioxide for 15 minutes. But in those which breathed 10 per cent carbon dioxide, the intensity of cough was significantly reduced.[82] The resting ventilatory activity was markedly increased at both the levels of hypercapnia. During 5 hours of hypercapnia (inhalation of hypercapnic/hyperoxic gas mixture: inspiratory carbon dioxide fraction = 0.1, $FIO_2 = 0.25$), the cough intensity was significantly decreased in healthy conscious cats. Depression of cough occurred immediately in the acute phase (15 minutes of hypercapnia), although the ventilatory parameters were markedly enhanced.[83]

Tissue hypercapnia induced by intraperitoneal acetazolamide resulted in hyperventilation in conscious cats and at the same time in inhibition of cough efforts.[82] In anaesthetised humans, an increase in carbon dioxide-induced ventilatory drive decreases the degree and duration of respiratory response to airway irritation.[84] A direct depressant effect of hypercapnia on the neural pathway relevant to cough reflex responses should be considered.

5.7 CONCLUSION

Our experimental studies have allowed us to conclude that a direct stimulation of cardiac, splanchnic, oesophageal and nasal sensory afferents do not give rise to a cough. However, extrapulmonary afferent inputs into the brainstem have an important role in the regulation of the cough reflex. A modulation of the intensity of cough response to mechanical or chemical stimulation of the lower airway mucosa, occurs as its main consequence.

Stimulation of cardiac afferent and splanchnic nerve endings and the block of peripheral chemoreceptor activity leading to depression of breathing is accompanied by marked inhibition of cough response to mechanical stimuli. Enhanced ventilation due to increased peripheral chemoreceptor input either by acute severe hypoxemia or-electrical stimulation of sinus nerve, and by stimulation of nasal sensory afferents in cats, are accompanied by an increased cough response to mechanical stimuli. There is no experimental evidence regarding the central control mechanisms modulating the activity of the cough generator for these inhibitory and excitatory inputs. Studies on the behaviour of medullary respiratory neurons have led to the conclusion that the same respiratory neurons involved in the generation of the eupnoic pattern of breathing also participate in the production in the cough motor pattern.[85]

We can speculate that sudden inhibitory and excitatory inputs into the brainstem may affect ventilatory and cough responses by the same mechanism. This gating mechanism is proposed so as to understand the regulation of the cough motor pattern and the duration over which, repetitive coughing is produced. It is also used to explain the magnitude of the expiratory motor drive.[86]

Abdominal and cardiac afferent inputs with inhibitory effect on inspiratory drive could either downregulate the gating mechanism neurons, which activate pre-motor expiratory neurons or exert a non-specific inhibitory effect on breathing. The pressure changes during vigorous coughing would contribute to morbidity of abdominal visceral disease,[87] so the effect of stimulation of splanchnic afferent receptor on the downregulation of cough may be a manifestation of a visceral, protective reflex.

Identical changes in the intensity of ventilation and cough response were not observed in all our experimental studies. Stimulation of the nasal mucosa in anaesthetised guinea pigs, led to an enhanced cough response to a mechanical stimulation, with a transient reduction in the respiratory rate. When hypoxia is prolonged, cough response to mechanical stimulation is reduced, but ventilation remains increased. Similarly, during hypercapnia, the response was a hyperventilation and a reduction in the intensity of cough. Thus, the mechanism responsible for modulation of the cough response by extrapulmonary afferent inputs is more complex. Since afferent nerve fibres from the nose project to the nucleus tractus solitarius, it is reasonable to speculate that they may facilitate the cough-related pathways in the brainstem by central sensitisation.[35] It is likely that the cough generator is less resistant to the direct inhibitory effect of hypoxia and hypercapnia, than mechanisms regulating central inspiratory activity.

Pathogenesis of chronic cough, when the pathological processes are outside the laryngeal and tracheobronchial regions, is not fully understood. Stimulation of afferent nerve endings in healthy as well as inflamed oesophageal mucosa cannot modulate cough intensity. It is likely that a decreased threshold of nerve endings mediating cough, due to chronic stimulation of oesophageal mucosal receptors and probably laryngeal and tracheal afferents are involved in the cough of patients suffering from gastro-oesophageal reflux disease (GERD). Increased cough sensitivity occurs in patients with seasonal allergic rhinitis. From our experimental data, it can be concluded that increased sensitivity of nerve endings in larynx and lower airways is mainly responsible for this effect. Cough reflex sensitivity could be increased either by microaspiration of inflammatory nasal secretion that sensitise cough-mediating sensory nerves in the lower airways or by a reflex effect arising from stimulation of nasal receptors.

REFERENCES

1. Irwin RS, Madison JM. Symptom research on chronic cough: a historical perspective. Annals of Internal Medicine 2001;134:809–14.
2. Irwin RS, Boulet L-P, Cloutier MM, Fuller R, Gold PM, Hoffstein V, Ing AJ, McCool D, O'Byrne P, Poe RH, et al. Managing cough as a defense mechanism and as a symptom: a consensus panel report of the American College of Chest Physicians. Chest 1998;44(Suppl):133S–181S.
3. Pratter MR, Bartter T, Akers S, DuBois J. An algorithmic approach to chronic cough. Annals of Internal Medicine 1993;49:977–83.
4. Mello CJ, Irwin RS, Curley FJ. The predictive values of the character, timing, and complications of chronic cough in diagnosing its cause. Archives of Internal Medicine 1996;156:997–1003.
5. Pratter MR, Hingston DM, Irwin RS. Diagnosis of bronchial asthma by clinical evaluation: an unreliable method. Chest 1983;84:42–7.
6. Irwin RS, French CL, Curley FJ, Zawacki JK, Bennett FM. Chronic cough due to gastroesophageal reflux: clinical, diagnostic, and pathogenetic aspects. Chest 1993;104:1511–7.

7. Korpas J, Tomori Z. Cough and other respiratory reflexes. Basel, Switzerland: Karger, 1979.
8. Karlsson J-A, Sant´Ambrogio G, Widdicombe JG. Afferent neural pathways in cough and reflex broncho constriction, Journal of Applied Physiology 1988;65:1007–23.
9. Fuller RW, Jackson DM. Physiology and treatment of cough. Thorax 1990;45:425–30.
10. Sant´Ambrogio G. Coughing: an airway defensive reflex. In: Andrews P, Widdicombe JG, editors. Pathophysiology of the gut and airways. Portland Press, London and Chapel Hill, 1993.
11. Widdicombe JG. Afferent receptors in the airways and cough. Respiration Physiology 1998;44:5–15.
12. Mazzone SB, Canning BJ, Widdicombe JG. Sensory pathways for the cough reflex. In: Chung F, Widdicombe JG, Boushey H, editors. Cough: causes, mechanisms and therapy. Blackwell Publishing, 2003.
13. Ishrat-Husain S. Rhinolith—a rare cause of chronic cough. Canadian Medical Association Journal 1967;7:540–1.
14. Wolff AP, May M. The tympanic membrane: a source of the cough reflex. Journal of the American Medical Association 1973;23:1269.
15. Widdicombe JG. Neurophysiology of the cough reflex. European Respiratory Journal 1995;8:1193–202.
16. Tatar M, Korpas J. Contribution to the problem of the influence of anaesthesia on experimental cough. Bratislavske lekarske Listy 1983;79:276–85. (In Slovakian).
17. Hanacek J, Brozmanova M, Tatar M, Karcolova D, Strapkova A, Szepe P. Effects of long-term high oxygen concentration breathing on defensive respiratory reflexes in guinea pigs. Pulmonary Pharmacology 1996;9:367–8.
18. Hutchings HA, Morris S, Eccles R, Jawad MSM. Voluntary suppression of cough induced by inhalation of capsaicin in healthy volunteers. Respiratory Medicine 1993;87:379–82.
19. Plaschke PP, Jansom CH, Nerrman E, Bjornsson J, Ellbjar S, Jarvholm B. Onset and remission of allergic rhinitis and asthma and relationships with atopic senzitization and smoking. American Journal of Respiratory and Critical Care Medicine 2000;162:920–4.
20. Levi CR, Tyler GR, Olson LG, Sanders NA. Lack of airway response to nasal irritation in normal and asthmatic subjects. Australian & New Zealand Journal of Medicine 1990;20:578–82.
21. Littel NT, Carlisle CC, Millman RP, Bramen SS. Changes in airway resistance following nasal provocation. American Review of Respiratory Diseases 1990;141:580–3.
22. Lamblin C, Brichet A, Perez T, Darras J, Tonnel AB, Wallert B. Long-term follow up of pulmonary function in patients with nasal polyposis. American Journal of Respiratory and Critical Care Medicine 2000;161:406–13.
23. Curley FJ, Irwin RS, Pratter MR, Stiress DH, Doern GV, Vernaglie PA, Larkin AB, Baker SP. Cough and the common cold. American Review of Respiratory Diseases 1988;138:305–11.
24. Corren, J. Allergic rhinitis and asthma: how important is the link? Journal of Allergy and Clinical Immunology 1997;99:781–6.
25. O´Connell F, Thomas VE, Pride NB, Fuller, RW. Capsaicin cough sensitivity decreases with successful treatment of chronic cough. American Journal of Respiratory and Critical Care Medicine 1996;150:374–80.
26. Pecova R, Vrlik M, Tatar M. Cough sensitivity in allergic rhinitis. Journal of Physiology and Pharmacology 2005;56(Suppl IV):171–8.

27. Karlsson J-A. The role of capsaicin-sensitive C-fibre afferent nerves in the cough reflex. Pulmonary Pharmacology 1996;9:315–21.
28. Tatar M, Pecova R, Karcolova D. Sensitivity of cough reflex in awake guinea-pigs, rats and rabbits. Bratislavske lekarske Listy 1997;98:539–43. (In Slovakian).
29. Namimatsu A, Okazaki R, Go K, Hata T. Relationship between density of muscarinic receptors and nasal hypersecretion in a nasal allergic model. Japanese Journal of Pharmacology 1992;59:427–34.
30. Tatar M, Karcolova D, Kollarik M. The effect of experimental rhinitis on chemically-induced cough in awake guinea pigs. European Respiratory Journal 1997;10(Suppl 25):182s.
31. Anbo X, Uchida Y, Nomura A, Iijima H, Dong F, Zhang M-J, Hasegawa S. Effects of airway inflammation on cough response in the guinea pig. Journal of Applied Physiology 1998;85:1847–54.
32. Tatar M, Karcolova D, Kollarik M. Role of superior laryngeal nerves in regulation of cough sensitivity in awake guinea-pigs with experimental rhinitis. European Respiratory Journal 1998;12(Suppl 28):57s.
33. Tatar M, Karcolova D. Role of repeated allergen challenge on cough reflex in awake guinea pigs with experimental rhinitis. European Respiratory Journal 1999;14(Suppl 30):223s.
34. Tatar M, Karcolova D, Pecova R, Kollarik M, Plevkova J, Brozmanova M. Experimental modulation of the cough reflex. European Respiratory Review 2002;12:264–9.
35. Mazzone SB, Canning BJ. Plasticity of the cough reflex. European Respiratory Review 2002;12:236–42.
36. Woodson GE, Sant´Ambrogio F, Anderson JW, Sant´Ambrogio G. Menthol induced hypopnea is greatly diminished by trigeminal nerve blockade. Physiologist 1991;34:266.
37. Karcolova D. The role of airway nerve endings in the cough reflex in awake guinea pigs. PhD Thesis Martin, 2000. (In Slovakian).
38. Plevkova J, Brozmanova M, Kollarik M, Revallo M, Varechova S, Tatar M. Modulation of experimentally induced cough reflex by the stimulation of nasal mucosa in cats and guinea pigs. Respiratory Physiology and Neurobiology 2004;142:225-35.
39. Sekizawa S, Tsubone H. Nasal receptors responding to noxious chemical irritants. Respiratory Physiology 1994;96:37–48.
40. Lung MA, Widdicombe JG. Lung reflexes and nasal vascular resistance in the anaesthetized dog. Journal of Physiology 1987;386:465–74.
41. Boscan P, Paton JF. Integration of cornea and cardiorespiratory afferents in the nucleus of the solitary tract of the rat. American Journal of Physiology: Heart and Circulatory Physiology 2002;282:H1278–87.
42. Undem BJ, Carr MJ, Kollarik M. Physiology and plasticity of putative cough fibres in the guinea pig. Pulmonary Pharmacology and Therapeutics 2002;15:193–8.
43. Kollarik M, Undem BJ. Plasticity of vagal afferent fibres mediating cough. In: Chung F, Widdicombe JG, Boushey H, editors. Cough: causes, mechanisms and therapy. Blackwell Publishing, 2003.
44. Plevkova J, Brozmanova M, Tatar M. The effect of intensified nasal breathing on the cough reflex intensity in guinea pigs with ovalbumin induced rhinitis. Acta Medica Martiniana 2004;4(2):3–4.
45. Ing AJ, Ngu MC, Breslin ABX. Chronic persistent cough and clearance of esophageal acid. Chest 1992;102:1668–71.

46. Ing AJ, Ngu MC, Breslin ABX. Pathogenesis of chronic persistent cough associated with gastroesophageal reflux. American Journal of Respiratory and Critical Care Medicine 1994;149:160–7.
47. Tatar M, Pecova R. The effect of experimental gastroesophageal reflux on the cough in anaesthetized cats. Bratislavske lekarske Listy 1996;97:284–8. (In Slovakian)
48. Kollarik M, Plevkova J, Brozmanova M, Revallo M, Varechova S, Bartos V, Plank L, Tatar M. The effect of chemical stimulation of esophageal mucosa on citric acid induced cough and specific airway resistance in guinea pig. Bratislavske Lekarske Listy 2005;106:101–6.
49. Sekizawa S, Ishikawa T, Sant'Ambrogio FB, Sant'Ambrogio G. Vagal esophageal receptors in anesthetized dogs: mechanical and chemical responsiveness. Journal of Applied Physiology 1999, 86:1231–1235.
50. Benini L, Ferrari M, Sembenini C, Olivieri M, Micciolo R, Zuccali V, Bulighin GM, Fiorino F, Ederle A, Lo Cascio V, Vantini I. Cough threshold in reflux oesophagitis: influence of acid and of laryngeal and oesophageal damage. Gut 2000;46:762–7.
51. Tatar M, Javorkova N, Demeter M, Dilova Z, Biringer K, Pecova R, Balaz D, Hyrdel R. Effect of acidification of distal esophagus on cough sensitivity in patient with gastroesophageal reflux disease. European Respiratory Journal 2003;22(Suppl 45):172s.
52. Sleight P, Widdicombe JG. Action potentials in fibres from receptors in the epicardium and myocardium of the dog's left ventricle. Journal of Physiology 1965;181:235–58.
53. Paintal AS. Impulses in vagal afferent fibres from specific pulmonary deflation receptors. The response of these receptors to phenyldiguanide, potato starch, 5-hydroxytryptamine and nicotine and their role in respiratory and cardiovascular reflexes. Quarterly Journal of Physiology 1955;40:89–111.
54. Silva-Carvalho L, Paton JFR, Rocha I, Goldsmith GE, Spyer KM. Convergence properties of solitary tract neurons responsive to cardiac receptor stimulation in the anesthetized cat. Journal of Neurophysiology 1998;79:2374–82.
55. Tatar M, Nagyova B, Widdicombe JG. Veratrine-induced reflexes and cough. Respiratory Medicine 1991;85(Suppl A):51–5.
56. Tatar M, Webber SE, Widdicombe JG. Lung C-fibre receptor activation and defensive reflexes in anesthetized cats. Journal of Physiology 1988;402:411–20.
57. Dawes GS, Comroe Jr JH. Chemoreceptors from the heart and lungs. Physiological Reviews 1954;34:167–201.
58. Tatar M, Nagyova B. Effects of lung inflation on airways defence reflexes. European Respiratory Journal 1990;3(Suppl 10):141s.
59. Tatar M, Sant´Ambrogio G, Sant´Ambrogio FB. Laryngeal and tracheobronchial cough in anesthetized dogs. Journal of Applied Physiology 1994;76:2672–9.
60. Lee L-Y, Kwong K, Lin YS, Gu Q. Hypersensitivity of bronchopulmonary C-fibers induced by airway mucosal inflammation: cellular mechanisms. Pulmonary Pharmacology and Therapeutics 2002;15:199–204.
61. Canning BJ. Interaction between vagal afferent nerve subtypes mediating cough. Pulmonary Pharmacology and Therapeutics 2002;15:187–92.
62. Holzer P. Capsaicin: cellular targets, mechanisms of action, and selectivity for thin sensory neurons. Pharmacological Reviews 1991;43:143–201.
63. Blackshaw LA, Page AJ, Partosoedarso ER. Acute effects of capsaicin on gastrointestinal vagal afferents. Neuroscience 2000;96:407–16.

64. Kirkup AJ, Brunsden AM, Grundy D. Receptors and transmission in the brain-gut axis: potential for novel therapies I. Receptors on visceral afferents. American Journal of Physiology: Gastrointestinal and Liver Physiology 2001;280:G787–G794.
65. Holzer P, Michl T, Danzer M, Jocic M, Schicho R, Lippe IT. Surveillance of the gastrointestinal mucosa by sensory neurons. Journal of Physiology and Pharmacology 2001;52:505–21.
66. Berthoud H-R, Neuhuber WL. Functional and chemical anatomy of the afferent vagal system. Autonomic Neuroscience 2000;85:1–17.
67. Neuhuber WL, Sandoz PA, Fryscak T. The central projections of primary afferent neurons of greater splanchnic and intercostal nerves in the rat. Anatomy and Embryology 1986;174:123–44.
68. Renehan, WE, Zhang X, Beierwaltes WH, Fogel R. Neurons in the dorsal motor nucleus of the vagus may integrate vagal and spinal information from the GI tract. American Journal of Physiology 1995;268:G780–G790.
69. Bean JW. Intestine in reflex chemical control of breathing. American Journal of Physiology 1952;171:522–7.
70. Siegelova J. The role of intercostal muscles in splanchnic ventilation reflexes in rabbits. Physiologia Bohemoslovaca 1975;24:466–7.
71. Tatar M, Nagyova B. Abdominal capsaicin-sensitive receptor activation and mechanically induced cough in anesthetized cats. Prague, International Union of Physiological Science, 1991;p98.
72. Tatar M, Korpas J, Polacek H, Zahradny V. Study of the respiratory defensive reflexes in conscious cats in the acute phase of deficient oxygen supply into the organism. Bratislavske lekarske Listy 1985a;84:157–64. (In Slovakian)
73. Forster HV, Pan LG, Lowry TF, Serra A, Wenninger J, Martino P. Important role of carotid chemoreceptor afferents in control of breathing of adult and neonatal mammals. Respiratory Physiology 2000;49:199–208.
74. Kara T, Narkiewicz K, Somers VK. Chemoreflexes—physiology and clinical implications. Acta Physiologica Scandinavica 2003;177:377–84
75. Sapru HN. Carotid chemoreflex: neural pathways and transmitters. Advances in Experimental Medicine and Biology 1996;410:357–64.
76. Tatar M. Effect of denervation of peripheral chemoreceptors on cough during hypoxia. Bulletin Européan de Physiopathologie Respiratoire 1987;23(Suppl 10):65s.
77. Tatar M, Nagyova B. Mechanically-induced cough is depressed by acute hyperoxia in anaesthetized cats. Abstracts of XXXI. International Congress of Physiological Sciences Helsinky July 9–14 1989;pp386–7.
78. Tatar M, Korpas J, Polacek H, Zahradny V. Changes induced by severe hypoxia in respiratory defence reflexes in anaesthetised cats. Respiration 1986a;49:114–21.
79. Cherniack NS, Edelman NH, Lahiri S. Hypoxia and hypercapnia as respiratory stimulants and depressants. Respiratory Physiology 1970;4:113–26.
80. Gautier H, Bonora M. Possible alterations in brain monoamine metabolism during hypoxia-induced tachypnea in cats. Journal of Applied Physiology 1980;49:769–77.
81. Tatar M, Korpas J, Polacek H, Zahradny V. Effects of hypoxia on respiratory defence reflexes. Effects of thirty hours´ oxygen deficiency on cough, the expiration reflex and sneezing in awake cats. Physiologia Bohemoslovaca 1985b;34:41–8.
82. Kulik AM, Tarakanov IA, Tatar M, Korpas J. Cough reflex in hypercapnia. Bulletin Européan de Physiopathologie Respiratoire 1987;23(Suppl 10):63s.

83. Tatar M, Polacek H, Pullmann R. Changes of airway defence reflexes in the course of five-hour hypercapnia in conscious cats. Bratislavske lekarske Listy 1986b;85:533–40. (In Slovakian)
84. Nishino T, Hiraga K, Honda Y. Inhibitory effects of CO_2 on airway defensive reflexes in enflurane-anesthetized humans. Journal of Applied Physiology 1989;66:2642–6.
85. Shannon R, Baekey DM, Morris KF, Li Z, Lindsey BG. Functional connectivity among ventrolateral medullary respiratory neurones and responses during fictive cough in the cat. Journal of Physiology 2000;525:207–24.
86. Bolser DC, Davenport PW. Expiratory motor control during the cough reflex. European Respiratory Review 2000;12:243–8.
87. Farkas GA, Schroeder MA, De Troyer A. Effect of midline laparotomy on the cough reflex in dogs. Neuroscience Letters 1989;107:120–4.

6 Central Control of Cough

J Jakuš

6.1 INTRODUCTION

Cough is an airway reflex that protects the lungs against aspiration of foreign particles and noxious substances. A high expiratory airflow removes them together with mucus from larynx, trachea and larger bronchi. Cough reflex has been described as the watchdog of the lungs.[1] Cough can also be performed voluntarily. Voluntary control results from cortical influences which bypass the respiratory central pattern generator (CPG), reaching the spinal and cranial motoneuron pools. Coughing is a reflex response being evoked by irritant stimulation (mechanical, chemical, electrical, thermal) of the two main tussive sites, i.e. the larynx (laryngeal cough) and the tracheobronchial tree (tracheobronchial cough). Cough reflex depends on vagal afferents.[2] A stimulation of external auditory canal, tympanic membrane, distal oesophagus or abdominal organs may trigger cough, because they are supplied by branches of the Xth or vagus nerve. Cough profoundly affects the timing and pattern of breathing, and thus cough and quiet breathing cannot co-exist. The most common cause of cough may be a respiratory tract infection, e.g. acute and chronic bronchitis, bronchial hyper-responsiveness or asthma, lung tumours or stimulation of sensory branches of the vagus nerve by neuropeptides (e.g. in patients treated with angiotensin converting enzyme inhibitors), but rarely by the acid of gastric content (gastro-oesophageal reflux).

Although a comprehensive review of cough is available as an excellent monograph by Korpáš and Tomori[3] and by several others,[2,4-7] and several have defined the basic features of the cough reflex, its peripheral nerve pathways and mechanisms; however the mechanisms of the central genesis of cough is almost unknown.

A decade (1990–2000) of research on brain has added extensive knowledge to the field of respiratory rhythmogenesis, but an intense search of the central control mechanisms of cough has just been initiated. There was a serious gap in understanding the basic biophysical and neurophysiological mechanisms of cough neurogenesis in contrast to the knowledge known worldwide, about using centrally acting antitussive drugs, which inhibit cough reflex at different brainstem sites.

6.1.1 Historical Background

The study of neural pathways of cough began in the early 19th century[8,9] after the discovery of medullary regions that control quiet breathing. However, they were not investigated comprehensively because of the prevalent use of morphine and opioids (that inhibit cough) and partly because of technical difficulties involved.[7] Nevertheless, using pharmacological lesions, or electrophysiological methods in anaesthetised and (or) paralysed animals, (in the 1950s–1970s) resulted in two main concepts of the cough 'centre'. The first concept corresponds to an older view, that within the medulla oblongata a separate, anatomically well localised and independent cough centre could exist. This idea resulted mainly from pioneering studies using electrophysiological and pharmacological studies as well as from experiments using central nervous system (CNS) transections. Hence, a variety of areas 'critically' involved in coughing were established in the dorsolateral upper part of the medulla oblongata,[10] in areas adjacent to the obex,[11] around the NTS,[12] or in the area dorsomedial to the trigeminal tract and nucleus,[13] as well as within the rostral pons.[14] Pharmacological studies[15-17] had highlighted findings that some drugs may have adverse effects on cough and quiet breathing. Kasé[18] reported that nucleus reticularis parvocellularis may play a role as a cough centre. These findings were generally regarded as evidence for the existence of an independent cough centre. However, no compelling evidence is available for such a suggestion, because distinct sets of neurons at several levels of the brainstem are involved in central integration of the cough reflex.

A functional concept of cough centre was proposed by Bucher,[19] and it was further adopted by Korpáš[20] and Ivanco[21] who proposed that both types of cough (laryngeal and tracheobronchial) as well as active expiration (e.g. expiration reflex, expiratory period of sneezing, expiratory efforts during increased ventilation, expulsive part of retching, vomiting, micturition, parturition, etc.) may share a common basic central mechanism. Recent advances in the understanding of neuronal mechanisms for the production of cough and other reflex motor behaviours, support the functional concept of a likely cough centre.

6.2 NEUROPHYSIOLOGY OF THE COUGH REFLEX

6.2.1 Types and Patterns of Cough

Cough is not a stereotype reflex, like hiccup or sneezing, but it may show a variety of forms.[7] It can be affected by voluntary action, by natural or artificial stimuli, or by the property of a particular tussive area from which the reflex is triggered (e.g. mechanical stimulation of the larynx results in laryngeal cough with stronger inspiratory efforts and smaller expiratory ones). Although the larynx is considered as the most sensitive area for cough,[3] yet a higher elicitability of the cough reflex is seen after stimulation of the tracheobronchial tree, in studies both on dogs[22] and cats.[23] In experiments on guineapigs,[24] the cold block of the superior laryngeal nerve enhanced the tracheobronchial (TB) cough, indicating that some laryngeal afferent pathways may inhibit cough. According to Korpáš and Tomori,[3] the maximal value of inspiratory intrapleural pressure (Ppl) during laryngeal cough was higher compared to this parameter in TB cough.[23] Plasticity of cough (i.e. coughing can be tuned by stimuli that affect both its sensory and central pathways) is of great importance. As proposed recently, the laryngeal and tracheobronchial coughs are controlled by regulatory elements called 'gates' that provide excitatory input to the cough CPG which serves both reflexes.[25] A high degree of dynamic plasticity within the common 'cough-respiratory' network may elucidate profound regulatory differences between cough and quiet breathing, or differences between the laryngeal and tracheobronchial coughs, reflex inhibition or enhancement of cough as well as some clinical aspects of cough response in disease.[26]

6.2.2 Phases of Cough

Cough is a fast and strong reflex which involves concurrent activation of several groups of respiratory chest wall (pump), and laryngeal and upper airway (valve) muscles. They are activated sequentially, creating a well coordinated and fixed pattern (Figs 6.1 and 6.2). There are three main phases of coughing which are as follows:

1. **Inspiratory Phase or Deep Initial Inspiration** (Inspiratory pump and upper airway abductor muscles contract, while glottis is open): It starts

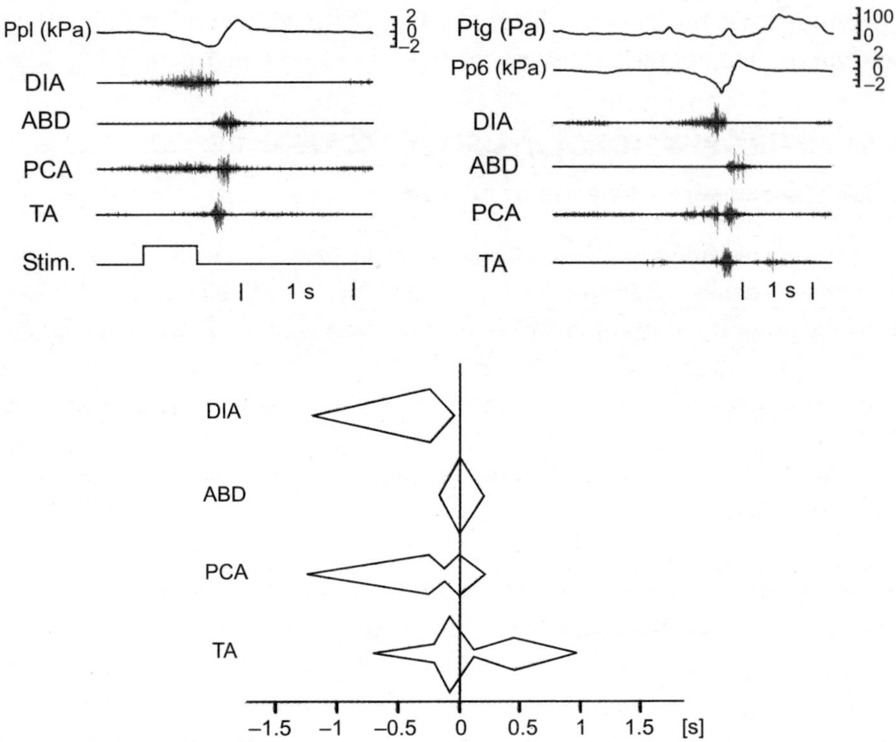

Time (ms)		Intensity (%)	Time (ms)		I ntensity (%)
– 1250 ± 40	onset of the PCA		– 55 ± 20	offset of the DIA	
– 1210 ± 40	onset of the DIA		– 5 ± 5	2.peak of the PCA	840 ± 100
– 710 ± 50	onset of the TA		0	peak of the ABD	810 ± 80
– 250 ± 10	1.peak of the PCA	800 ± 100	200 ± 10	offset of the PCA	
– 240 ± 35	peak of the DIA	560 ± 30	205 ± 15	offset of the ABD	
– 170 ± 10	onset of the ABD		450 ± 30	2.peak of the TA	670 ± 110
– 80 ± 10	1.peak of the TA	1600 ± 250	980 ± 60	offset of the Ta	

Fig. 6.1 Tracheobronchial cough. *Upper part:* Records of pleural pressure (Ppl), electromyographic activities in the diaphragm (DIA), abdominal muscles (ABD), posterior cricoarytenoid muscle (PCA) and thyroary tenoid muscle (TA) with moment of stimulation (Stim.) on the left side and with a record of transglottic pressure (Ptg) on the right side. *Lower part:* Diagram of electromyographic activities in DIA, ABD, PCA and TA during tracheobronchial cough indicating the time relations and maximal intensities compared to baseline values. (For details, see Poliacek et al., 2003, Ref. [23]).

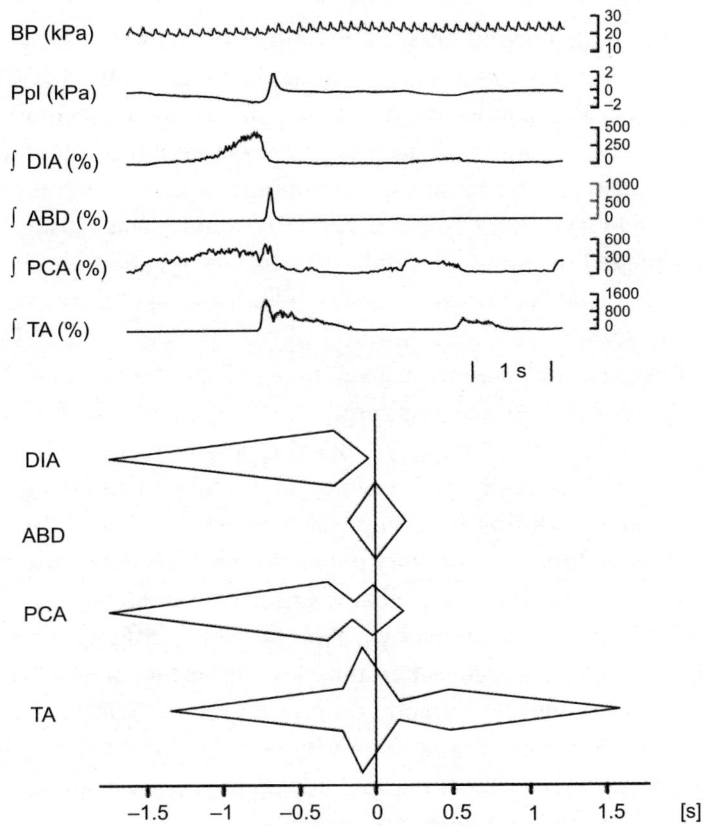

Time (ms)		Intensity (%)	Time (ms)		Intensity (%)
– 1750 ± 60	onset of the PCA		– 45 ± 20	offset of the DIA	
– 1740 ± 60	onset of the DIA		– 15 ± 7	2 peaks of the PCA	1110 ± 170
– 1350 ± 70	onset of the TA			0 peak of the ABD	860 ± 100
– 315 ± 15	1 peak of the PCA	1240 ± 260	180 ± 20	offset of the PCA	
– 275 ± 50	peak of the DIA	660 ± 40	190 ± 10	offset of the ABD	
– 180 ± 10	onset of the ABD		480 ± 30	2 peaks of the TA	900 ± 200
– 80 ± 10	1 peak of the TA	2700 ± 400	1590 ± 80	offset of the TA	

Fig. 6.2 Laryngeal cough. *Upper part:* Records of blood pressure (BP), pleural pressure (Ppl), integrated electromyographic activities in diaphragm (òDIA), abdominal muscles (òABD), posterior cricoarytenoid muscle (òPCA) and thyroarytenoid muscle (òTA) during laryngoph aryngeal cough immediately following a period of previous reflex elicited mechanically. *Lower part:* Diagram of electromyographic activities in DIA, ABD, PCA and TA during laryngeal cough indicating the time relations and maximal intensities compared to the baseline values. (For details, see Poliacek et al. 2003, Ref. [23]).

with a strong prolonged burst of electric discharges in diaphragm (DIA), external intercostal muscles and auxiliary inspiratory muscles. Contraction of inspiratory pump muscles (with upper airway abductors that enlarge the upper airways) results in a deep negative deflection of pleural (Ppl) and intrapulmonary (PP) pressures, which in turn enables a strong inspiratory airflow and rise in lung volume. The DIA activity was closely associated with a preceding burst of discharges in laryngeal abductor- posterior cricoarythenoid (PCA) muscle, and later with a burst of activity in laryngeal adductor-thyreoarythenoid muscle (TA).[23,27] Hence, in most instances, a ramp-like expiratory activity in abdominal (ABD) and laryngeal TA muscles was observed during late inspiratory phase of cough. Such pre-expulsive muscle contraction can amplify ABD muscles during rapid descent of DIA at the end of inspiratory phase of cough, thereby maximising the muscle force generation during the compressive phase.[25]

2. **Compressive Phase** (Expiratory pump-ribcage and ABD muscles contract, while glottis is closed): It is characterised by a sudden drop of activity in DIA and PCA, accompanied by a short but very strong electric activity in expiratory ABD and laryngeal TA muscles. This in turn breaks the inspiratory airflow, closes the glottis and compresses the air within the lungs and airways. High values of intrapulmonary pressure (about 40 kPa in humans) can decrease the patency of intrapulmonary airways and stimulate a variety of receptors within the lungs and airways.
3. **Expulsive Phase** (The glottis opens abruptly and sudden decompression creates a turbulent flow of air which is blown out at a very high flow rate): During this brief phase, there is a strong contraction of ABD, ribcage expiratory muscles and laryngeal abductor (PCA muscle), together with a decrease in activity of laryngeal adductor (TA). The velocity of air within the trachea may reach 50–120 $m.s^{-1}$, due to high pressure gradients and concomitant bronchoconstriction.

In addition to the above phases of cough, a phase of subsequent glottal constriction occurs occasionally. It is characterised by prolonged activation of laryngeal adductor (TA), that results in narrowing of the glottis and increase of transglottic pressure. The role of this phase is not clear. It may prevent propulsion of the stimuli from the glottal region into the lungs acting as post-inspiratory breaking mechanism on expiratory airflow in eupnoeic breathing. In recent experiments,[23,27] the 4th phase was observed in 96 per cent of cough responses, which had been analysed from electromyograms of laryngeal adductor (TA). Similarly, this phase was also detected in enhanced lumbar motoneuron activity in the last phase of cough in spontaneously breathing cats.[28] The 4th phase also showed as a prolonged depolarisation of medullary laryngeal (moto) neurons in fictive cough in decerebrate, paralyzed animals.[29,30]

6.3 NEUROGENESIS OF COUGH

6.3.1 Role of Central Respiratory Network

Recent findings support the functional concept of the cough centre, indicating that the basic central respiratory network (central respiratory rhythm and pattern generator—CPG) consisting of respiratory neurons in rostral, ventrolateral medulla [BÖT or rostral (VRG—ventral respiratory group)] may configure both breathing and cough motor patterns.[31-33] The caudal VRG of medulla which contains both silent and spontaneously active expiratory pre-motoneurons[34,35] may transmit the excitatory motor drive to spinal motoneurons in coughing,[36] sneezing[37] or vomiting.[38,39] Pools of silent respiratory and the non-respiratory related neurons in the caudal VRG are responsible for strong expiratory efforts in cough,[40] and they take part in forced expirations of many motor behaviours related to breathing (e.g. expiration reflex, retching, sneezing, vomiting, etc.).

6.3.1.1 Respiratory Neurons: Morphology and Function

It is generally accepted that pools of respiratory neurons within the brainstem are responsible for precise control of respiratory movements during three neuronal phases of quiet breathing: inspiratory, post-inspiratory (stage I) and expiratory (Stage II). Each phase (Fig. 6.3) corresponds to the phasic activities of respiratory neurons, which display the phase-locked discharge activity and interact synaptically with each other using chemical neurotransmission.[41] Specific neurotransmitters (excitatory or inhibitory) and intrinsic membrane properties of neurons (such as voltage-dependent currents of K^+, Na^+, Cl^-, Ca^{2+}) determine the particular discharge pattern of each type of respiratory neurons involved in respiratory rhythm and pattern generation (Fig. 6.4).

The brainstem contains several anatomically distinct areas with distinct groups of neurons (Fig. 6.5) involved in various aspects of the neural control of

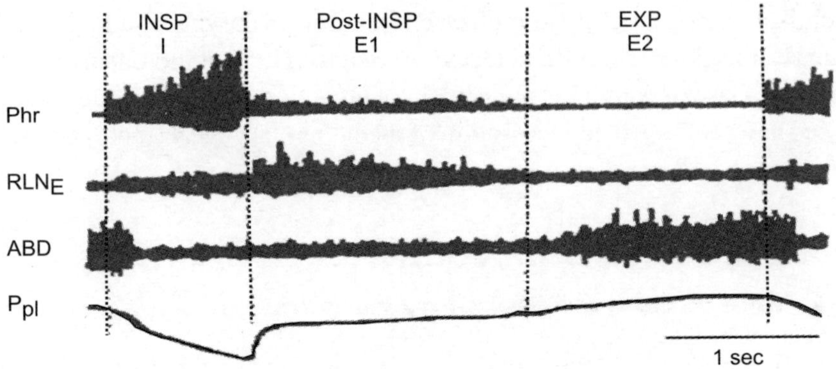

Fig. 6.3 A montage of multipotential efferent discharge activities recorded in phrenic nerve (Phr), expiratory fibres of recurrent laryngeal nerve (RLN_E), and abdominal lumbar nerve (ABD) completed by pleural pressure (Ppl) deflections. Respiratory cycle consists of 3 phases: inspiratory phase (INSP I), post-inspiration (Post-INSP) or passive expiration phase (E1), and expiration (EXP) or late expiration phase (E2). The activity in Phr, RLN_E and ABD, and the P_{pl} swings may be noted indicating the phases (bounded by dotted lines) of quiet breathing in cat. (Adapted from Bianchi et al., 1995, Ref. [69]).

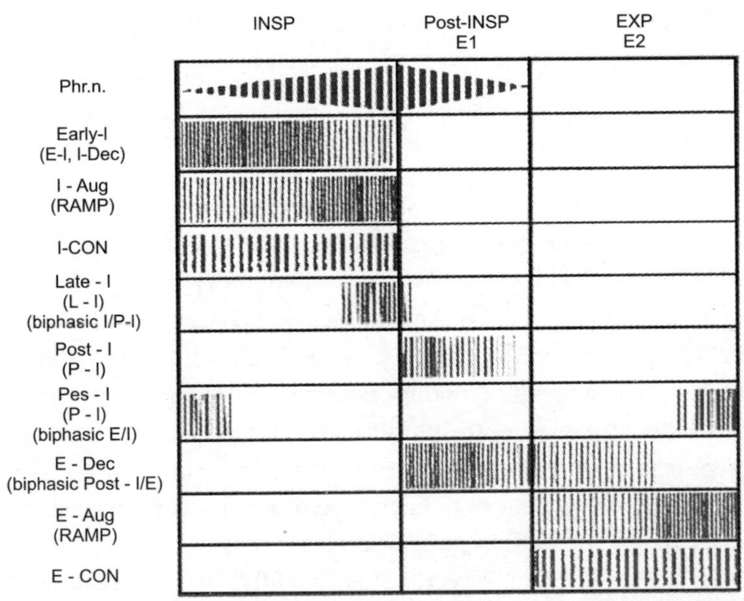

Fig. 6.4 Diagrammatic representation of 9 patterns of action potential discharge from medullary respiratory neurons with phrenic nerve (Phr.n.) activity. (For nomenclature, definitions and details see Bellingham, 1998; or Jakuš et al., 2004, Ref. [72]).

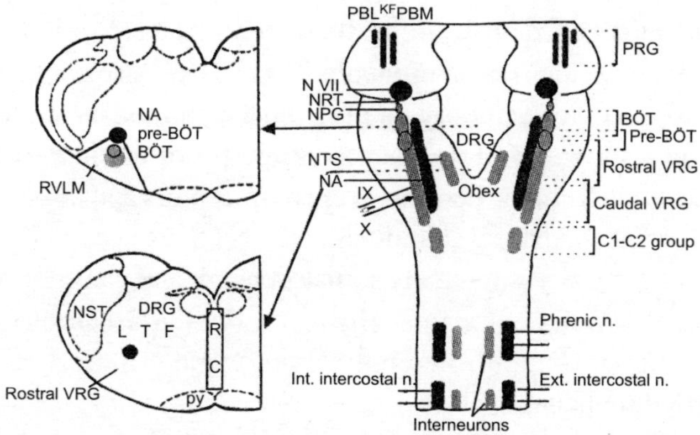

Fig. 6.5 Schematic representation of main brainstem areas containing pools of respiratory and respiratory-related neurons in cat. Transverse sections on left were drawn from two rostrocaudal levels of dorsal medullary view at right, indicating the location of neuronal structures within the medulla. NA, nucleus ambiguus; N VII, facial nucleus; VRG, ventral respiratory group; Caudal VRG, nucleus retroambigualis; Rostral VRG, nucleus para-ambigualis; NTS, nucleus tractus solitarii; NST, spinal trigeminal nucleus; BÖT, Bötzinger complex; pre-BÖT, pre-Bötzinger complex; DRG, dorsal respiratory group; LTF, lateral tegmental field; NRV, ventral reticular nucleus; RC, rostral and caudal raphe nuclei; NRT, retrotrapezoid nucleus; NPG, paragigantocellular nucleus; Obex, anatomic reference point; PRG, pontine respiratory group (consisting of PBL, KF and PMB, parabrachial lateral, Kölliker-Fuse and parabrachial medial nuclei, respectively); py, pyramidal tract; RVLM, rostral ventrolateral medulla; IX and X, glossopharyngeal and vagus cranial nerves; C1 and C2, segments of the spinal cord. (For nomenclature and details, see Jakuš et al., 2004, Ref. [72]).

breathing, e.g. in afferent signal processing, central chemoreception, respiratory rhythm generation, and motor pattern formation. Hence, the respiratory neurons (RN) are concentrated in two main areas of the medullary reticular formation, the dorsal (DRG) and ventral (VRG) respiratory groups.

The DRG lies bilaterally in the dorsomedial medulla around the obex.[42] It corresponds mostly to the ventrolateral nucleus of the solitary tract (vl NTS) and the surrounding reticular formation. The vl NTS contains a morphologically uniform group of respiratory neurons whose action potentials occur in a bursting pattern during inspiration. The majority of neurons are inspiration augmenting or I-Aug neurons and about 75 per cent of them, send their axons down to the contralateral spinal cord, the remaining axons are homolateral.[43] The I neurons of the vl NTS are mostly reticulospinal, driving the phrenic motoneurons and diaphragm as well as the intercostal motoneurons and muscles monosynaptically.

In addition to spinal cord projections, these neurons have ipsilateral, collateral projections to the nucleus retroambigualis.[44] The DRG also comprises P (pump) neurons (which receive excitatory inputs from the pulmonary stretch and irritant receptors) and a subgroup of non-augmenting (proprioreticular) neurons with afferent projections from the peripheral chemoreceptors and laryngeal receptors. The medial, dorsal and lateral subnuclei of the NTS are accepted as a brainstem integrative area for processing many somatosensory and viscerosensory afferent inputs entering medulla oblongata. However, the DRG neurons having some modulatory role in shaping the central motor pattern are not essential for respiratory rhythmogenesis.

The VRG[45,46] corresponds to a bilateral longitudinal column of I and E neurons, extending from the 1st cervical segment of the spinal cord rostrally up to the medullary facial nucleus, including the nucleus ambiguus (NA) and nucleus retroambigualis (NRA). The VRG can be functionally divided into three subdivisions: caudal VRG (cVRG], rostral (para-ambigual, intermediate) VRG, and most rostral VRG containing pre-Bötzinger and Bötzinger complexes.

The *caudal VRG,*[47] sometimes referred to as NRA, is located below the obex and caudally to nucleus ambiguus. This part contains a high density of reticulospinal E-Aug neurons, although I neurons are intermingled. The E-Aug neurons have axons descending along the contralateral spinal cord to the thoracic level without giving off any axon collateral in the medulla, extensively arborising at the thoracic and lumbar levels and supplying the spinal expiratory neurons (abdominal muscles). The caudal VRG extends caudally to the spinal cord C1-C2 level, where respiratory interneurones are also found (C1-C2 group).[48]

The *rostral VRG*[47] is located in the ventrolateral medulla at the same rostrocaudal level as the DRG, containing a density, predominantly of I-Aug neurons. The majority of them are reticulospinal premotoneurons (output neurons of respiratory CPG), driving the phrenic and intercostal motoneurons which in turn drive the diaphragm and external (inspiratory) intercostal muscles. In addition to spinal projections, these I neurons have collateral projections to both homolateral and contralateral NRA, although they do not project to the nucleus tractus solitarius (NTS). Both I neurons of rostral VRG and vl NTS make up the pre-motor population, driving the spinal inspiratory motoneurons (finally supplying the diaphragm and external intercostal muscles). The rostral VRG includes the nucleus ambiguus and para-ambigual regions. Both regions contain a variety of glossopharyngeal and vagal motoneurons which innervate the pharyngeal and laryngeal valve muscles. These motoneuron pools receive a drive from the respiratory CPG, hence they show either I, post-I, or E firing activity, but they do not contribute to the generation of respiratory rhythm. Similar upper airway motoneurons were recorded in Bötzinger area and in caudal VRG.

The *most rostral VRG* is located near the rostral end of the VRG, just behind the facial nucleus. It contains Bötzinger (BÖT) and pre-Bötzinger (pre-BÖT) complexes, which are a continuation of rostral VRG. Hence, they are sometimes treated together and designed as BÖT/rostral VRG area.

The *BÖT complex*[49] contains mostly E-Aug reticulospinal neurons, which are distributed in the area ventromedial to the retrofacial nucleus. However, they do not make a morphologically distinct nucleus. E-Aug neurons of BÖT complex have extensive bilateral collaterals among the medullary nuclei and send contralateral projections down the contralateral spinal cord. Thus, they appear to have a wide bilateral inhibitory influence upon BÖT, VRG, DRG neurons and also phrenic motoneurons. In addition to E-Aug neurons, the BÖT/VRG area contains some proprioreticular (inter)neurons with E -Dec, I-Dec and I-CON patterns as well as vagal and glossopharyngeal motoneurons. The vagal and glossopharyngeal motoneurons send their axons into the superior laryngeal nerve (SLN) or the glossopharyngeal branches of the Xth and IXth nerves. Motoneurons of the SLN are located in the retrofacial nucleus and show mostly I activity. The IXth nerve that innervates the pharyngeal muscles shows exclusively I activity. Hence, it seems reasonable to suppose that motoneurons with E firing activity, which are frequently recorded in BÖT, send their axons to pharyngeal branches of the Xth nerve.

The *pre-BÖT complex*[50] is hypothesised to contain neuronal circuits generating the basic respiratory rhythm. This area, (approximately 450 μm) localized between the Bötzinger complex and the rostral VRG (in neonatal rat) contains very few reticulospinal neurons, but a 100 per cent proprioreticular (inter)neurons. Amongst them are included mostly: Pre-I (biphasic, phase spanning neurons), Early-I (I-Dec), and postinspiratory (P-I) neurons, i.e. all classes of cells proposed to be involved in respiratory phase transitions. In comparison, the adjacent Bötzinger complex contains 20 per cent, and the rostral VRG, no proprioreticular units.[51] It is believed that the pre-Bötzinger complex is a source of pacemaker neurons with specific intrinsic properties (relatively slow oscillations of membrane potential by cyclic activation and inactivation of intrinsic conductances or intracellular messengers). These pacemaker neurons with voltage-dependent oscillatory membrane potentials have their electrical activity synchronous with rhythmic motor activity in hypoglossal nerves.[50] Hence, the pre-BÖT complex is postulated as the kernel of respiratory rhythm oscillator and as a target of many convergent inputs, including those from modulatory afferent circuits, which crucially affect the genesis of respiratory rhythm.[52] In addition, the neurons of the pre-BÖT complex may provide an important link for central chemoreceptor-related respiratory drive.[53]

In addition to DRG and VRG, there are various medullary structures which play at least a modulatory role in neural control of quiet breathing. Budznski et al[54] and Connelly et al.[55] suggests that in adult animals the nucleus paragigantocellularis lateralis (NPGL) and nucleus retrotrapezoideus (NRT), which are located at the level of the facial and retrofacial nuclei in the most rostral part of VRG, respectively, could be a part of respiratory CPG. However, there is still no clear evidence that the NPGL or NRT are identical with the pre-Bötzinger complex—the proposed kernel for respiratory rhythmogenesis. Axons of neurons (mostly the phase-spanning type) localised in both nuclei project extensively into the DRG, VRG, PRG or rostrally toward the hypothalamic nuclei. In addition to their respiratory function, they seem to be involved in cardiovascular tasks,[56] probably mediating the signals from central chemosensitive areas toward the medullary neurons controlling respiration and circulation. In addition, neurons in the subretrofacial nucleus situated just caudally to the NPGL play a vital role in controlling sympathetic vasomotor outflow, peripheral vascular resistance and blood pressure.[57]

In the rostral pons, a density of respiration-related (tonic and phase spanning) neurons have been reported bilaterally in the areas of nucleus parabrachialis medialis (NPBM), nucleus parabrachialis lateralis (NPBL) and Kölliker-Fuse (KF) nucleus.[58-60] The neuronal clusters shown in Figure 6.5 are often designated as the pontine respiratory group (PRG). It is accepted as an integrative brainstem area that receives afferent projections from the NTS, area postrema, lateral tegmental field, and ventral surface of the medulla, which are related to the control of respiratory, cardiovascular, visceral and gustatory functions. Thus, neurons subserving these functions may interfere with respiration at the pontine level. This could provide an explanation for the strong modulatory influence of PRG neurons on the breathing pattern promotion of inspiratory termination in the absence of pulmonary afferent feedback.[61] However, the precise mechanism and the role of PRG neurons for such an influence on the inspiratory phase remains obscure. It seems that projections from PRG neurons to the medullary respiratory neurons are indirect, mostly toward the raphe and reticular nuclei.[62]

The PRG neurons are not essential for respiratory rhythm generation per se, but they may stabilise the respiratory pattern, slow down the rhythm, and influence the timing of respiratory phases, e.g. during sleep or general anaesthesia. In addition, the PRG could be a part of the pathway transmitting information from the respiratory CPG to suprapontine structures such as diencephalon, mesencephalon or amygdala or vice versa from the hypothalamus to the rostral pons.

Very little is known about the suprapontine respiration-related areas localised in the cortex, thalamus, hypothalamus, or even the mesencephalon. These regions are known to be involved mainly in adjusting respiration to alterations elicited by exercise, locomotion, postural changes, hypoxia, hypercapnia and thermal changes. The cortical neurons supplying the phrenic and intercostal motoneurons at the level of the spinal cord (corticospinal-pyramidal pathways) originate in area 4 of motor cortex.[63] In addition, cortical inputs impinging upon midbrain neurons arise from the prefrontal cortex. The limbic inputs are likely to be involved in the ventilatory changes during different emotional and arousal states. The major cortical inputs into the caudal hypothalamus originate from areas 4 and 6 of the motor cortex. Both motor and limbic areas of the cortex are connected with the major medullary regions (DRG, VRG) involved in respiratory outflow. The axons from neurons located in the caudal hypothalamus project to the midbrain periaquaductal grey (PAG) and ventrolateral medulla.[64] The PAG receives inputs from the caudal hypothalamic neurons and then projects to pontine nuclei (NPBM, KF) and rostral VRG and DRG.[65]

6.3.1.2 Basic Principles of Respiratory Rhythm and Pattern Generation

Respiratory rhythmogenesis is driven by complex interactions that reflect both synaptic interactions between the synaptic inputs to brainstem neurons as well as intrinsic voltage-dependent membrane properties of those neurons. On the basis of current knowledge, the following principles underlie respiratory rhythmogenesis in adult respiratory CPG:

1. A reciprocal synaptic inhibition is important for respiratory rhythmogenesis in mature respiratory network.
2. An external source of tonic excitation is also of vital importance.
3. Decrementing respiratory neurons are mutually inhibitory.

4. Late inspiratory (expiratory) neurons are important in terminating their respective phases.
5. Augmenting neurons show a discharge pattern that may be shaped by the decreasing inhibition of decrementing neurons and by an increasing excitation from recurrent collaterals of incrementing neurons of the same phase.
6. At least one type of respiratory neurons involved in respiratory rhythmogenesis, must display a property of accommodation.
7. Synaptic inhibition of incrementing inspiratory neurons occurs at the expiratory stage 2 when a low voltage-dependent calcium current is activated, providing initial depolarisation to subthreshold level.
8. Recurrent synaptic excitation and possibly a slow depolarising persistent sodium current depolarise the neuron to its threshold.
9. Action potentials activate high voltage-dependent calcium currents, increasing synaptically generated depolarisation.
10. Entry of calcium through these channels as well as glutamate-gated N-methyl-D-aspartate NMDA channels activate the calcium-dependent potassium currents, hence slowing down both depolarisation and firing.
11. Post-I neurons are sufficiently disinhibited to fire and rapidly inhibit ramp I neurons.
12. Synaptic hyperpolarisation activates the IH current, which tends to repolarise the neuron until the onset of the respiratory cycle.

The respiratory pattern (i.e. duration of I and E neuron bursts, number of spikes in a burst or recruitment of I or E units) may result from activation of pattern formation network, consisting of excitatory and inhibitory propriobulbar (propriobrainstem) interneurons. The pattern generator affects the activity of the primary respiratory network (in adults) or the activity of the basic oscillator (in prenatal and newborn periods), thus shaping the respiratory pattern into either eupnoeic, apneustic or gasping neural patterns. The excitatory transmission of rhythmic drive in the respiratory CPG is mediated by excitatory amino acids (mostly through non-NMDA receptors), including those at the site of pre-motoneuron to motoneuron synapses.

Generation of respiratory rhythm has three models:

1. Network models (where inhibitory synaptic interactions are essential for rhythmogenesis).
2. Pacemaker models (where neurons with pacemaker properties underlie rhythmicity),
3. Hybrid models (Fig. 6.6) as a fusion of the two former models.

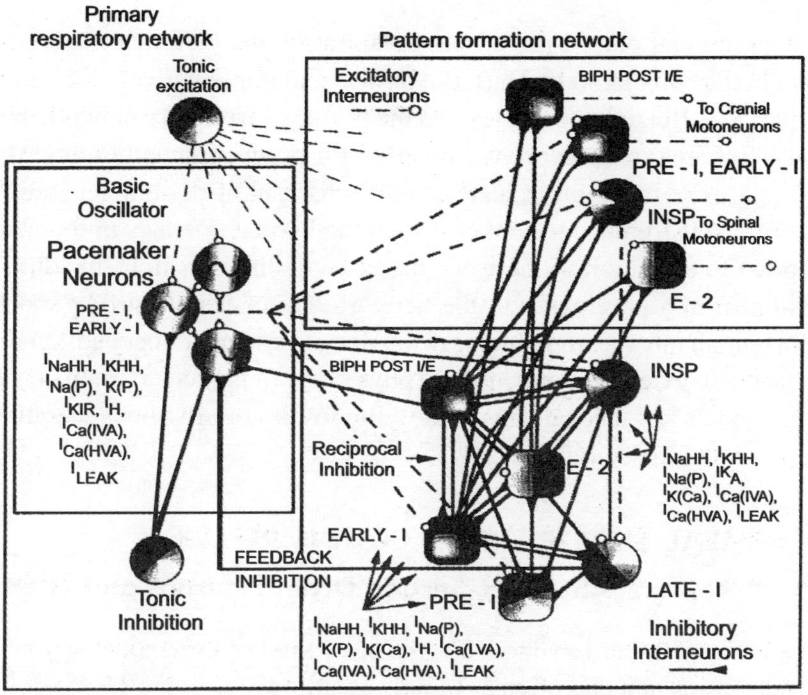

Fig. 6.6 Tentative hybrid model of respiratory rhythm and pattern formation networks in ventrolateral medulla, that represents the kernel for rhythm and pattern generation. Interneurons are based on their spiking patterns in relation to inspiratory (I) and expiratory (E) phases of respiratory cycle. Each neuron type is distributed bilaterally in the medulla. Connections are postulated from patterns of spike discharge and synaptic activation in *vitro* and in *vivo*. Tentative conductances for each class of neuron are indicated; excitatory and inhibitory subpopulations are postulated to have similar currents. Afferent circuits active *in vivo* are not included. Conductance abbreviations: INaHH, fast Na^+; INa(P), persistent Na^+; IKHH, delayed rectifier K^+; IKIR, inwardly rectifying K^+; IK(P), slowly activating, persistent K^+; IKA, hyperpolarisation-activated K^+; IK(Ca), Ca^{2+}-dependent K^+; ICa(LVA), low-voltage-activated Ca^{2+}; ICa(HVA), high-voltage-activated Ca^{2+}; ICa(IVA), intermediate-voltage-activated Ca^{2+}; IH, hyperpolarisation-activated, mixed cation conductance. For nomenclature of neurons and the model function. (Modified from Smith 1997, see Ref. [70 and 72]).

However, till now a realistic model of respiratory CPG and its basic mechanisms are only tentative. Nevertheless, it seems that the generation of respiratory rhythm in prenatal or newborn animals, results predominantly from activity of a basic oscillator which may consist of neurons (Pre-I, Early I) with pacemaker properties. Such a basic oscillator probably undergoes a process of maturation during ontogenesis. Hence, in mature animals, the basic oscillator can be an integral part of the primary respiratory network that may normally operate in the adult as well. Thus, the basic oscillator tentatively located in the medullary pre-Bötzinger complex and the primary respiratory network in BÖT/ rostral VRG area might represent a kernel for production and timing of three neural phases of breathing. Clearly, the mechanism of rhythm generation can transform itself from a pacemaker-driven mode (that operates in foetuses and newborns) to an inhibitory network-based mode that functions in adults. The transition from a pacemaker to the network dominance occurring soon after birth in human infants might increase the risk of sudden infant death syndrome. (For excellent reviews on anatomy and physiology of particular group of neurons and the models and mechanisms underlying respiratory rhythm generation and pattern formation see references[66-72]).

6.4 NEURAL SUBSTRATE OF COUGH REFLEX

6.4.1 Receptors, Afferents, Second Order Neurons and Efferents

Receptors for TB and laryngeal coughs are a kind of polymodal sensors with rapid adaptation and classified as rapidly adapting receptors (RARs) or irritant receptors.[3,73] They are a kind of thin myelinated sensory nerve fibres with small diameter (A) located within and under the airway epithelium of larynx, carina and main bronchi. In cats, they are mostly localised at the level of carina (trachea), a site most sensitive for eliciting cough. The receptors are either scanty or absent in the smaller airways and alveoli, consistent with the weakness of cough reflex from these areas.[73] RARs are not specific cough receptors, but are rather a subtype.[74] However, they are very sensitive to direct mechanical stimuli, hence a probing of the lower trachea and main bronchi (by inhalation of irritants, chemical substances, or inflation and deflation of lungs) may result in TB and laryngeal coughs (also under specific occasions in tachypnoea, augmented breaths, laryngeal and bronchial constriction, vasodilation, mucus secretion or Hering-Breuer deflation reflex).

However, activation of C-fibre receptors in the airways may evoke cough, reflexly[75] by release of sensory neuropeptides, which cause a neurogenic inflammation. This in turn may stimulate RARs to produce coughing. However, the reflex inputs from bronchial and pulmonary C-fibre receptors are expected to inhibit the strength of the cough reflex in cats.[76] The reflex inputs from slowly adapting pulmonary stretch receptors are known to play modulatory but permissive role in production of cough reflex,[3,7,77] probably by central facilitation of expiratory motoneurons.[78] Pulmonary stretch receptors do not affect the inspiratory amplitude and inspiratory/expiratory phase timing during cough episodes,[79] however they are necessary for expression of cough motor pattern. As documented in TB cough, the tonic activity of SARs reaches its maximal frequency 110.8 ± 6.3 imp/s during the inspiratory phase, preceding the peak inspiratory volume by 50 ms. The lowest frequency (1.3 ± 0.1 imp/s) was present during the expulsive phase, when a part of the expiratory reserve volume (ERV) (below the level of functional residual capacity (FRC) had been expelled from the lungs.[80,81] Other reflex inputs from extrapulmonary afferents (cardiac, abdominal and skin) are known to inhibit the strength of cough reflex.[82,83]

For TB cough, the afferent information from pulmonary RARs (including the inputs from C-fibre receptors and SARs) is conveyed by myelinated branches of the Xth nerve, terminating in different subnuclei of NTS, where they make synaptic contact on cough second-order relay neurons.[84] In particular, second-order neurons of pulmonary RARs are localised within the commissural subnucleus and in the caudal portion of the medial subnucleus of NTS. Thus, tracheobronchial RARs do not project directly to the DRG.

For laryngeal cough, the internal branch of the superior laryngeal nerve is the main afferent pathway. For the TB cough too, the laryngeal afferent fibres project to various commissural subnuclei of the caudal NTS,[85,86] providing a possible convergence site for both types of coughs.[87] However, most laryngeal receptor afferents project to areas of the NTS rostral to the obex and medial to the DRG.[88,89] Caudal VRG and BÖT/rostral VRG may receive afferent information from the larynx via multiple synaptic pathways.[90]

It was established that one-fourth of the neurons recorded from the commissural nuclei (caudal to obex) contained most of cough (RAR)-second order relay neurons[91] and several units arising from them increased their firing activity, but a 10 per cent of them decreased their firing following mechanical tracheal stimulation.[87,92] While a some of the neurons underwent only weak or no respiratory modulation, other units (which were silent during control period) were recruited. The authors hypothesised that the airway cough receptors and their second-order NTS relay neurons are silent during eupnoea. In addition, these units may receive inputs from the DRG and (or) BÖT-rostral VRG, but not from airway receptors. A similar behaviour of neurons from the NTS/DRG region (rostral to obex) was also observed. Most laryngeal afferent fibres project to the NTS area rostral to the obex[88] and some neurons were excited and others inhibited by stimuli that produce cough. One may speculate that some unknown pool of interneurons in the central cough reflex pathway may receive convergent afferent information related to both laryngeal and tracheobronchial cough. Such a pool of interneurons may serve as a proposed functional gate through which cough afferent information passes. Cough (RAR) second-order relay neurons may further project to pontine and medullary regions containing neuronal circuitries involved in respiratory control.[93-95]

Higher-order central projections of cough, i.e. second-order relay neurons from other inputs are not well established, but they may affect the pontine or medullary respiratory neurons too.[84]

Efferent pathways in both types of cough (and also in sneezing, expiration reflex, and quiet breathing) carry central motor command from the pre-motor DRG and VRG neurons to spinal expiratory motoneurons, and then via the phrenic, intercostal and lumbar nerves to expiratory pump muscles. Only one report on cats[96] demonstrated that the efferent motor pathways for coughing might be separated from the spinal pathways driving rhythmic breathing. The central motor command from pre-motoneurons is also transmitted via the cranial motoneurons (which supply the pharyngeal and laryngeal valve muscles) and by sympathetic or parasympathetic nerves (that supply the airway smooth muscles and glands). The increase in inspiratory motoneuron activity during cough is probably due to inspiratory drive from BÖT or rostral VRG neurons and second-order relay NTS neurons.

6.4.2 Central Intramedullary Pathways (Experimental Findings)

6.4.2.1 Pontine and Medullary Transections

Transection experiments in cats[11,14] showed that neurons in the rostral pons may have modulatory effects on the cough reflex. Hence, in our early experiments on non-paralysed cats[97] and using the method of successive, rostral-to-caudal transections at the level of pons, ponto-medullary border and rostral medulla, we tried to define such pontine and medullary regions that would be essential for cough (Fig. 6.7). Transection of the rostral pons (8 mm above the obex) regularly abolished the expiratory signs of TB cough, while leaving intact, its inspiratory components. Similarly, a transection at the level of rostral medulla (5 mm) actually stopped rhythmic breathing, and tracheobronchial stimulation was not effective. In addition to profound effects on breathing, this study proved the modulatory role of pontine neurons on cough reflex, indicating that the rostral

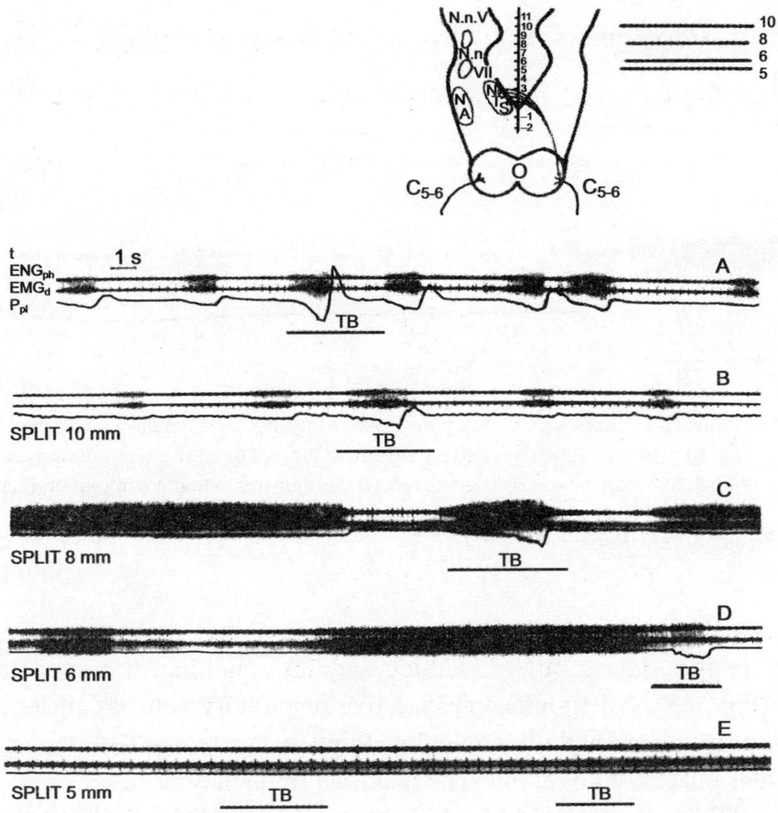

Fig. 6.7 Electroneurogram of the right phrenic nerve (ENG_{ph}), electromyogram of the left half of the diaphragm (EMG_d), and pleural pressure (P_{pl}) changes in a spontaneously breathing cat during mechanical stimulation (Stim.) of the tracheobronchial mucosa (TB) before (record A); and after brainstem transections (SPLIT) 10 mm (record B); 8 mm (record C), 6 mm (record D); and 5 mm (record E) rostrally to the obex. Abbreviations: N.n.V, nucleus nervi trigemini; N.n.VII, nucleus nervi facialis; NTS, nucleus tractus solitarii; NA, nucleus ambiguus; C5-6, cervical roots of the phrenic nerve. (For details, see Ref. [97])

pontine structures are responsible for expression of strong expiratory efforts in cough, although its basic central structures might be localised in medulla oblongata.

6.4.2.2 Recording Experiments

Transection experiments yielded some findings in some earlier recordings of experiments in the medulla on cats.[34,98] We recorded the single-unit activity of

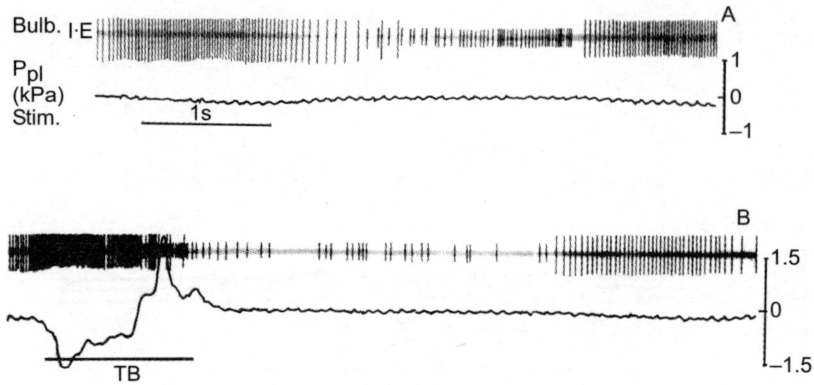

Fig. 6.8 Changes in bulbar inspiratory and expiratory neurons ($Bulb_{I-E}$: Inspiratory—higher spikes, expiratory—lower spikes) as well as in pleural pressure (Ppl) during cough elicited from tracheobronchial (TB) region (record B) after mechanical stimulation (Stim.) of airways in comparison with control breathing (record A). (Reproduced from Ref. [34] with permission from Publisher).

inspiratory and (or) expiratory neurons from medullary VRG, parallely with pleural pressure changes during quiet breathing and TB coughing in non-paralysed cats[34,99] (Fig. 6.8). All spontaneously active respiratory neurons (inspiratory and expiratory) recorded during quiet breathing had increased their firing rates in particular phases of coughing. The maximal frequency of single expiratory neurons in TB cough reached 132 ± 13.9 imp/s (as evaluated from 17 neurons in 20 tests), while the frequency of inspiratory neurons was 192.0 ± 33.8 imp/s (14 neurons in 20 tests).

No recruitment of inspiratory units from VRG during the inspiratory phase of cough was found. In addition, silent expiratory units were regularly recruited during the expulsive phase of coughing (with a maximal frequency 158.7 ± 16.2 imp/s). Similar recruitment of originally silent neurons was observed during expiratory efforts in sneeze and expiration reflexes, indicating that the neurons involved were not specific for coughing. This study indicated that: (a) the respiratory neurons which take part in the genesis of quiet breathing may be involved in coughing; (b) a pool of originally silent expiratory neurons from VRG may take part in configuration of the cough motor pattern; (c) the idea of anatomically localised independent cough centre in the medulla was considered improbable.

Oku et al[35] studied the behaviour of respiratory neurons from VRG BÖT area during fictive laryngeal cough induced by electrical superior laryngeal nerve stimulation in decerebrate, paralysed and artificially ventilated cats. As was shown on spontaneously breathing cats with TB coughs,[34] similar types and patterns of inspiratory and expiratory activities had been seen in particular phases of fictive laryngeal coughing. As the duration of E-Aug neurons (of both caudal VRG and BÖT) did not correspond to the duration of burst in lumbar motoneurons, the authors speculated that another unknown source of descending drive to spinal motoneurons might be involved in laryngeal coughing.

During the last decade, experimental models of fictive cough reflex were introduced.[100,101] Studies were conducted on decerebrate, thoracotomised, paralysed, and artificially ventilated cats. Either fictive laryngeal or fictive TB cough was elicited either by an electrical SLN stimulation[100,101] or by a mechanical stimulation of tracheal mucosa.[101,102,103] Neuron spike-trains were recorded simultaneously from multiple brainstem structures by arrays of 60 individually adjustable tungsten microelectrodes, especially for studying cough and the expiration reflex.[36,103] In addition, a functional interaction (connectivity) among a variety of respiratory neurons of the network was detected with cross-correlation methods and neuron to nerve interactions with spike-triggered averaging, using modern computer simulation techniques.[29,86] Hence, new experimental methods brought substantial amount of data, that enabled the development of plausible models of cough motor pattern generation[32,33,103] (see, section 6.6).

6.4.2.3 Immunohistochemical and Synaptic Blockade Experiments

In order to localise the neurons that are functionally related to the fictive laryngeal cough, the expression of immediate-early gene C-Fos, a marker of neuronal activation, was employed in acute experiments on decerebrate, paralysed and artificially ventilated cats.[104] Laryngeal cough was elicited frequently by repeated electrical stimulation of the superior laryngeal nerve. The c-Fos immunoreactivity was found bilaterally enhanced (Fig. 6.9) at two levels of the brainstem: (a) at the medullary level the highest density of c-Fos labelling was detected within the nuclei of the solitary tract (especially in the interstitial and ventrolateral subdivisions of NTS) in the medial part of lateral tegmental field, internal division of lateral reticular nucleus, the retro- and para-ambigual regions, and around the retrofacial nucleus, and (b) within the pons an enhanced labelling was found in

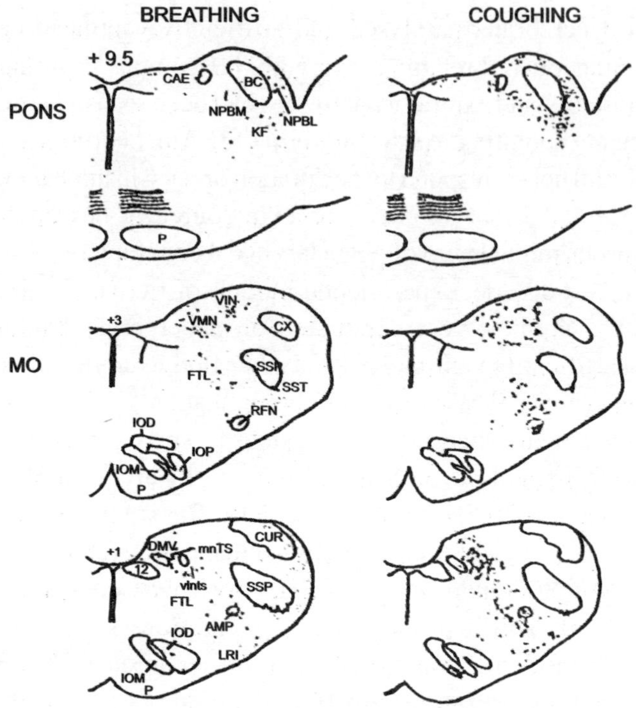

Fig. 6.9 Distribution of brainstem c-Fos neuroimmunoreactivity in control BREATHING and fictive laryngeal COUGHING at the level of PONS (6.5 mm rostrally to obex) and medulla oblongata—MO (3 mm and 1 mm rostrally to obex, respectively). Each dot represents one Fos-positive neuron. 12, nucleus hypoglossus; 5SP, spinal trigeminal nucleus; 5ST, spinal trigeminal tract; AMB, para-ambigual region; BC, brachium conjunctivum; CAE, locus caeruleus; CUR, CX, rostral and external cuneate nuclei; DMV, dorsal motor nucleus of the vagus; FTL, lateral tegmental field; IOM, IOD, IOP, medial, dorsal and principal nuclei of the inferior olivae; KF, Kölliker-Fuse nucleus; LRI, lateral reticular nucleus; NPBL, NPBM, lateral and medial parabrachial nuclei; RFN, retrofacial nucleus; mnTS, vlnTS, medial and ventrolateral subnuclei of the nucleus tractus solitarius; VIN, VMN, inferior and medial vestibular nuclei; P, pyramidal tract (Modified from Gestreau et al., 1997).[104]

the medial and lateral parabrachial nuclei and below the caudal border of brachium conjunctivum affecting the Kölliker-Fuse nucleus.

These experiments revealed that Fos-like immunoreactivity overlaps the dorsal and ventral medullary areas, which contain a dense population of respiratory neurons (being normally involved in central integration of quiet breathing). In addition, the pontine parabrachial nuclei, medullary lateral tegmental field and lateral reticular nucleus were displayed, indicating that all the above-mentioned structures were activated in fictive laryngeal cough in cats.

Synaptic blockade experiments are based on the irreversible inhibitory effect of kainic acid microinjections (chemical lesions) on synaptic neurotransmission. As a neurotoxin, kainic acid, functionally, mainly destroys the neuronal cell bodies in the target regions, while sparing terminals and fibres of passage.[105] Based on c-Fos findings from recording and transection experiments, we were concerned with the question: whether the medullary midline raphe nuclei, the ventral medullary reticular nucleus of the lateral tegmental field as well as the pontine respiratory group neurons were involved in modulation (configuration) of cough and other airway reflexes? In order to make a functional synaptic blockade within the particular areas, kainic acid lesions in pentobarbitone or chloralose anaesthetised, non-decerebrate, spontaneously breathing cats were performed. Coughing was elicited by mechanical stimulation of the laryngeal and tracheal regions.

Kainic acid microinjections into the obscurus and pallidus raphe nuclei and the surrounding medial medullary reticular formation (Fig. 6.10) regularly and completely removed signs of both the tracheobronchial and laryngeal coughs seen in phrenic and lumbar motoneurons as well as the signs of expiration reflex induced from the glottal area. In addition, the lesions had significantly prolonged the post-inspiratory and expiratory periods of quiet breathing and decreased the arterial blood pressure.[106] The mechanisms by which the midline raphe neurons influence cough reflex, breathing or sympathetic outflow are unclear (refer, section 6.7.1).

Furthermore, we also tested the hypothesis that neurons of both the nucleus reticularis ventralis and the adjacent parts of lateral tegmental field could be involved in motor pathways associated with cough and other airway reflexes. Experiments showed that uni- and bilateral microinjections of kainic acid into the medullary lateral tegmental field (LTF) above the obex (Fig. 6.11) had removed all signs of the presence of cough reflexes, altered the eupnoeic breathing pattern and decreased systemic arterial blood pressure.[107] The critical injection site for suppression of reflexes was located between DRG and VRG. It seems that the LTF could be a part of the relay network for afferent information to the respiratory cough CPGs. However, the specific synaptic interactions and proper mechanisms are still tentative (see, section 10.7.2).

The effect of kainic acid injections into the pontine respiratory group (PRG) was similar (Fig. 6.12).

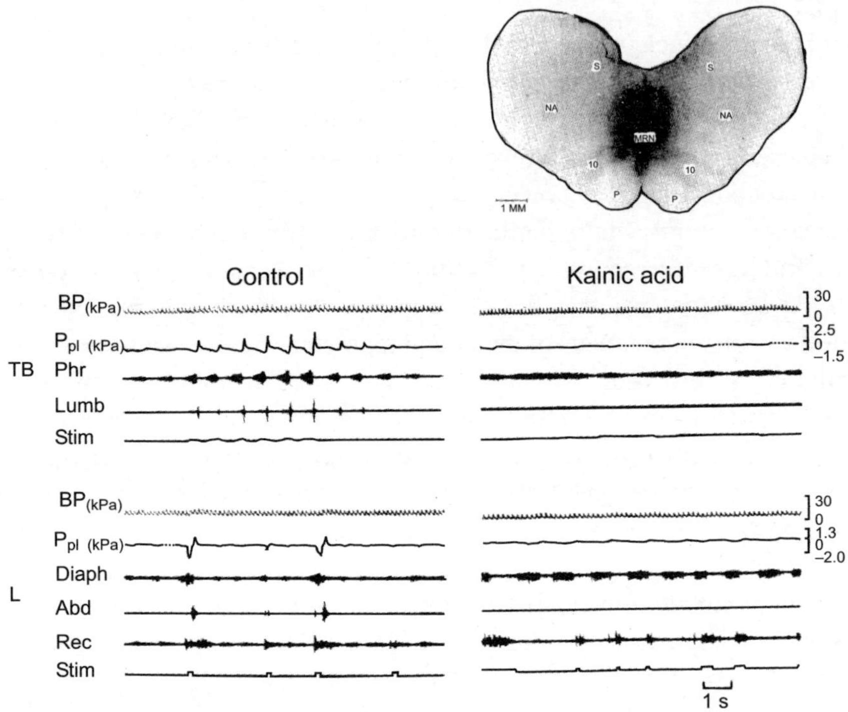

Fig. 6.10 Tracheobronchial cough (TB) and laryngeal cough (L) in cats under pentobarbitone anaesthesia in control condition (CONTROL) and after kainic acid injections (KAINIC ACID). BP—systemic arterial blood pressure; P_{pl}—pleural pressure; Phr—electroneurogram of the phrenic nerve, Diaph—electromyogram of the diaphragm; Lumb—electroneuro-gram of the lumbar nerve, Abd—electromyogram of the obliquus abdominis, Rec—electroneurogram of the recurrent laryngeal nerve, Stim—mechanical stimulation. Transverse medullary section at the level of 2.6 mm rostral to the obex showing the extent of the kainic acid lesion (dark area) to the medullary midline. Abbreviations: P, pyramidal tract; IO, inferior olivae; MRN midline raphe nuclei; S, solitary tract; NA, nucleus ambiguus (For details, see Jakuš et al., 1998)[106]

Destruction of PRG neurons abolished all signs of TB and laryngeal cough and expiration reflex, it altered the eupnoeic breathing pattern and decreased the arterial blood pressure.[108] The pontine respiratory group was considered an important source of facilitatory input into the brainstem circuitry that mediates cough and expiration reflexes. The findings are consistent with the known effects of PRG on quiet breathing and coughing (see section 6.4.1.1).

Since there are specific signs of a destructive effect of kainic acid on neuronal somata,[109] we suppose that all the three regions mentioned above

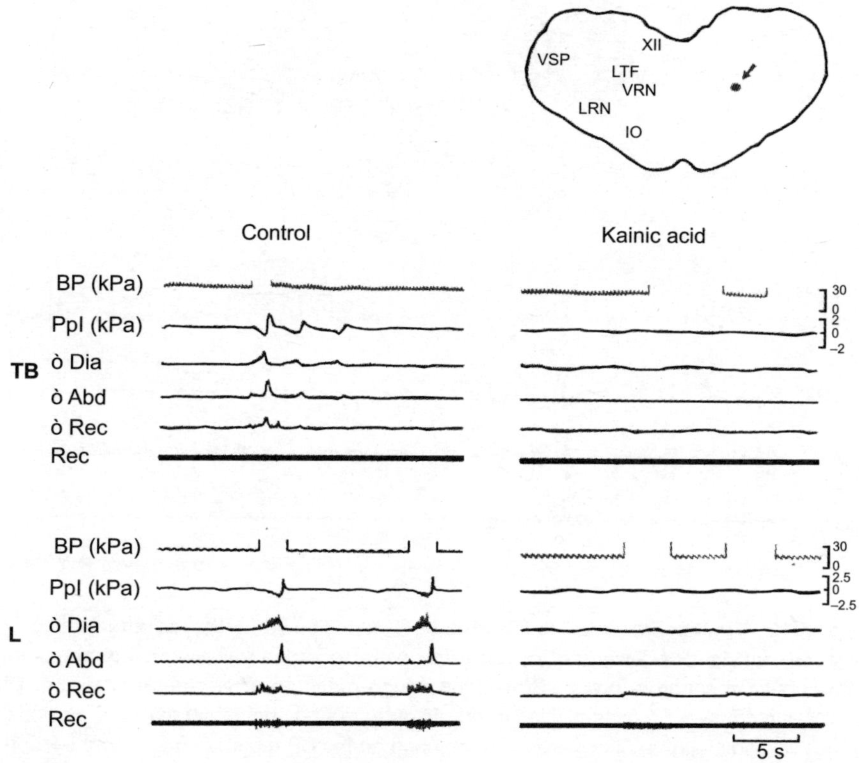

Fig. 6.11 Tracheobronchial (TB) cough and laryngeal (L) cough in control conditions and after KAINIC ACID injections to the ventral reticular nucleus (VRN) and the adjacent part of medullary lateral tegmental field (LTF) applied unilaterally (shown by *arrow*). Transverse medullary section at the level of 2.5 mm rostral to the obex. Interruption in blood pressures indicate the moment of mechanical stimulation. Abbreviations: XII, hypoglossal nucleus; VSP, spinal tract of the trigeminal nerve; LRN, lateral reticular nucleus; IO, inferior olivae (For details, see Jakuš et al, 2000)[107]

(belonging to rapheal, medial and lateral parts of reticular formation) may play an essential role in the modulation of cough and expiration reflexes. They may serve as an important source of facilitation for basic neuronal circuit(s) which produce or mediate cough and expiration reflexes in cats.

Since the central pathways and synaptic connections among neurons of NTS, BÖT/VRG, Raphe nuclei, LTF, PRG or cerebellum are not established still, there is no reason to exclude the possibility of yet another unknown brainstem areas altering the cough motor pattern (see section 10.7).

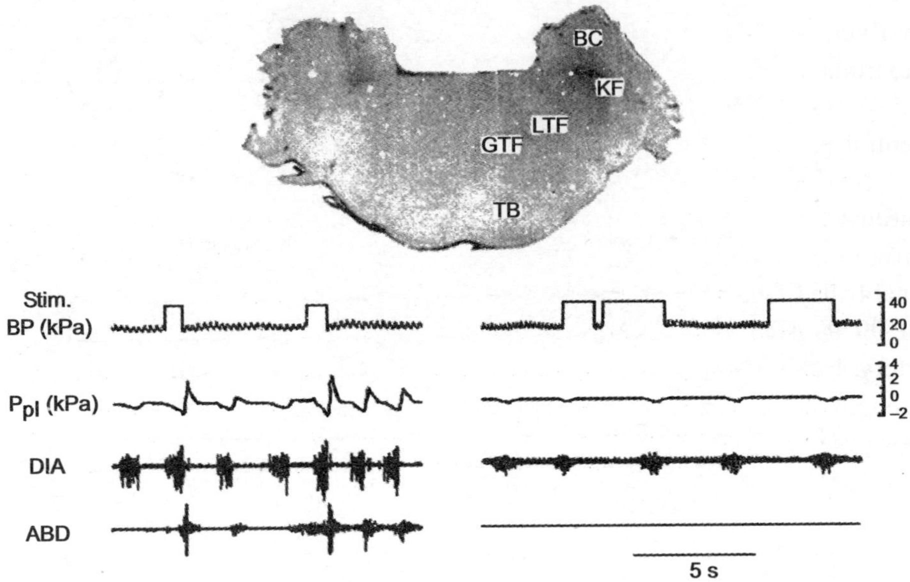

Fig. 6.12 Tracheobronchial cough in control condition (on left) and after kainic acid injection (at right). No signs of cough reflex were recorded following bilateral lesion of the pontine respiratory group. BP—blood cough pressure; P_{pl}—pleural pressure, DIA, ABD—electromyographic activities in the diaphragm and abdominal muscles. Periods of repeated stimulations (Stim.) are superimposed on the BP records. Transverse section of the pons 10.5 mm rostrally to the obex with bilateral kainic acid injections (darker areas). Abbreviations: BC, brachium conjunctivum; KF, Kölliker-Fuse nucieus; LTF, pontine lateral tegmental field; GTF, pontine gigantocellular tegmental field; TB, trapezoid body (For details, see Poliacek et al, 2004)[108]

6.4.2.4 Experiments with Antitussive Drugs

Older pharmacological experiments in cats and dogs, using antitussive drugs[11,13,110-112] introduced new methods for their systemic and non-systemic applications, and brought the first modern view of their effects on cough, respiration and sympathetic outflow. Many techniques and routes of application were used to determine the site of action of antitussive drugs. As a result, a variety of areas critically involved in coughing were established, e.g. areas adjacent to the obex,[11] and areas dorsomedial to the trigeminal tract and nucleus[13] or within the nucleus reticularis parvocellularis.[18] Such, more or less circumscribed medullary areas were regarded as playing the role of a cough centre. Since codeine was the only antitussive drug available until 1950s, these investigations evolved a new research and development of antitussive drugs such as dextromethorphan, noscapine, benzonatate, baclofen, substances CP 99, 994, SR 48, 968, BW 443C, levodropropizine, moguisteine, with either peripheral or central effects.

Novel experimental work of Bolser and his colleagues on the influence of antitussive drugs on cough and respiration[33, 40, 113, 114] have brought considerable progress in search for central mechanisms of cough reflex. The authors established that centrally acting drugs (codeine, dextromethorphan, baclofen, CP 99, 994 and SR 48, 968), when administrated in low doses via the vertebral artery, had reduced cough number (number of cough/stimulus trial) and the strength of cough (evaluated as a decrease of rectus abdominis burst amplitude). However, no effect of antitussives on cough cycle timing or diaphragm amplitude in cough was determined. The authors concluded that: (a) central antitussive drugs primarily suppress cough by inhibition of the expiratory motor drive and cough number, and (b) timing of cough cycle and intensity of inspiratory motor drive can be controlled independently from the cough number.[114] Recent data from this laboratory indicate that antitussive drugs do not inhibit TB cough by suppression of the entire cough CPG, but may have specific effects on its particular components. The authors presumed that suppresion of cough expulsion by central antitussive drugs resulted from inhibition of a specific TB gating system.[25] Such inhibition of TB gate by antitussives may block the activity of expiratory neurons of caudal VRG, which are responsible for expiratory motor drive in coughing (see, Role of Botzinger Complex). However, the pool of neurons participating in gating mechanism responsible for excitation of caudal VRG neurons remains unknown as yet. Currently under debate is the, excitatory effect of E-Aug early neurons from BÖT/rostral VRG on caudal VRG pre-motoneurons on coughing. But, the effects of antitussive drugs on activity of E-Aug early neurons as well as their effects on pool of neurons located outside the VRG are still not known.

6.5 MODELS OF COUGH PATTERN GENERATOR AND UNDERLYING MECHANISMS

The central part of cough reflex arc is generally believed to consist of the medullary input neurons, the central coordinating network, the pre-motor and motor outputs, and the possible modulatory inputs. The above-mentioned experiments have identified certain particular brainstem loci as important parts of cough motor pattern generator. However, the question whether the cough motor pattern is produced by the same pools of neurons that generate normal respiratory rhythm or by a separate cough centre have only been answered recently. The systemic and comprehensive work of Shannon and his colleagues[32] resulted in the development of an original cough model and then a revised cough network model (Fig. 6.13).[103] A cough network model (Fig. 6.14) was introduced recently by Bolser and his colleagues;[33] all previous models were based on real patterns of recorded respiratory neurons while taking into account the character (excitatory and inhibitory) of their synaptic interactions.

6.5.1 Role of Bötzinger Complex/Ventral Respiratory Group

The respiratory network within the ventrolateral medulla that generates the eupnoeic pattern of breathing also takes part in producing cough motor pattern.[29,31,34-36,86,97,99,102,103] Thus, respiratory and cough motor patterns are generated by the same network of medullary Bötzinger complex/ventral respiratory group neurons (referred here as common respiratory-cough network, or the cough CPG). This common CPG conveys pre-motor drive to the inspiratory (expiratory) pre-motor cells, and specific respiratory muscles. The dorsal respiratory group—DRG (associated with nucleus tractus solitarii) also sends pre-motor drive to spinal (phrenic and intercostal) inspiratory motoneurones. The rise in DRG inspiratory neuronal activity during cough may result from inspiratory drive from BÖT/VRG neurons and from NTS cough receptor relay neurons. Experiments showed that most of VRG and BÖT/VRG neurons have discharge patterns that could be considered appropriate for contributing to the cough motor pattern.[29,31,32,34,35,103] Respiratory neurons in BÖT/VRG area mutually interact with other respiratory or non-respiratory neurons in the medulla, pons and cerebellum to create a larger dynamic network.[33] The Bötzinger complex E-Aug neurons are certainly involved in the generation of eupnoeic and cough motor patterns,[115] hence, lignocaine blockade and kainic acid lesions within the Bötzinger complex area in spontaneously breathing rabbits had suppressed the spontaneous rhythmic expiratory activity in abdominal muscles as well as the inspiratory and expiratory components of TB cough. It was also established that the Bötzinger complex E-Aug neurons convey (at least partly) an excitatory drive to the caudal E-VRG neurons, and thus to expiratory motor neurons.[31] This excitatory drive is mediated by ionotropic excitatory amino acids—EAA (mainly non-NMDA) receptors during both eupnoeic breathing

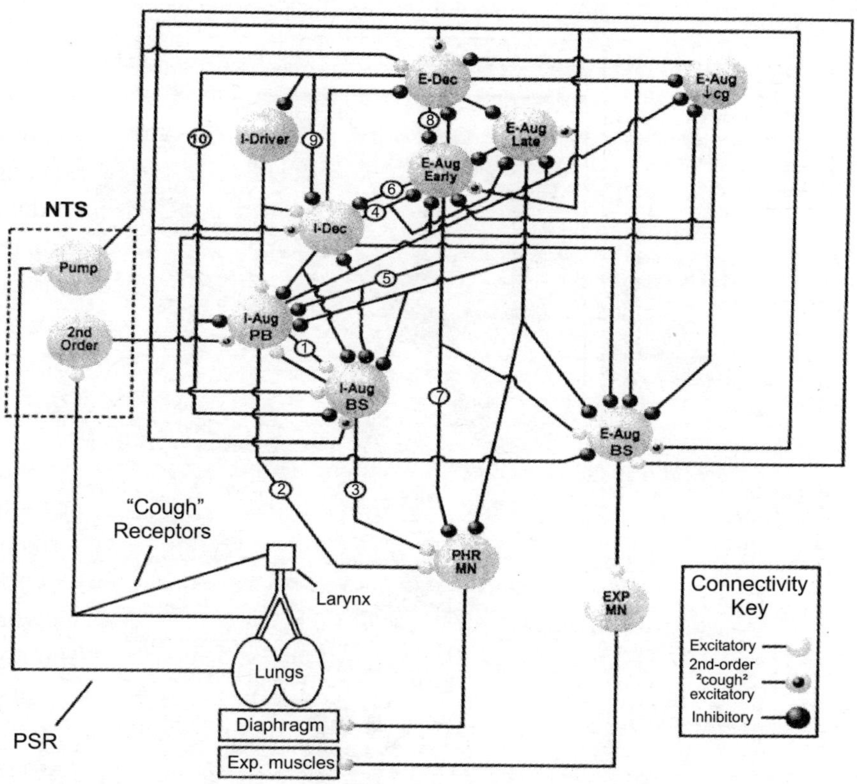

Fig. 6.13 Revised cough network model with illustration of respiratory neuronal network connections in ventrolateral medulla and inputs from nucleus tractus solitarius (NTS) cough receptor second-order neurons and pulmonary stretch receptor (PSR) pump cells. EXP MN, spinal expiratory motoneuron; PHR MN, phrenic motoneurone; E-Aug Early and E-Aug Late, neurons that begin fire prior to and during expiratory phase 2, respectively. E-Aug (⁻cg), neuron that decreased firing rate during cough; I-Driver, inspiratory neuron also active before the expiratory-inspiratory phase transitions (I-E/I) and with a constant firing rate throughout the inspiratory phase; definition specifically limited to BÖT/r. VRG neurons with excitatory functional links to other inspiratory neurons; I-Dec and E-Dec, inspiratory and expiratory modulated neurons with decrementing patterns (For other abbreviations and description of the model see Shannon et al, 2000).[103]

and coughing. Hence, the caudal E-VRG neurons (equipped with ionotropic EAA receptors) cannot be considered a simple output pre-motor system, but these neurons may affect the pattern of quiet breathing through axon collaterals, especially when activated strongly (e.g. during coughing, sneezing, expiration reflex or vomiting).

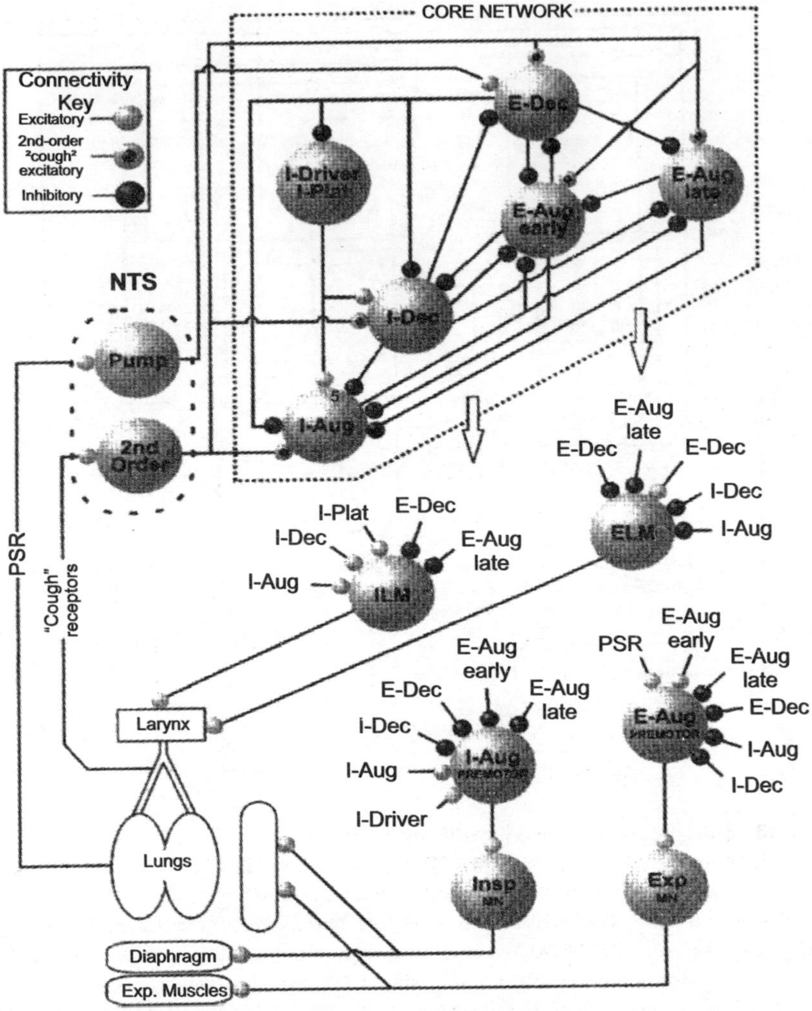

Fig. 6.14 The recent cough network model illustrates BÖT/VRG respiratory neuronal network connections and inputs from nucleus tractus solitarius (NTS); cough receptor 2nd-order neurons and pulmonary stretch receptor (PSR) pump cells. Neuronal connections onto respiratory bulbospinal premotor neurons (I-Aug, E-Aug) and laryngeal motoneurons (ILM, ELM) arise from the CORE NETWORK (demarcated by dotted liner). Other explanations and abbreviations as in Figure 6.13 (For more details and function of the model see Bolser et al, 2003).[33]

6.5.2 Neuronal Inspiratory Phase

According to the revised cough model (Fig. 6.13),[103] the airway cough receptors activate second-order neurons in the NTS, which start to distribute the afferent information concurrently to neurons within the BÖT/VRG area, the rostral and caudal parts of VRG. During the inspiratory phase of cough, all propriobulbar neurons (i.e. I-Driver, I-Aug PB, and I-Dec) and pre-motor bulbospinal I-Aug (BS) neurons are excited by NTS cough afferent second-order neurons, resulting in an increase of inspiratory phrenic motor nerve (PHR) activity. Inspiratory laryngeal motoneurons (not included in the scheme) increase their activity during this phase.[29] Expiratory neurons are inhibited, at least during early inspiration by I-Dec neurons. The neuronal inspiratory phase of cough is terminated by the inhibitory actions of propriobulbar E-Dec and early E-Aug neurons. The increased E-Dec and E-Aug neuronal activities are due to decrease in I-Dec inhibition. Such excitation is caused by increased PSR (via pump cells) and cough receptor activity.

In the model of Bolser et al[33] (Fig. 6.14) phrenic and intercostal spinal motoneurons are driven by I-Aug pre-motor neurons, whose discharge pattern is determined by excitatory inputs from core I-Aug and I-Driver neurons and inhibitory inputs from I-Dec neurons. Inspiratory laryngeal motoneurons (ILM) are under excitatory influence from core I-Aug, I-Dec and I-Plat (not shown) neurons, resulting in glottal abduction. The duration of inspiratory phase results from the activity of I-Driver and I-Dec neurons. This phase terminates, by the inhibitory actions of core E-Dec and early E-Aug neurons.

6.5.3 Neuronal Compressive Phase

In the revised model, there is a large increase in the activity of pre-motor bulbospinal E-Aug (BS), expiratory motoneurons and the laryngeal motoneurons (not included in the scheme) at the end of the inspiratory phase.[29] E-Aug (BS) increase their activity primarily because of excitation by cough receptors and pulmonary stretch receptors (PSR). The expiratory activity is promoted by disinhibition of I-Dec neurons and a post-inspiratory rebound.

As shown in the model of Bolser et al[33] (Fig. 6.14), the intercostal and abdominal spinal motoneurons receive excitatory drive at this phase from pre-motor E-Aug (BS) neurons. Their firing rate increases rapidly due to an enhanced excitation from core early E-Aug neurons. However reduced inhibition from core I-Dec and I-Aug neurons (postinspiratory rebound) and/or reduced inhibition from PSR may promote the activity of E-Aug (BS) neurons. A short burst of expiratory laryngeal motoneuron (ELM) activity, being followed by glottal adduction, resulting from an excitatory input of core pre-motor E-Dec neurons. During the compressive phase of cough, there is an inhibition of inspiratory laryngeal motoneurons by E-Dec and E-Aug neurons.

6.5.4 Neuronal Expulsive Phase

As seen in the revised model, the activity of E-Aug (BS) neurons and expiratory motoneurons (EXP MN) continues to increase immediately after the compressive phase. As the expiratory phase of cough progresses, the activities in E-Aug (BS) (and also in EXP MN and the expiratory muscles) surprisingly do not display an augmented pattern of activity (as seen during the expiratory period of quiet breathing and indicated by a dotted line (i), but it changes into a decrementing pattern (line) (Fig. 6.15).

This pattern is believed to be shaped by the inhibitory actions of propriobulbar E-Aug (late) neurons, I-Dec neurons, I-Aug neurons, and by a decrease in PSR activity.

As seen in the model of Bolser and his colleagues,[33] (Fig. 6.14) at the onset of this phase, the glottis quickly opens due to a rapid decline in expiratory laryngeal motoneuron activity. This motoneuron pattern results from a reduced excitation by core premotor E-Dec neurons and from inhibition by other E-Dec and E-Aug neurons. The firing rate of the premotor E-Aug neurons and thus the spinal expiratory motoneurons continue to increase. However, as the expiratory phase continues, the discharge rate of E-Aug neurons decreases in a pattern shaped by a decline in excitation from core early E-Aug and by an increasing inhibition from the late E-Aug neurons. The neuronal expulsive phase is terminated by enhanced activity of inspiratory Dec and Aug neurons having escaped from inhibition by the expiratory neurons.

The general conclusions from Shannon´s models are as follows: (a) the cough motor pattern is produced by the same BÖT/VRG medullary neuronal circuits involved in the production of the eupnoeic pattern of breathing; (b) the same pre-motor and motor (inspiratory and expiratory) neurons convey the descending drive during coughing and breathing, and (c) the same pre-motor neurons help to shape the laryngeal (inspiratory and expiratory) patterns during eupnoea and coughing.

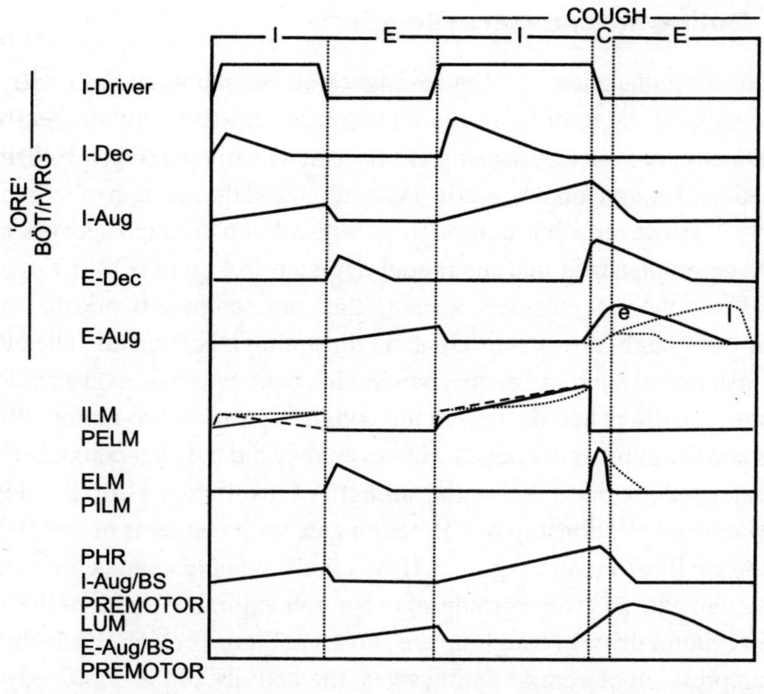

Fig. 6.15 Diagrammatic representation of major respiratory neurons from "CORE" BÖT/r.VRG network, and their discharge profiles, estimated from integrated signals *in vivo* during particular phases of breathing (inspiratory—I, expiratory-E) and coughing (inspiratory—I, compressive—C, expiratory—E). Each profile includes neurons with similar firing patterns, but different peak rates and duration of activities. PILM, PELM, premotor inspiratory and expiratory laryngeal neurons; LUM, lumbar motor nerve to abdominal expiratory muscles; PHR, phrenic motoneurones. Notice the sharp decline in ELM activity during coughing (full line) compared to breathing (dotted line). For other abbreviations see Fig. 6.13. (Reproduced from Ref. [33] with permission from Publisher).

A similar but more complex cough network model of Bolser and his colleagues incorporates Shannon´s ideas, from new data. This data has been obtained from experiments in which antitussive drugs were used[114,116] and in which it was found that cough and breathing was regulated differently by afferents from pulmonary stretch receptors[79,114] It was also based on several earlier reports about how TB and L cough even influenced differently by chemoreceptors inputs.[117,18] But our understanding of both the current cough network models and the underlying mechanisms of cough production is still inadequate.

6.5.5 Gating Mechanism in Cough

Bolser and his colleagues[25,33,40] had brought forth an important piece of evidence that in cough the excitability of the common BÖT/VRG network neurons can be additionally controlled by a gating mechanism which could (Fig. 6.16A) regulate the initiation of cough motor pattern, its duration, and the strength of its expiratory effort.[25,33,40] However, while comparing it with the above cough network models, it should be emphasized that the model depicted in Figure 6.14, i.e. the pump cells, NTS cough receptor neurons, and the core cough network that controls the timing of cough, do not participate in the gating mechanisms. The evidence for an existence of such gating mechanism in cough was based on a finding that the antitussive drugs had decreased the cough expiratory pre-motor and motor patterns and the number of coughs. However, they did not alter cough inspiratory or expiratory phase durations or the strength of inspiratory effort in cough.

A proposed relationship of TB cough gate with elements of cough pattern generator are illustrated in Figure 6.16A. Likely synaptic connections between the TB cough gate and some groups of pre-motor expiratory neurons that control expiratory motor drive in coughing are shown in Figure 6.16B. While the gate is under suppression of central antitussives, the activity of pre-motor expiratory E-Aug BS neurons decreases. It, however, does not affect the activity of the three neuronal groups (E-Dec, E-Aug late, E-Aug early neurons) that participate in regulation of both breathing and cough expiratory phase durations. Furthermore, the antitussive drugs do not inhibit cough receptor interneurons in NTS.[33] The gating mechanism is presynaptic to medullary expiratory neurons.[25,33] This means that a decrease in the expiratory pre-motor activity is accomplished by inhibition of the gating neurons, which then prevent the excitatory effects of cough receptor inputs on pre-motor expiratory cells. In other words, the TB gate mechanism is presynaptic to E-Aug and caudal VRG pre-motor neurons. In addition, it is possible, that the laryngeal and tracheobronchial coughs are controlled by two separate functional gates. The laryngeal gate seems to be less sensitive to central antitussive drugs compared to the tracheobronchial gate, since an intravertebral administration of codeine suppresses expiratory muscle activation during TB cough, but had no effect on the response of expiratory threshold loading in anaesthetized cats.[33,79]

The gating mechanism is presumed to control the start of cough network by raising its elicitability above a threshold level. Hence, a single cough effort results from transient excitation of the gating mechanism, while cough attack may continue as long as the cough threshold is exceeded. This gating mechanism

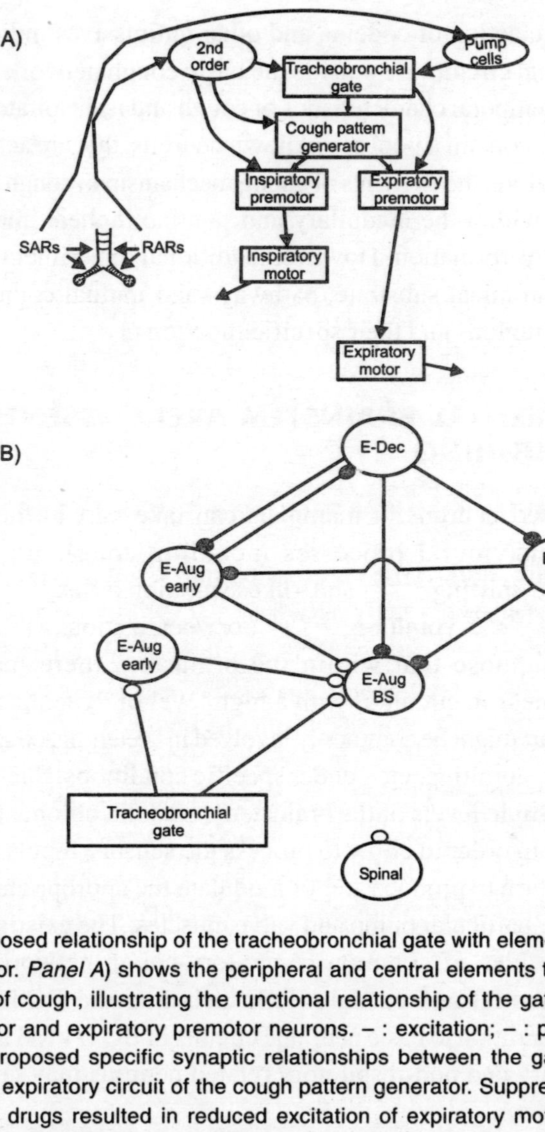

Fig. 6.16 Proposed relationship of the tracheobronchial gate with elements of the cough pattern generator. *Panel A*) shows the peripheral and central elements that participate in the production of cough, illustrating the functional relationship of the gate with the cough pattern generator and expiratory premotor neurons. – : excitation; – : permissive. *Panel B*) shows the proposed specific synaptic relationships between the gate and selected elements of the expiratory circuit of the cough pattern generator. Suppression of the gate with antitussive drugs resulted in reduced excitation of expiratory motor pathways but leaved the three neuronal groups that participate in regulation of expiratory phase duration (i.e. E-Dec, E-Aug late), and a subset of expiratory neurons with augmenting discharge patterns during breathing, but decrementing patterns during cough (E-Aug early), relatively unaffected. O, excitation; inhibition; Spinal, spinal expiratory motoneurons. Other abbreviations as in Figure 6.13. For explanation, see the text. (Reproduced from Bosler et at, 2003; with permission).

controls the strength of cough expiratory effort[33] too. However, a morphological substrate of such a gate, its location and mechanism is as yet unknown.

The selective action of codeine and other antitussives indicated that their effects on neuronal circuits are outside the basic cough network (i.e. on circuits that regulate the temporal characteristics of cough and its inspiratory magnitude). Such circuits may contain a pool of unknown neurons, that are active only during coughing.[33] Therefore, the elements of gating mechanism in cough might comprise neurons located within the medullary and pontine rapheal, medial, lateral or cerebellar reticular formation. However, additional experiments are needed to elucidate the anatomical substrate, pathways and mutual connections among these suspicious regions and their specific functions.

6.6 SUPPLEMENTAL BRAINSTEM AREAS ESSENTIAL FOR COUGHING

Respiration-related neurons in mammals can take part in the generation of a number of behavioural processes including coughing,[33,34,36,72,103,113] sneezing,[119,120,121] sniffing,[122,123] sniff-like aspiration reflex,[124,125,126] expiration reflex,[3, 20, 29, 127, 128, 129] vomiting,[38, 39, 130] or vocalization,[61,131,132] Hence, it is reasonable to suppose that within the brainstem there may exist some multifunctional neuron circuit(s) with a high level of dynamic plasticity, from which at least a part might be commonly involved in breathing, coughing, sneezing, expiration reflex, vomiting, etc., under specific conditions. Such circuit(s) may be located at multiple levels of the brainstem (medulla oblongata, pons varolii, mesencephalon) in order to allow to process the sensory inputs from particular receptors and in turn to produce and/or modulate the appropriate pre-motor and motor outputs for particular pump and valve muscles. The existing experimental data support the idea of common respiratory-cough network composed by neurons of the rostral and caudal VRG, including the BÖT/VRG neurons. Nevertheless, in addition to basic neuronal circuits in BÖT/VRG neurons, another pool of respiratory and non-respiratory related neurons may greatly affect the cough motor pattern.

Recording and lesion experiments in cough (briefly discussed in 6.5.2.2 and 6.5.2.3), had brought forth evidence consistent with a possible modulatory role of midline reticular neurons within and around the area of obscurus and pallidus raphe nuclei, the ventral reticular nucleus, pontine respiratory group and adjoining reticular formation as well as in cerebellum, generating the cough motor pattern.[34,97,99,106,107,133,134,135]

6.6.1 Medullary Midline and Raphe Nuclei

There are several lines of evidence that the rapheal system of medullary reticular formation[136] consisting of the midline raphe nuclei and the surrounding reticular formation is important for coughing,[106,129] expiration reflex,[29,106] vomiting,[137] sympathetic cardiovascular outflow,[138] postural tonus of skeletal muscles[139] and breathing.[140,141,142,143] As has been established, the caudal raphe neurons are influenced by arterial baroreceptors[144,145] and carotid body chemoreceptors,[146] both known to alter breathing. The midline portion of the brainstem contains respiratory-related neuronal assemblies with mostly tonic, phase-spanning activity, similar to PRG neurons.[129,138,147] Similarly, this area contains a number of non-respiratory modulated cells. Both types of neurons were seen to change their burst activity during coughing; however, the activity of non-respiratory cells overlapped cough episodes.[129] The raphe nuclei might be affected directly by inputs from the BÖT/VRG[148] and PRG.[149] However, no direct connections between NTS and raphe midline neurons were established.[150] DRG inspiratory neurons do not project to the raphe nuclei.[66] Also the projections and functional relationships between raphe midline neurons, LTF and cerebellar nuclei are presently unknown.

In our experiments, kainic acid destruction of cells in raphe midline resulted in the disappearance of both TB and L cough motor responses and the motor signs of expiration reflex, alterations in eupnoeic breathing and fall in arterial blood pressure in anaesthetized non-paralyzed cats.[106]. The mechanisms by which midline neurons influence cough reflex are not known. Midline neurons send their projections to phrenic motoneurones,[51,151] and intercostal and abdominal motor pool.[63,152,153] Therefore, we speculated that the elimination of cough and expiration reflex by kainic acid lesions had been due to the removal of an important source of facilitatory input to the spinal motoneurons to the brainstem circuitry that mediate cough and expiration reflex. Furthermore, the raphe midline neurons might be involved, at least partly, in cough gating mechanism.

6.6.2 Lateral Tegmental Field and Ventral Reticular Nucleus

The medullary lateral tegmental field represents the medial system of reticular formation[136] known to modulate and integrate a variety of respiratory, respiratory-related and cardiovascular reflexes.The following studies have demonstrated an important integrative role of LTF in mediation of gasping[154] and gasp-like aspiration reflex,[125] vomiting ,[155] sneezing,[121] sympathetic and baroreceptor control,[156] and production of vestibulo-sympathetic reflexes.[157] In contrast, the LTF neurons appear to play no significant role in the neurogenesis of eupnoeic breathing.

This quite large area of medullary reticular formation contains weakly modulated respiratory neurons[158] as well as non-respiratory modulated units, the later with projections to the spinal cord.[159] The medial part of the lateral tegmental field contain neurons which participate in fictive laryngeal coughing, as revealed by c-fos immunoexpression technique.[104]

We documented that kainic acid lesion in ventral reticular nucleus and the adjacent rostral medullary LTF (at the site between DRG and VRG) removed the motor patterns of both TB and L coughs and expiration reflex, altered the eupnoeic breathing pattern and decreased the systemic arterial pressure in anaesthetized non-paralysed cats[107]. The pathways and mechanisms by which the lateral tegmental field neurons influence cough, quiet ventilation and systemic arterial blood pressure are currently unknown. One explanation is that the lateral tegmental field may modulate cough reflex (also expiration reflex) by facilitation of the afferent cough information to cough CPG, thus increasing the sensitivity of the BÖT/VRG network to afferent inputs. Furthermore, the LTF neurons can form or at least contribute to the gating mechanism in coughing.

6.6.3 Pontine Respiratory Group

Pontine respiratory group (pneumotaxic centre) consists of neurons located within and around the medial and lateral parabrachial nuclei and the Kölliker-Fuse nuclei, representing the lateral system of the reticular formation.[136] Pontine respiratory group is known to modulate eupnoeic respiration.[69,160] Most PRG neurons are tonically active with a 'phase-spanning' pattern. Neurones of the PRG project to raphe nuclei[149] and thus may provide a modulatory drive in coughing. Baekey et al[133] documented the participation of pontine neurons in production of fictive cough motor pattern. Most PRG neurons showed changes in their firing pattern during fictive cough and eupnoea.[29] The observed changes in pontine neuronal activity probably reflect inputs from NTS,[161] mutual interactions of pontine respiratory neurons[162] and reciprocal interactions with BÖT/rostral VRG.[69,160,163] However, direct influences from the medullary lateral tegmental field, raphe midline or cerebellum to the PRG in the rostral pons are presently unknown. Similarly, the mechanism by which the pontine respiratory group interacts with BÖT/rostral VRG to modulate coughing is not yet established.

Our findings in cats showed that successive surgical transections at the level of rostral pons to the pontomedullary junction removed the motor signs of cough and ER in anaesthetized non-paralyzed cats[97] However, it was still not clear if the effects of transections resulted from destruction of cell bodies, neuronal pathways, or both. In our recent experiments, we documented that kainic acid injections given to the PRG of the pons completely abolished the motor signs of TB and L coughs and expiration reflex and decreased the systemic arterial blood pressure.[108] The pathways and underlying modulatory mechanisms by which the PRG may interact with the BÖT/VRG are not well known. These findings are in accordance with the activation of neurons within the rostro-dorsal lateral pons revealed by C-Fos immunoreactive method during fictive laryngeal cough reflex.[104] We assume that the PRG neurons could be an important source of facilitation for neuronal networks which mediate cough and expiration reflexes in a manner similar to the role of medullary midline raphe nuclei and LTF neurons.

6.6.4 Cerebellum

Several reports indicate that the cerebellum can influence respiratory CPG,[164] affecting more, the expiratory than the inspiratory muscle response to resistive respiratory load.[165] Discrete electrical stimulation within the rostral fastigial nucleus increased the rate of breathing with premature termination of VRG neuron activity. These effects disappeared after injections of kainic acid into the rostral fastigial nucleus, indicating that medullary VRG neurons may be influenced from this nucleus.[166] Other similar experiments in which bilateral electrolytic lesions to BÖT complex had been carried out, had revealed that cerebellar modulation of respiratory phrenic motor output depends on the integrity of this area too.[167] The interposed and lateral cerebellar nuclei seem to participate in pulmonary reflexes, whereas the fastigial nucleus may take part in responses to chemical stimulation. These nuclei contain cells with respiratory modulation due to their inputs from the pulmonary stretch receptors and BÖT/VRG area. The pathways and connections between the cerebellum and BÖT/VRG are not known. Interactions between the interposed nuclei and PRG are also unknown. As documented by Xu and Frazier,[168] radio-frequency lesions of the nucleus interpositus or total removal (cerebellectomy), resulted in suppression of expiratory cough intensity and the number of coughs per stimulus trial, but it had not eliminated coughing. Destruction of the fastigial nucleus had no effect on cough parameters. The infracerebellar nucleus affects the medullary expiratory neurons, spinal expiratory motoneurons and respiratory rate.[168] Thus, it seems that the cerebellum may be one of another cough modulators. In addition, cerebellum may be involved in the permissive role of PSR in the production of cough, since it appears to attenuate their facilitatory effects on the pump expiratory muscles during increased lung volume.[165] However, the mechanisms and pathways by which the particular cerebellar and brainstem respiratory circuits mutually interact, are presently obscure and need further detailed study.

6.7 CONCLUSION

There is compelling evidence for the presence of a common respiratory-cough network in the rostral medulla (BÖT/VRG area) that is able to generate both a basic respiratory rhythm and breathing motor pattern as well as the motor pattern of cough and expiration reflexes. A common respiratory-cough network conveys pre-motor drive to the inspiratory (expiratory) pre-motor cells, and the particular pump and valve respiratory muscles. The dorsal respiratory group—(DRG), associated with the nucleus tractus solitarii (NTS), also conveys pre-motor drive to spinal inspiratory motoneurons.

Cough receptor relay neurons for TB and L coughs are localised in NTS, probably within the commissural subnucleus in the caudal portion of medial subnucleus of the NTS.

Excitability of the common respiratory-cough network seems to be additionally controlled by a gating mechanism, presumed to control both the startle of cough by rising its elicitability above a threshold and the strength of cough expiratory effort. Morphological substrate of such cough gate, its location, mechanisms and relationship to the common respiratory-cough network are unknown.

The midline raphe nuclei, lateral tegmental field and pontine respiratory group are indispensable for expression of cough and expiration reflexes. The Cerebellum appears to be an important cough modulator. The pathways and mutual interaction of neurons in these regions during cough and other airway reflexes are still, almost unknown. Thus, in addition to current advances in understanding of basic motor circuits involved in the genesis of cough and other airway reflexes, a search for other neurons and circuits located outside VRG/BÖT needs to be performed.

APPENDIX OF ABBREVIATIONS

ABD	abdominal muscle
BÖT	Bötzinger complex
BS	bulbospinal (reticulospinal)
CPG	central pattern generator
cVRG	caudal part of medullary ventral respiratory group
DIA	diaphragm
DRG	dorsal respiratory group
E-Dec	expiratory neuron with decrementing firing rate
E	expiratory (neuron)
EAA	ionotropic excitatory amino acids
E-Aug (early)	expiratory neuron with augmenting discharge pattern
E-Aug (late)	activity limited primarily to late part of expiratory interval (stage-2 expiration)
ELM	expiratory laryngeal motoneuron
ERV	expiratory reserve volume
EXP MN	expiratory motoneuron
FRC	functional residual capacity
I	inspiratory (neuron)
I-Aug	inspiratory neuron with augmenting firing rate during the phase
I-CON	inspiratory neuron with continual firing
I-Dec	inspiratory neuron with decrementing firing rate during the phase
I-Driver	inspiratory neuron with a relatively constant discharge rate throughout the I phase (I-Plat)
ILM	inspiratory laryngeal motoneuron
I-Plat	inspiratory neuron with continual firing (plateau) activity
KF	Kölliker-Fuse nucleus
L	laryngeal
LTF	lateral tegmental field
NA	nucleus ambiguus
NMDA	N-methyl-D-aspartate
NPBL	nucleus parabrachialis lateralis
NPBM	nucleus parabrachialis medialis
NPGL	nucleus paragigantocellularis lateralis

NRA	nucleus retroambigualis
NTS	nucleus tractus solitarii
P	pump (neurons)
PAG	periaquaductal grey
PB	propriobulbar
PCA	posterior cricoarythenoid muscle
PHR	phrenic motor nerve
P-I	postinspiratory
PP	intrapulmonary pressure
Ppl	pleural pressure
pre-BÖT	pre-Bötzinger complex
PRG	pontine respiratory group
PSRs	pulmonary stretch receptors
RARs	rapidly adapting pulmonary stretch receptors
RN	respiratory neurons
RTN	retrotrapezoideus nucleus
SARs	slowly adapting pulmonary stretch receptors
SLN	superior laryngeal nerve
TA	thyreoarythenoid muscle
TB	tracheobronchial
vl. NTS	ventrolateral nucleus of the solitary tract
VRG	medullary ventral respiratory group
IXth nerve	glossopharyngeal nerve
Xth nerve	vagus nerve

REFERENCES

1. Leith DE. Cough. In: Brian JD, Proctor DF, Reid LD, editors. Respiratory defense mechanisms. Part II. New York-Basel: M. Dekker, 1977;545–92.
2. Karlsson JA, Sant´Ambrogio G, Widdicombe JG. Afferent neural pathways in cough and reflex bronchoconstriction. Journal of Applied Physiology 1988;65:1007–23.
3. Korpáš J, Tomori Z. Cough and other respiratory reflexes. In: Herzog H, editor. Basel: Karger, 1979;1–356.
4. Coleridge HM, Coleridge JCG. Pulmonary reflexes: neural mechanisms of pulmonary defense. Annual Review of Physiology 1994;56:69–91.
5. Sant´Ambrogio G. Coughing: an airway defensive reflex. In: Andrews P, Widdicombe JG, editors. Pathophysiology of the gut and airway. London-Chapel Hill: Portland Press, 1993;89–96.

6. Widdicombe JG. Reflexes from the upper respiratory tract. In: Cherniack NS, Widdicombe JG, eds. Handbook of Physiology; section 3, The respiratory system, Vol II, Control of breathing, Part I. Bethesda: American Physiological Society, 1986;363–94.
7. Widdicombe JG. Neurophysiology of the cough reflex. European Respiration Journal 1995;8(7):1193–1202.
8. Muller J. In: Elements of Physiology. London: Taylor and Walton, 1838;343–58.
9. Williams CJB. In: The pathology and diagnosis of diseases of the chest. 4th edn. London: Churchill, 1840;43–75.
10. Borison HL. Electrical stimulation of the neural mechanism regulating spasmodic respiratory acts. American Journal of Physiology 1948;154:55–62.
11. Kasé Y, Wakita Y, Kito G, Miyata T, Yuizono T, Kataoka M. Centrally induced coughs in the cat. Life Sciences 1970;9:49–59.
12. Mori M, Sakai Y. Re-examination of centrally-induced cough in cats using a micro-stimulation technique. Japanese Journal of Pharmacology 1972;22(5):635–43.
13. Chou DT, Wang SC. Studies on the localization of central cough mechanisms: site of action of antitussive drugs. Journal of Pharmacology & Experimental Therapeutics 1975;194:499–505.
14. Dubi A. Zur Bedeutung pontiner Atmungssubstrate fûr den Husten. Helvitica Physiologica Pharmacologica Acta 1959;17:166–74.
15. Koreckў B, Paleèek F. The assessment of respiratory response curves to carbon dioxide in drug evaluation. In: Aviado DM, Paleèek F, editors. Drugs and respiration. Oxford, Praha; Pergamon Press, Med Press, 1964;27–30.
16. Günthner W, von Krieger E, editors. Husten und Auswurf. Deisenhofen; Dustri Verlag, 1972;1–215.
17. Pozzeto H, Traimer J. Physiologie et physiopathologie de la toux. Poumon 1962;18:393–406.
18. Kasé Y. Antitussive agents and their sites of action. Trends in Pharmacological Sciences 1980;237–9.
19. Bucher K. Pathophysiology and pharmacology of cough. Pharmacological Reviews 1958;10:43–58.
20. Korpáš J. The expiration reflex from vocal cords. Physiologica Bohemoslovakia 1972;21:408–9.
21. Ivanco I. Functional-morphological organization of respiratory and cough centres. Studia Pneumol Phtiseol Cechoslov 1973;33:153–6. (In Slovak).
22. Tatár M, Sant´Ambrogio G, Sant´Ambrogio F. Laryngeal and tracheobronchial cough in anesthetized dogs. Journal of Applied Physiology 1994;76:2672–9.
23. Poliacek I, Stránsky A, Jakuš J, Baráni H, Tomori Z, Halašová E. Activity of laryngeal abductor and adductor muscles during cough, expiration and aspiration reflexes in cats. Physiological Research 2003;52(2):749–62.
24. Forsberg K, Karlsson JA, Zackrisson C, Persson CGA. Selective inhibition of cough and bronchoconstriction in conscious guinea pigs. Respiration 1992;59:72–6.
25. Bolser DC, Davenport PW. Expiratory motor control during the cough reflex. European Respiratory Review 2002b;12(85):243–8.
26. Mazzone SB, Canning BJ. Plasticity of the cough reflex. European Respiratory Review 2002;12(85):236–42.
27. Poliacek I. Electrophysiological analysis of mechanisms underlying the laryngeal motor control in cats. PhD Thesis. Martin; JLF UK, 2000;1–158.

28. Stránsky A, Szereda-Przestaszewska M, Widdicombe JG, Tomori Z. The activity of laryngeal motoneurones and laryngeal resistance during defensive reflexes from the respiratory tract. Physiology Bohemoslov 1976;25(5):471.
29. Baekey DM, Morris KF, Gestreau Ch, Li Z, Lindsey BG, Shannon R. Medullary respiratory neurones and control of laryngeal motoneurones during fictive eupnoea and cough in the cat. Journal of Physiology (London) 2001;534(2):565–81.
30. Shiba K, Satoh I, Kobayashi A, Hayashi F. Multifunctional laryngeal motoneurons: an intracellular study in the cat. Journal of Neurosciences 1999;19(7):2717–27.
31. Bongianni F, Mutolo D, Fontana GA, Pantaleo T. Discharge patterns of Bötzinger complex neurons during cough in the cat. American Journal of Physiology 1998;274:1015–24.
32. Shannon R, Baekey DM, Morris KF, Lindsey BG. Ventrolateral medullary respiratory network and a model of cough motor pattern generation. Journal of Applied Physiology 1998;84:2020–35.
33. Bolser DC, Davenport PW, Golder FJ, Baekey DM, Morris KF, Lindsey BG, Shannon R. Neurogenesis of cough. In: Boushey H, Chung KF, Widdicombe JG, editors. Oxford: Blackwell Science, 2003;173–80.
34. Jakuš J, Tomori Z, Stránsky A. Activity of bulbar respiratory neurones during cough and other respiratory tract reflexes in cats. Physiology bohemoslov 1985;34(2):127–36.
35. Oku Y, Tanaka I, Ezure K. Activity of bulbar respiratory neurons during fictive coughing and swallowing in the decerebrate cat. Journal of Physiology (London) 1994;480(2):309–24.
36. Shannon R, Baekey DM, Morris KF, Lindsey BG. Brainstem respiratory networks and cough. Pulmonary Pharmacology 1996;9:343–7.
37. Wallois F, Macron JM, Jounieaux V, Duron B. Influence of trigeminal nasal afferents on bulbar respiratory neuronal activity. Brain Research 1992;599(1):105–16.
38. Miller AD, Nonaka S, Siniaia MS, Jakuš J. Multifunctional ventral respiratory group: bulbospinal expiratory neurons play a role in pudendal discharge during vomiting. Journal of Autonomic Nervous System 1995a;54:253–60.
39. Miller AD, Yamaguchi T, Siniaia MS, Yates BJ. Ventral respiratory group bulbospinal inspiratory neurons participate in vestibular-respiratory reflexes. Journal of Neurophysiology 1995b;73(3):1303–7.
40. Bolser DC, Davenport PW. Functional organization of the central cough generation mechanism. Pulmonary Pharmacology & Therapeutics 2002;15(3):221–5.
41. Richter DW. Generation and maintenance of the respiratory rhythm. Journal of Experimental Biology 1982;100:93–107.
42. Bianchi AL. Localization and study of respiratory medullary neurons. Antidromic starting by spinal cord or vagal stimulation. Journal of Physiology (Paris) 1971;63(1):5–40.
43. Berger AJ, Averill DB, Cameron WE. Morphology of inspiratory neurons located in the ventrolateral nucleus of the tractus solitarius of the cat. Journal of Comparative Neurology 1984;224(1):60–70.
44. Merrill EG. Where are the real respiratory neurones? Federation Proceedings 1981;40:2389–94.
45. Batsel HL. Localization of bulbar respiratory center by microelectrode souding. Experimental Neurology 1964;9:410–26.
46. Bianchi AL. Antidromic activation of bulbar respiratory neurons. Journal of Physiology (Paris) 1969;61(1):91.

47. Feldman JL. Neurophysiology of breathing in mammals. In: Bloom FE, editor. Handbook of physiology. The nervous system. IV. Intrinsic regulatory systems of the brain. Bethesda: American Physiological Society, 1986;463–524.
48. Aoki M, Mories S, Kawahara K, Watanabe H, Ebata N. Generation of spontaneous respiratory rhythm in spinal cats. Brain Research 1980;202:51–63.
49. Lipski J, Merrill EG. Electrophysiological demonstration of the projection from expiratory neurones in rostral medulla to contralateral dorsal respiratory group. Brain Research 1980;197(2):521–4.
50. Smith JC, Ellenberger HH, Ballanyi K, Richter DW, Feldman JL. Pre-Bötzinger complex: a brainstem region that may generate respiratory rhythm in mammals. Science 1991;254:726–9.
51. Dobbins EG, Feldman JL. Brainstem network controlling descending drive to phrenic motoneurons in rat. Journal of Comparative Neurology 1994;347(1):64–86.
52. Rekling JC, Feldman JL. Pre-Bötzinger complex and pacemaker neurons: hypothesized site and kernel for respiratory rhythm generation. Annual Review of Physiology 1998;60:385–405.
53. McCrimmon DR, Monnier A, Hayashi F, Zuperku EJ. Pattern formation and rhythm generation in the ventral respiratory group. Clinical & Experimental Pharmacology & Physiology 2000;27(1–2):126–31.
54. Budzinska K, von Euler C, Kao FF, Pantaleo T, Yamamoto Y. Effects of graded focal cold block in rostral areas of the medulla. Acta Physiologica Scandavia 1985;124(3):329–40.
55. Connelly CA, Ellenberger HH, Feldman JL. Respiratory activity in retrotrapezoid nucleus in cat. American Journal of Physiology 1990;258(2):33–44.
56. Feldman JL, Ellenberger HH. Central coordination of respiratory and cardiovascular control in mammals. Annual Review of Physiology 1988;50:593–606.
57. Dampney R. The subretrofacial nucleus: its pivotal role in cardiovascular regulation. News in Physiology 1990;5:63–7.
58. Cohen MI, Wang SC. Respiratory neuronal activity in pons of cat. Journal of Neurophysiology 1959;22:33–5.
59. Bertrand F, Hugelin A. Respiratory synchronizing function of nucleus parabrachialis medialis: pneumotaxic mechanisms. Journal of Neurophysiology 1971;34(2):189–207.
60. Bianchi AL, St.John WM. Medullary axonal projections of respiratory neurons of pontile pneumotaxic center. Respiration Physiology 1982;48(3):357–73.
61. von Euler C. Brain stem mechanisms for generation and control of breathing pattern. In: Cherniack NS, Widdicombe JG, editors. Handbook of physiology, the respiratory system, Vol.2; Control of breathing. Bethesda: American Physiological Society, 1986;1–67.
62. Gang S, Mizuguchi A, Kobayashi N, Aoki M. Descending axonal projections from the medial parabrachial and Kölliker-Fuse nuclear complex to the nucleus raphe magnus in cats. Neuroscience Letters 1990;118(2):273–275.
63. Rikard-Bell GC, Bystrzycka EK, Nail BS. The identification of brainstem neurones projecting to thoracic respiratory motoneurones in the cat as demonstrated by retrograde transport of HRP. Brain Research Bulletin 1985;14(1):25–37.
64. Vertes RP, Crane AM. Descending projections of the posterior nucleus of the hypothalamus: phaseolus vulgaris leucoagglutinin analysis in the rat. Journal of Comparative Neurology 1996;374(4):607–31.

65. Cameron AA, Khan IA, Westlund KN, Cliffer KD, Willis WD. The efferent projections of the periaquaductal gray in the rat: a Phaseolus vulgaris-leucoagglutinin study. I. Ascending projections. Journal of Comparative Neurology 1995;351(4):568–84.
66. Ezure K. Synaptic connections between medullary respiratory neurons and considerations on the genesis of respiratory rhythm. Progress in Neurobiology 1990;35:429–50.
67. Richter DW, Jordan D, Ballantyne D, Meesmann M, Spyer KM. Presynaptic depolarization in myelinated vagal afferent fibres terminating in the nucleus of the tractus solitarius in the cat. Pflügers Archives 1986;406:12–19.
68. Richter DW, Spyer KM. Studying rhythmogenesis of breathing: comparison of in vivo and in vitro models. Trends in Neurosciences 2001;24(8):464–72.
69. Bianchi AL, Denavit-Saubie M, Champagnat J. Central control of breathing in mammals: neuronal circuitry, membrane properties, and neurotransmitters. Physiological Reviews 1995;75(1):1–45.
70. Smith JC. Integration of cellular and network mechanisms in mammalian oscillatory motor circuits: insights from the respiratory oscillator. In: Stein PSG, Grillner S, Selverston AI, Stuart DG, editors. Neurons, Networks and Motor Behavior. London: The MIT Press, 1997;97–104.
71. Bellingham MC. Driving respiration: the respiratory central pattern generator. Clinical & Experimental Pharmacology & Physiology 1998;25(10):847–56.
72. Jakuš J, Tomori Z, Stránsky A. Neuronal determinants of breathing, coughing and related motor behaviours. Wist, Martin, 2004;334.
73. Widdicombe JG. Sensory neurophysiology of the cough reflex. Journal of Allergy & Clinical Immunology 1996;98(5):84–90.
74. Widdicombe J. Neuroregulation of cough: implications for drug therapy. Current Opinions in Pharmacology 2002;2(3):256–63.
75. Widdicombe JG. Afferent receptors in the airways and cough. Respiration Physiology 1998;114:5–15.
76. Tatár M, Webber SE, Widdicombe JG. Lung C fibre receptor activation and defensive reflexes in anaesthetized cats. Journal of Physiology (London) 1988;402:411–40.
77. Hanácek J, Davies A, Widdicombe JG. Influence of lung stretch receptors on the cough reflex in rabbits. Respiration 1984;45:161–8.
78. Sant'Ambrogio G, Widdicombe J. Reflexes from airway rapidly adapting receptors. Respiration Physiology 2001;125(1–2):33–45.
79. Bolser DC, Davenport PW. Volume-timing relationships during cough and resistive loading in the cat. Journal of Applied Physiology 2000;89(2):785–90.
80. Jakuš J, Tomori Z, Stránsky A, Smutná M. To the function of the pulmonary stretch receptors during defensive airway reflexes. Cs Fysiol 1981;30: 247–9. (In Slovak)
81. Jakuš J, Stránsky A, Tomori Z. Aktivität der Lungendehnungsrezeptoren während intrapulmonaler Umfang und Druckveränderungen bei Respirationsreflexen. Folia Med Martiniana 1983;9(1):85–101.
82. Tatár M, Nagyová B, Widdicombe JG. Veratrine-induced reflexes and cough. Respiration Medicine 1991;85:51–5.
83. Yoshihara S, Abe T, Fukuda N, Ando T, Asai H, Ichimura T. Skin stimulation with cold water inhibits capsaicin-induced cough and decreases substance P-like immunoreactivity in guinea-pig lungs. Biomedical Research 1996;17:271–8.
84. Jordan D. Central nervous pathways and control of the airways. Respiration Physiology 2001;125:67–81.

85. Bellingham MC, Lipski J. Morphology and electrophysiology of superior laryngeal nerve afferents and postsynaptic neurons in the medulla oblongata of the cat. Neuroscience 1992;48(1):205–16.
86. Shannon R, Bolser DC, Lindsey BG. Neural control of coughing and sneezing. In: Miller AD, Bianchi AL, Bishop BP, eds. Neural control of the respiratory muscles. Boca Raton: CRC, 1997;213–22.
87. Bolser DC, Reier PJ, Davenport PW. Responses of the anterolateral abdominal muscles during cough and expiratory threshold loading in the cat. Journal of Applied Physiology 2000;88(4):1207–14.
88. Kalia M, Mesulam MM. Brainstem projections of sensory and motor components of the vagus complex in the cat: II. Laryngeal, tracheobronchial, pulmonary, cardiac, and gastrointestinal branches. Journal of Comparative Neurology 1980;193(2):467–508.
89. Lucier GE, Egizii R, Dostrovsky JO. Projections of the internal branch of the superior laryngeal nerve of the cat. Brain Research Bulletin 1986;16(5):713–21.
90. Jiang C, Lipski J. Synaptic inputs to medullary respiratory neurons from superior laryngeal afferents in the cat. Brain Research 1992;584(1–2):197–206.
91. Lipski J, Ezure K, Wong She RB. Identification of neurons receiving input from pulmonary rapidly adapting receptors in the cat. Journal of Physiology (London) 1991;443:55–77.
92. Shannon R, Morris KF, Li Z, Lindsey BG. Medullary raphe neuronal responses during fictive cough. Society of Neuroscience Abstracts 1995;21:1879.
93. Ezure K, Manabe M, Otake K, Sasaki H. Synaptic connections from decrementing and constant inspiratory neurons in cat medulla. Neuroscience Research Supplement 1990;11:21.
94. Kubin L, Davies RO. Central pathways of pulmonary and airway vagal afferents. In: Dempsey JA, Pack AI, editors. Lung Biology in Health and Disease: Regulation of Breathing. New York: Marcel Dekker, 1995;219–84.
95. Otake K, Ezure K, Lipski J, Wong She RB. Projections from the commissural subnucleus of the nucleus of the solitary tract: an anterograde tracing study in the cat. Journal of Comparative Neurology 1992;324(3):365–78.
96. Newsom Davis J, Plum F. Separation of descending spinal pathways to respiratory motoneurones. Experimental Neurology 1972;34:78–94.
97. Jakuš J, Tomori Z, Bošelová L, Nagyová B, Kubinec V. Respiration and airways reflexes after transversal brainstem lesions in cats. Physiologica Bohemoslov 1987b;36(4):329–40.
98. Engelhorn R, Weller E. Zentrale Repräsentation hustenwirksamer Afferenzen in der Medulla oblongata der Katze. Pflûgers Archives ges Physiol 1965;284:224–239.
99. Jakuš J, Tomori Z, Stránsky A. Bulbar respiratory activity during defensive airway reflexes in cats. Acta Physiologica Hungaria 1987a;70(2–3):245–254.
100. Grélot L, Milano S. Diaphragmatic and abdominal muscle activity during coughing in the decerebrate cat. Neuroreport 1991;2(4):165–8.
101. Bolser DC. Fictive cough in the cat. Journal of Applied Physiology 1991;71:2325–31.
102. Shannon R, Bolser DC, Lindsey BG. Medullary neurons mediating the inhibition of inspiration by intercostal muscle tendon organs? Journal of Applied Physiology 1988;65(6):2498–505.
103. Shannon R, Baekey DM, Morris KF, Li Z, Lindsey BG. Functional connectivity among ventrolateral medullary respiratory neurones and responses during fictive cough in the cat. Journal of Physiology 2000;525(1):207–24.

104. Gestreau Ch, Bianchi AL, Grélot L. Differential brainstem Fos-like immunoreactivity after laryngeal-induced coughing and its reduction by codeine. Journal of Neuroscience 1997;17(23):9340–52.

7 Breathing and Airway Reflexes in Ontogenesis

K JAVORKA

7.1 FOETAL BREATHING AND BREATHING MOVEMENTS

In the foetus, the exchange of blood gases, i.e. absorption of oxygen (O_2) and removal of carbon dioxide (CO_2), takes place via the maternal lungs, blood, circulation and through the placenta. In other words, the alveolar air is replaced with the mother´s blood. In the placenta, the blood gas exchange is regulated by a special doubled (maternal and foetal) mechanism that controls blood gases values (Fig. 7.1), blood flow and gas transfer.

Blood flow in the non-innervated organ, i.e. the placenta, is controlled by humoural agents such as catecholamines, angiotensin II, vasopressin, oestrogens, and progesterone and also by PO_2 and PCO_2. The blood flow in placenta is coordinated by mechanisms similar to those that optimise ventilation or perfusion

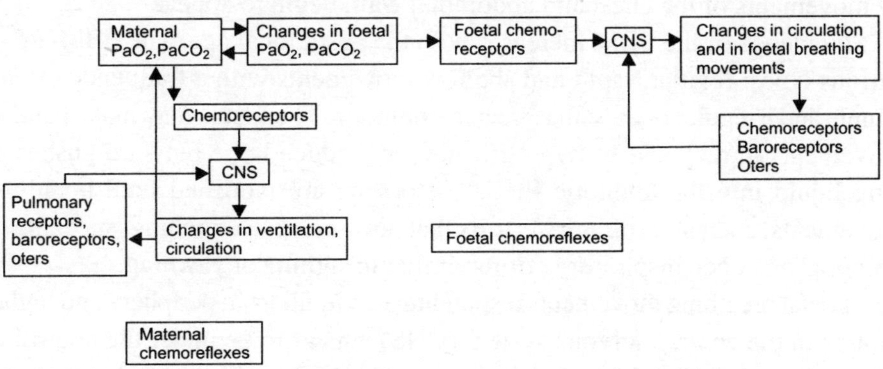

Fig. 7.1 Chemoreflex pathways as seen in the faeto-maternal placental unit

ratios in the lungs during postnatal life. If PaO_2 and oxygen content in the placental tissue fall, a reversible vasoconstriction in the relevant part of placental circulation (hypoxic foetoplacental vasoconstriction), is elicited. This vasoconstriction is similar to the well-known hypoxic pulmonary vasoconstriction as seen later during postnatal life. The role of this vasoconstriction is to shunt the fetal blood away from the hypoxic area in the placenta to areas with higher PaO_2. This regulatory phenomenon is common for both prenatal placenta and postnatal lungs.

Other important well-known mechanisms that help in transporting oxygen and carbon dioxide during foetal life are the presence of foetal haemoglobin with greater O_2 affinity than adult haemoglobin, a modified Haldane effect and the presence of a Bohr effect which appears doubled with respect to the two blood circulations: As maternal blood gains CO_2 and metabolic products from foetus, its increased acidity results in a shift of the oxygen-haemoglobin dissociation curve to the right (lowered affinity for O_2). This effect promotes loss of oxygen from maternal blood to the foetus. On the other hand, the foetus, by releasing CO_2 and acid metabolites to the maternal blood decreases the acidity of its own blood and the foetal blood becomes more alkaline. It results in a shift of the dissociation curve of the foetal blood to the left (increased affinity for O_2). These effects operate concurrently promoting transfer of O_2 from maternal to foetal bloodstreams.[1]

While activities like growth, maturation, differentiation of lung tissues and metabolic activities, continue to be seen all along as a functional entity, the foetal respiratory system may be considered virtually inactive till the 14th week of gestation, after which the foetal breathing movements (FBM) or rhythmic contractions of respiratory muscles (particularly of the diaphragm), accompanied by movements of the chest and abdominal wall, begin to appear.

Incidence of the FBM increases with the gestational age. The FBM are of various types: regular, rapid and shallow movements with a frequency 60-90/ minute and irregular ones with a greater amplitude. The foetus may make panting movements in response to hyperthermia, or produce large outward gushes of lung liquid into the amniotic fluid.[2] Also seen are modified fetal breathing movements, such as expiratory efforts that are similar to coughing, sneezing or grunting, and deep inspiratory efforts similar to sighing or yawning.

Foetal breathing movements responding to stimuli from periphery and higher centres in the central nervous system (CNS) appear to be under the control of the respiratory areas of the medulla oblongata.[3,4] These findings, that the fetus has an active respiratory centre and that it can carry out breathing movements, has changed the generally held view about the mechanism of initiation of the first breath and regulation of breathing in early postnatal period. It may be concluded that birth does not initiate breathing but only modifies it. It acquires a new and the inevitable physiological function.

7.2 VENTILATION AND ITS REGULATION IN NEWBORNS

7.2.1 Ventilation in Newborns

The dominant inspiratory muscle in newborns and children is the diaphragm. Its position is higher than in adults, but this advantage is offset by the presence of a soft and compliant chest and low tone of the intercostal muscles. Since the ribs are still soft (due to insufficient mineralisation of bones), this taken together with a low intercostal muscle tone, are responsible for the high chest wall compliance. Compliance of thoracic wall (C_w) in newborns is five times higher than compliance of the neonatal lungs (C_L). The C_L in newborns, as compared to that of adults, in absolute values, is very small. In healthy newborns, its value is 3 to 6 ml/cmH_2O, and in adults, 150 to 250 ml/cmH_2O.

However, if we compare the specific lung compliances (per TLC), they are not different in newborns and adults.

Airway resistance in newborns (R_{aw}) is very high (10 times higher than in adults) as a result of the airways' small diameter. The higher values of R_{aw}, appear to result in an increase in the work of breathing and a rapid development of respiratory muscle fatigue.

Frequency of breathing in newborns is about 40/minute on the first postnatal day. Transient tachypnoea in the first days can be caused by an increased pulmonary interstitial pressure due to slow elimination of pulmonary fluid and stimulation of juxtapulmonary capillary (J) receptors. Tidal volume (V_T) in newborns is 5 to 7 ml/kg body weight and ventilation is 200 to 280 ml/kg/min on an average.

7.2.2 Regulation of Ventilation in Early Postnatal Period

Chemical, neural and integrative regulation of ventilation in newborns, especially in the preterm ones, has many peculiarities that are unique in their control of ventilation. The specific responses of the ventilation to different stimuli (such as hypoxia, hypercapnia, distension of the lungs and changes in intrapulmonary pressure) may reflect gradual maturation of the ventilatory control for continuous

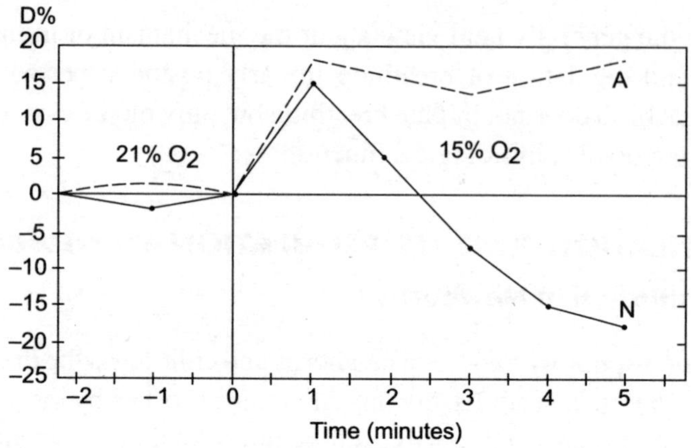

Fig. 7.2 The biphasic reaction of ventilation (expressed as percentage of control), to breathing hypoxic gas mixtures (15%) in newborns (N) as compared to that in adults (A).

breathing after birth, as opposed to the intermittent process of foetal breathing movements *in utero*.

7.2.2.1 Chemical Regulation in Newborns

Term newborns during the first week of life, and preterm newborns for the first 2–3 weeks of life, typically show a biphasic reaction to inhalation of low O_2.[5,6] The primary reaction under hypoxic conditions is hyperventilation replaced by an inhibition of breathing (Fig. 7.2). The hyperventilatory phase is influenced by the ambient temperature. When temperature is below the thermoneutral zone (e.g. less than 25°C), only a decrease in ventilation is observed and the initial hyperventilation is eliminated. The cause of this biphasic reaction is not known so far, but it has been suggested that hypoxia affects ventilation in two different ways: a stimulatory effect through peripheral chemoreceptors and a direct depressive effect on the respiratory areas in the brainstem. This second depressive phase of hypoxia on breathing, may be evoked by a predominant central depressive action over the relatively immature stimulatory mechanism of the peripheral chemoreceptors in the newborns.

Newborns also respond to changes in CO_2 and pH; to an increase in PCO_2 or hypercapnia, the response is hyperventilation. The response of newborns to

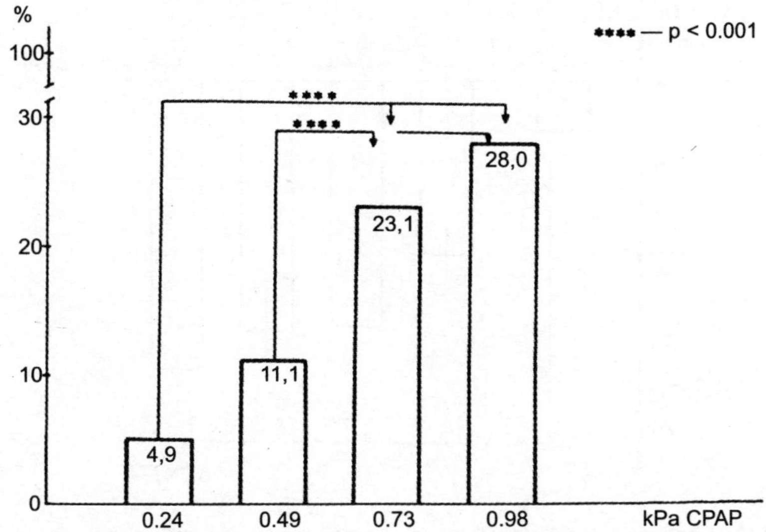

Fig. 7.3 Incidence of apnoeic responses during elevation of airway pressure to 0.24, 0.49, 0.73 and 0.98 kPa expressed as a percentage of [continuous positive airway pressure (CPAP)] applications.It may be noted that higher the pressure, the greater the incidence of apnoea. (Reproduced from Ref. [9] with permission from Publisher).

inhaled CO_2 appears greater than that of the adults, with its CO_2 response curve shifted to the left of the adult, and with resting $PaCO_2$ lower than the adult.[7] Although the ventilatory response to hypercapnia is more pronounced than to hypoxia in newborns, it is only 3–4 times higher compared to that in adults (an increase 10–20 times). Preterm newborns respond less to hypercapnia than term newborns and the decreased response is likely to be centrally mediated.[6]

A decrease in arterial pH stimulates ventilation in newborns just as it does in adults, i.e. independently of PCO_2, even in situations when $PaCO_2$ has fallen as in metabolic acidosis. This reaction is expected to be mediated via active central chemoreceptors.

7.2.2.2 Neural Regulation in Newborns Reflexes of Slowly Adapting Stretch Receptors

Slowly adapting stretch receptors (SARs) located in smooth muscle throughout the tracheobronchial tree, are responsible for the Hering-Breuer reflex (HBR). This reflex is one of the best studied lung reflexes in human ontogenesis. An

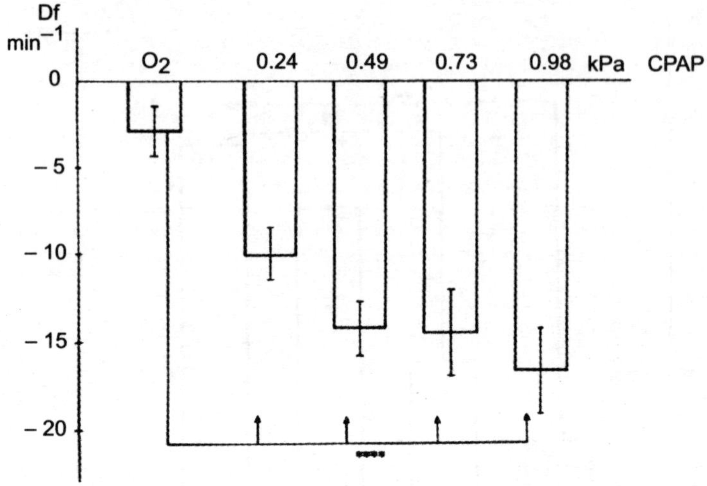

Fig. 7.4 Changes in respiratory frequency during the administration of oxygen at normal ambient pressure and on raising the pressure in the airways and lungs [continuous positive airway pressur (CPAP)] to 0.24, 0.49, 0.73 and 0.98 kPa. The differences were significant. (Reproduced from Ref(9) with permission from Publisher).

increase in the lung inflation and airway pressure produces an inhibition of inspiration and promotion of an expiration resulting in a fall in the respiratory rate, or in a transient expiratory apnoea.

In the early 1960s, Cross and his colleagues[8] showed that lung inflation in newborns who were between 1 and 124 hours old, caused a depression in breathing or an apnea; its duration depending on the volume of air used.

The inflation reflex in 32 preterm newborns was studied by our group for up to 3 days after birth.[9] The CPAP (continuous positive airway pressure) device was used to induce short-term (10 s) pressure increase in the airways. Elevation of pressure in the airways and lungs to 2.5, 5.0, 7.5 and 10.0 cmH_2O (0.25, 0.49, 0.73 and 0.98 kPa) produced an apnoea with the occurrence in relation to the height of CPAP. The incidence of apnoea increased proportionately to the increase in applied pressure (Fig. 7.3).

Increase in lung volume during inspiration leads to shortening of inspiratory period, which results in the acceleration of breathing. We have found not only a depression of breathing during administration of oxygen at normal ambient pressure indicating active function of peripheral chemoreceptors but also a decrease in respiratory frequency depending on the pressure in the airways and lungs[9] (Fig. 7.4).

The strength of this reflex can also be studied through occlusion of respiratory airways at the end of expiration. Olinsky et al,[10] measured the duration of inspiratory effort after occlusion of airways in newborns. They found, as did Kirkpatrick et al,[11] that in preterm newborns this reflex is stronger, and that its strength declines with age. On the other hand, Thach et al,[12] found, using the same occlusion technique, that the HBR strength is the same in both preterm and full term neonates, and that it keeps increasing up to the 35th day of postnatal life and after which it gradually begins to decrease.

The HB reflex appears stronger in infants than in adults. Shortening of inspiratory period in adult humans begins only when tidal volume at rest has increased twice as much.[13] According to these findings, HBR plays a certain role in the regulation of breathing patterns in newborns even during eupnoea. Cyclically repeated HBR shortens the inspiratory time in each respiratory cycle; and thereby, the respiratory rate increases. This may be one of the reasons why respiratory rate in newborns is relatively high. The HBR, as a simple control system working on the principle of negative feedback, may be used as a temporary regulator of breathing in neurologically premature neonates.[10]

Reflexes of Rapidly Adapting Vagal Receptors

Rapidly adapting receptors (RARs, formerly irritant receptors) located in the trachea and the main bronchi are sensitive to mechanical and chemical stimuli. With the activation of RARs different responses may be evoked. Stimulation of the RARs in the small airways can evoke the Hering-Breuer deflation reflex.[14,15] The RARs reflexely shorten the duration of expiration, and activate inspirations.

In newborn rabbits, kittens and monkeys,[16,17] deflation of lungs produced an increase in the respiratory frequency and an augmentation of phrenic activity. Fleming et al,[18] supposed the RARs to be immature before 35 gestational weeks. Many authors, however, quote evidence that the receptors are already mature before this term[19,20] and that they may play a role in initiating the first breath after delivery.[8] They may also be one of many possible sources of irregular patterns of breathing in newborns.

The RARs are also attributed with playing an important role in the origin of augmented breaths[14,21] as well as in the occurrence of deep and rapid inspirations, (the so-called gasp reflex) which were observed in newborns at the beginning of lung inflation.[8,9] The sighs occur also occasionally during spontaneous quiet breathing at about intervals of 10 minutes, and they consist of slow deep inspiration followed by slow and passive expiration.[21]

According to Thach and Taeusch,[22] sighs occur in newborns in as many as 93 per cent of cases. Periodically repeated deep breaths are relatively more frequent in preterm infants, who respond this way to uneven ventilation or chest wall distortion. The augmented breaths disappear after increasing functional residual capacity (FRC) by the application of CPAP or CNP (continuous negative chest wall pressure). This suggests that the augmented breaths are a reflex response to a small FRC.[23] Such reflex sighs are very important for lung health. The augmented breath (in adults, and during artificial ventilation too) help to prevent pulmonary atelectasis from occurring.

We studied the occurrence and characteristics of deep inspirations at the onset of the application of CPAP, in preterm newborns up to 3 days after birth.[9] Out of 73 CPAP applications, forced respiratory efforts occurred in 37 cases (51%). Percentage of this occurrence was increased due to increasing inflation pressure. The great majority (92%) of these rapid and deep inspiratory efforts occurred at the onset of pressure increase, the rest at the end of CPAP. We found that the intensity of inspiratory efforts in contrast to the occurrence did not depend on inflation pressure. These rapid and deep inspiratory efforts were charaterised by a drop in the intrathoracic (oesophageal) pressure to a mean value of -2.0 ± 0.2 kPa and with a mean duration of 169 ± 8 ms. During these inspiratory efforts, the airflow increased by 280 per cent as compared to that at rest. The inspiratory reactions were doubled in 74 per cent of the cases, and the response resembled sighs, gasps or an aspiration reflex (Fig. 7.5).

The origin of these responses in response to rapid application of positive pressure to the airways and lungs remains unclear. The gasp reflex may be elicited by stimulation of RARs of airways by mechanical deformation, by receptors in the thoracic wall, or by stimulation of the naso- and oropharyngeal receptors responsible for the aspiration reflex.

Reflexes of C-fibre Endings and Juxtapulmonary Capillary Receptors (J-receptors)

Non-myelinated vagal fibres found throughout the tracheobronchial tree, located within the airway and alveolar epithelium, activated by irritants, such as capsaicin are identified as C-fibre endings. They may be divided to the bronchial and pulmonary groups with a special subtype of the J-receptors.

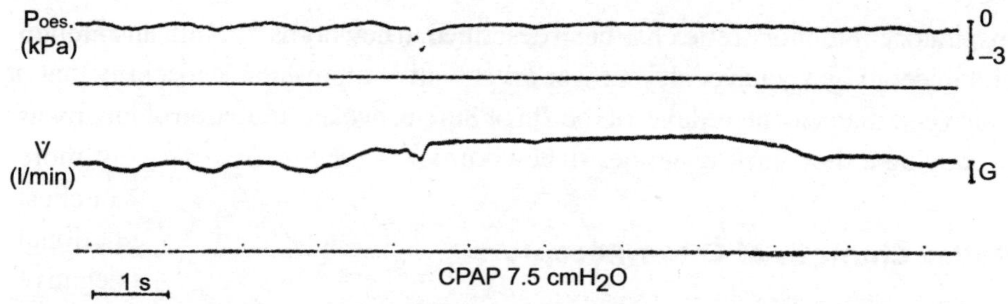

Fig. 7.5 Oesophageal pressure (P_{eos}.) and inspiratory airflow (V) in a forced respiratory effort in a newborn during elevation of the pressure in the airways and lungs [continuous positive airway pressur (CPAP)] to 0.73 kPa. (Modified from Ref. [9]).

Bronchial C-fibre endings innervating the airway mucosa[24] can be stimulated by a variety of different stimuli,[25] such as mechanical stimulation, chemical irritants and inflammatory mediators. Pulmonary C-fibre endings located in alveolar and possibly in the bronchoalveolar walls[21] are stimulated by the same agents that activate the bronchial C-fibre endings but with some difference in timing with reference to the route of injection of these substances.

Non-myelinated vagal fibres — a subtype of vagal C-fibre endings found in the lung interstitium close to capillaries are juxtapulmonary capillary receptors.[26] The J-receptors respond to increase in pressure and flow in pulmonary circulation and interstitium and they are are stimulated during pulmonary congestion and oedema,[27] e.g. by microembolisation of the pulmonary vascular bed, extreme physical exercise, or by application of some chemical agents. Responses are apnoea followed by rapid shallow breathing, bradycardia and hypotension, and somatomotor inhibition (J-reflex).[26,27]

Reflex responses from J-receptors in newborn animals were studied by Kalia[28] and Schleman et al,[29] Kalia observed that during the first week of their postnatal life, phenyldiguanide does not evoke the responses seen typically in kittens. However, the newborn piglets responded to the phenyldiguanide since 2nd postnatal day by apnoea, bradycardia and hypotension indicating on the activity of the C-fibres receptors in this early phase of life.

Reflexes of Thoracic Wall Receptors

In vagotomised cats, it was found that chest wall compression inhibits inspiration through pathways other than the vagus nerve.[30] An *intercostal-to-phrenic*, inspiratory-inhibitory reflex has been described in newborns by Knill and Bryan[31] and in detail by Hagan et al,[32] Lower chest wall compression, especially that of transverse diameter at the level of the 7th or 8th rib, evokes inhibition of inspiration producing a short-lasting apnoea in newborns.[31]

Reflex Changes of Other Receptors

Apart from the reflexes described above, there are other sensory pathways that could influence the pattern of breathing in newborns. For example, there are the visual, acoustic and vestibular receptors about whose influence on the respiratory patterns, very little is known. However, much is known about the influence of the tactile and cold receptors of the skin on changes in breathing patterns.

Even *in utero,* an influence on the foetal breathing movements (FBM) can be elicited either by directly cooling the skin of the foetus or by introduction of cold fluids into the amniotic sac.[33] Regular FBM may be evoked by the stimulation of peripheral somatic nerves and by electrical and mechanical stimulation of the skin of the foetus (somatic-respiratory reflex).[34,35] After such a stimulation, the foetus can continue its breathing movements upto several hours.

In preterm newborns too, apnoea can be interrupted by mechanical stimulation of the skin (pain or tactile stimuli) or of the airway mucosa (e.g. suction from pharynx) to evoke reflex breathing. The effect produced by stimulation of skin and mucosa exceeds the stimulus period and persists for several minutes. On the basis of these observations, Kattwinkel et al,[36] recommended that in premature newborns suffering from frequent apnoeic pauses, mechanical stimulation of the skin every 20–30 minutes helped prevent the apnoeic pauses.

Investigating Ashner´s oculocardiac reflex (OCR) in pre term newborns, changes in heart and respiratory rate evoked by pressure on eyeballs, were studied by our group.[37] On average, the heart rate decreased significantly from 132 to 122/minute. Beside this bradycardic response, there was a respiratory inhibition (a fall of the frequency of breathing from 48 to 35/minute on average) as a part of OCR which is active even in premature newborns.

A similar respiratory depression and bradycardia however, were elicited by applying pressure on the large fontanelle of the premature newborn´s head.[38] We can speculate about the physiological role of these responses. The inhibition of breathing evoked by a squeezing of the head may be important to a foetus or a newborn at birth. Inhibition of breathing during the passage of the foetus through the birth canal is also supported by the OCR and by the intracranial pressure increase (Cushing's reflex), and the concomittant bradycardia improves coronary flow.

7.3 PROTECTIVE AND DEFENSIVE AIRWAY REFLEXES IN NEWBORNS

Protective and defensive reflexes of airways are considered as those special mechanisms by which an organism can overcome the influence of exogenous harmful factors, on the respiratory system.

7.3.1 Protective Airway Reflexes in Newborns

The Kratschmer´s apnoeic reflex elicited by chemical irritation of the nasal mucous membrane and mediated through trigeminal nerve endings, is an example of a protective airway reflex. Apnoea and laryngoconstriction provoked by chemical stimulation of the nasal mucosa prevents harmful gases or irritant liquids from reaching the lungs. Stimulation of the nasal mucosa by water, accompanied by stimulation of cold receptors on face, especially in the perinasal region, elicits the *diving reflex.* Its respiratory and cardiovascular characteristics are the same as those of the Kratschmer's reflex (apnoea, laryngoconstriction, bradycardia, redistribution of blood, increase of peripheral vascular resistance and systemic blood pressure).

These reflexes were studied mainly in experimental animals. In adult humans, Allen[39] found that chemical irritation of the upper airways is followed by cessation of breathing, while the heart rate changes were not significant. Since cortical inhibition of trigeminal activity increases with age, it could be considered that trigeminal innervation in younger subjects will be of greater importance.[40] Actually, in newborn monkeys, apnoea elicited by immersion of face in cold water persists for a while in contrast to older monkeys who start normal breathing almost immediately.[41]

Sarnat[42] studied olfactory reflex response in human newborns to the inhalation of peppermint odour. He found that neonates, as early as 28–32 weeks of gestational age, are sensitive to this irritation and produce sucking movements or an arousal reaction. Allen et al.[43] stimulated the trigeminal area of preterm neonates by cold air (25°C). This stimulation resulted in an increase in heart rate; although bradycardia was observed in a small percentage (3%) of cases.

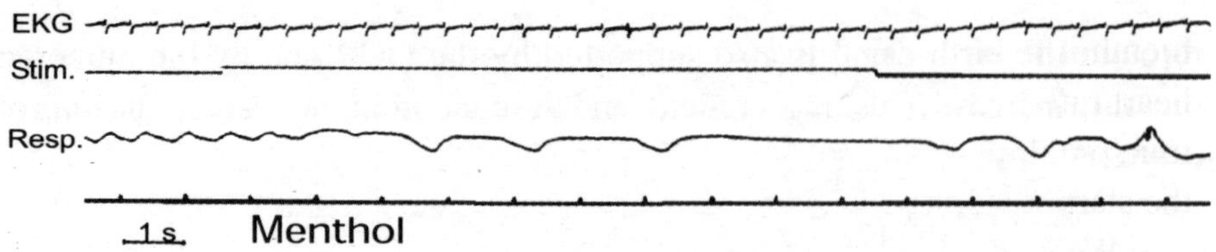

Fig. 7.6 ECG curve (EKG), time of chemical stimulation of the airways (Stim.), and respiration curve (Resp.) of a newborn infant before, during and after inhalation of menthol vapours; s, second.

According to Allen et al.[43] infants with abnormal responses may be in jeopardy of cardiorespiratory dysregulation and of the sudden infant death syndrome.

We studied protective and defensive airway reflexes[44] including Kratschmer´s reflex in 44 newborn infants of mean gestation age of 34 weeks (range 19–37 weeks) and mean birth weight of 1.9 kg (range 1.1–2.45 kg). Their average age at examination was 47 hours (range 9–92). We recorded intrathoracic pressure changes (in the thoracic segment of the oesophagus), using an electromanometer via a saline-filled catheter with terminal as well as side openings and ECG. The respiratory rate was calculated from oesophageal pressure recordings, or from chest movements recorded with a piezocrystal and instantaneous heart rate from the R-R interval of the ECG. Chemical stimulation of airways was performed by spontaneous inhalation of menthol fumes from the crystals which were held for 10 seconds in an open container about 1 cm from their nostrils, or the intranasal adminstration of 1–2 drops of the nasal drops (Mukoseptonex SPOFA, Carbaethopendicinium).

Respiratory reactions: Inhalation produced an apnoea lasting for a mean duration of 4.7 ± 0.4 s in 43 per cent of cases (Fig.7.6). In three cases it provoked sneezing, and in the rest the mean respiratory rate fell on an average of 55.6 to 31/min ($p < 0.05$). The application of nasal drops caused an immediate respiratory arrest in 50 per cent of the cases that lasted for 7.4 ± 2.3 s. In the rest, respiration rate fell on average from 57/min to 36/min ($p<0.02$).

Cardiac reactions: In anaesthetised rabbits, stimulation of the nasal mucosa by xylol vapours produced strong bradycardia and ventricular extrasystoles.[45] Contrary to these results seen in adult anaesthetized rabbits was the finding of an unchanged heart rate by the application of nasal drops, or of an increased heart rate in premature newborns without cardiac arrhythmias. The resulting heart rate changes were studied for 20 seconds from the onset of menthol fumes application; averaged values showed the greatest increase in heart rate in the 12th second and (increasing from 123 ± 1.8/min to 131.4 ± 1/min; $p<0.01$). This tachycardia response was significant in the 7th second from the start of stimulation and persisted up to the 20th second of observation.

We suggest that the tachycardia resonse occurs due to a general arousal reaction, despite simultaneous cessation of breathing movements. Additional reflexes such as sucking, licking and stretching movements, opening of the eyes, grimacing (expression of displeasure) and other signs of arousal reaction also appeared.

7.3.2 Defensive Airway Reflexes in Newborns

7.3.2.1 Defensive Airway Reflexes in Healthy/Premature Newborns

Defensive airway reflexes include reflexes such as sneezing, coughing, expiration and aspiration, which can actively eliminate irritants from the organism.[45] Various authors[46] have found that in experimental animals respiratory reactions to mechanical stimulation of the airways are either completely absent on the first day of life or are replaced by a different (mainly apnoeic) reaction. It is not certain whether newborn humans possess the ability to eliminate irritants from their airways actively, or not. Some authors,[47] for example, claim that human newborns, mainly premature ones are unable to cough effectively, with the consequent danger of aspiration because of neurological immaturity. Others[48,49] found that the newborn infants possess mechanisms for removing harmful substances from their airways.

We studied the effect of a mechanical stimulation of the nose, oropharyngeal and laryngeal region.[44] In 23 premature newborns (mean gestation age of 34 weeks, a mean birthweight of 1.9 kg, mean postnatal age 47 hours) while adapting to extrauterine life. For stimulation, we used a nylon fibre, which deforms the mucosa and can thus also stimulate deeper level receptors as during clearing and aspiration of the mucus in upper airways. Mechanical stimulation of the nasal mucosa elicited in our study an expulsive reaction (sneezing) in 67 stimulations out of 71, (i.e. 95%). It is generally known that sneezing begins with a deep inspiration. In our studies on premature newborns, we found that expiratory efforts evoked by mechanical stimulation of the nasal mucosa were not preceded by an initial deep inspiration (Fig. 7.7). Our speculation about this phenomenon is as follows. In adults, a sneeze starts with a deep inspiration,

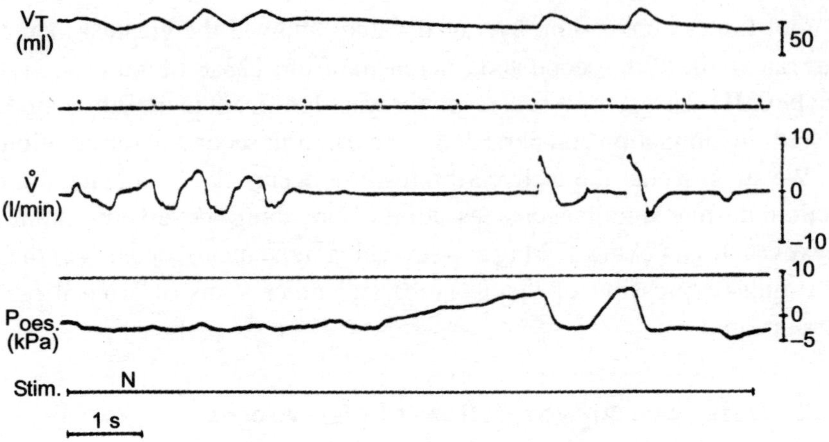

Fig. 7.7 Tidal volume (V_T), airflow (V) and oesophageal pressure (P_{oes}.) in sneezing elicited by mechanical stimulation (Stom.) of nasal mucosa in a premature newborn. (Reproduced from Ref. [56] with permission from Publisher).

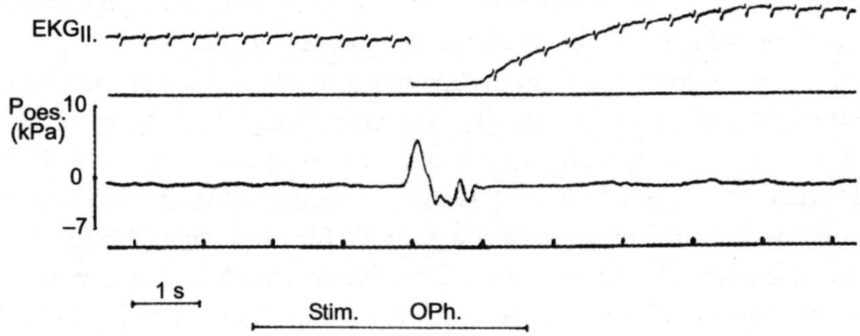

Fig. 7.8 ECG (EKG) and oesophageal pressure (P_{oes}.) in the expiratory-inspiratory reaction provoked by stimulation of the oropharyngeal region (Stim. OP.) in a premature newborn. (Reproduced from Ref. [44] with permission from Publisher).

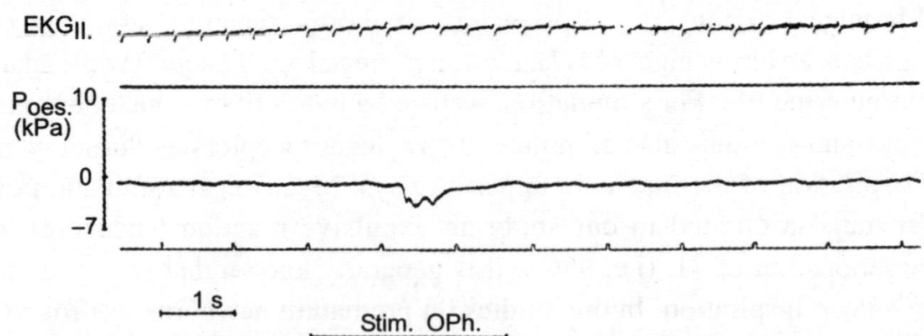

Fig. 7.9 ECG (EKG) and oesophageal pressure (P_{oes}.) in the inspiratory reaction elicited by stimulation of the oropharyngeal region (Stim.OPh.) in a premature newborn. (Reproduced from Ref. [44] with permission from Publisher).

Table 7.1 Intensity of the maximum effort (IME), the total intensity of the attack (TIA) and the mean intensity of the attack (MIA) given as inspiratory (i) and expiratory (e) values during sneezing, coughing and expiratory (ER) and inspiratory (IR) reaction. The values (in kPa) were calculated from the oesophageal pressure values and are given as mean and standard error of mean (x ± SEM).

	IMEi	*TIAi*	*MIAi*	*IMEe*	*TIAe*	*MIAe*
Sneezing	0.97 ± 0.11	3.04 ± 0.35	0.94 ± 0.11	5.57 ± 0.33	22.3 ± 2.2	5.12 ± 0.25
Coughing	3.38 ± 0.58	9.99 ± 2.27	2.07 ± 0.33	5.36 ± 0.37	23.7 ± 6.0	4.36 ± 0.41
ER				4.84 ± 0.65		
IR	3.43 ± 0.39					

usually through the mouth. It is known that the newborn infants have great difficulty in breathing through their mouths and a deep inspiration through the nose could drive a harmful substance further into the airways. Therefore, the sneeze reflex appears to be modified in them, appearing without a pronounced deep inspiration and this modification may thus serve a useful purpose.

Stimulation of the oropharyngeal region evoked transient respiratory arrest in 25 per cent and in others (75%) forced respiratory reactions develop. Expiratory reactions without preceding inspiratory effort (18%) which sometimes continue into a deep inspiration (Fig.7.8), intensified inspiratory reactions (in 33%; Fig. 7.9), and inspiratory-expiratory reactions, or coughing (in 25%).

The mean intensity of the maximum inspiratory and expiratory efforts, the total expiratory and inspiratory intensity of the attack (the sum of all efforts) and the mean intensity of the attack (obtained by dividing the intensity of the attack by the number of efforts) are given in Table 7.1.The mean intensity of a maximum number of inspiratory effort before an expulsive attack did not differ ($p > 0.05$) from mean oesophageal pressure value during the last three inspirations before the attack. Mean intensity of maximum an expiratory efforts was significantly greater ($p < 0.01$) than the values of oesophageal pressure during the last three expirations before the attack. Mean intensity of the maximum inspiratory effort in complex inspiratory-expiratory cough reaction was significantly greater (p <

0.001) than in nasal reaction. Mean intensities of the maximum expiratory efforts in reactions from nose and oropharynx were virtually the same.

In our study, we found that mechanical stimulation of the oropharyngeal and laryngeal regions produced forced respiratory reactions in 75 per cent of cases. However, during laryngoscopy, Miller et al[50] found that cough could be elicited in 49 per cent of full-term infants and 27 per cent of premature infants. The difference between the results, i.e. a better elicitability of responses seen in our study, may be related to the different characteristics of the stimuli. Mechanical stimulation accompanied by focussed deformation of the mucosa by a nylon fibre can thus also stimulate receptors in deeper layers of the respiratory mucosa.

In animals and adult humans, touching the vocal folds can elicit an expiration reflex consisting of a short, active expiratory effort without a preceding inspiration.[51] We were able to elicit brief expiratory reflexes similar to the expiration reflex. The short duration of the reaction (on average 175 ms) supports the view that this reflex in premature infants is a functional expiration reflex. Expiratory reactions were sometimes followed by deep inspirations. These successive inspirations in newborn infants are probably the outcome of an active Hering-Breuer reflex and indicates that such expirations are effected at the expense of expiratory reserve volume.

In experimental animals, stimulation of oropharynx can elicit an *aspiration reflex*[52] characterised by fast, deep inspirations without a subsequent expiratory effort, while stimulation of the laryngopharyngeal region can produce laryngopharyngeal cough, which has a very pronounced inspiratory component.[45,53] Inspiratory components of the reactions to stimulation of the oropharynx (cough) were also intensified in the present study. Independent deep inspiratory reactions observed during this study were in most cases doubled or trebled (60%), and their duration was longer than that of typical aspiration reflex in cats (150 ms).[52]

Mechanics of Breathing During Sneezing and Crying in Premature Newborns

During forced respiratory manoeuvres, marked changes in the mechanics of breathing may occur. Experiments on animals and adult humans[54,55] indicate marked changes in various mechanics of breathing. Therefore, we have studied ventilation and mechanics of breathing in premature newborns during sneezing.[56]

Twenty-two premature newborns, with no signs of cardiorespiratory disease, and of mean gestational age of 35.5 (32–37) weeks and mean birth weight of

Table 7.2 Frequency of breathing (f), inspiratory ($P_{oes.i}$) and expiratory ($P_{oes.e}$) oesophageal pressure, volume tidal (V_T), peak inspiratory flow (PIF), peak expiratory flow (PEF), ventilation (V), dynamic compliance (C) and total respiratory resistance (Rtot) during quiet breathing, sneezing and crying in premature newborns. The values are given as mean and standard errors of the mean, p = probability level, n = number of tests.

	Eupnoea *n = 68, x_1*	*Sneezing* *n = 104, x_2*	*Crying* *n = 59, x_3*	$p\ x_1 : x_2$	$p\ x_1 : x_3$
f/min	53.0 ± 4.1		35.8 ± 2.4		0.01
$P_{oes.i.}$ (kPa)	–0.55 ± 0.01	–2.73 ± 0.23	–2.89 ± 0.39	0.001	0.001
$P_{oes.e.}$ (kPa)	–0.19 ± 0.01	7.0 ± 0.27	3.69 ± 0.23	0.001	0.001
V_T (ml)	12.0 ± 0.02	27.1 ± 1.8	43.1 ± 2.6	0.001	0.001
PIF (l/s)	0.022 ± 0.001	0.063 ± 0.004	0.118 ± 0.004	0.001	0.001
PEF (l/s)	0.019 ± 0.001	0.126 ± 0.005	0.091 ± 0.008	0.001	0.001
V (ml/min)	497 ± 38		1763 ± 176		0.001
C (ml/kPa)	28.9 ± 0.5	19.3 ± 2.2	13.9 ± 1.8	0.01	0.001
Rtot (kPa/l/s)	7.9 ± 1.0	50.0 ± 0.7	26.5 ± 2.4	0.001	0.001

2.1 kg (1.5–2.5 kg) were investigated. The mean postnatal age at examination was 36 hours (10–66 h). Sneeze reflex was evoked by the mechanical stimulation of nasal mucosa. Pressure in the thoracic segment of the oesophagus was recorded using an electromanometer through a fluid-filled polyethylene catheter inserted via the mouth to the mid-oesophageal region. Airflow and tidal volume were recorded through a fixed mask by means of a pneumotachograph. In addition to pressure, flow and volume changes, even ventilation, dynamic compliance and total pulmonary resistance were determined. The value of resistance at peak expiratory flow during cough expulsion is called 'cough index'.[54,55] It is considered an important indicator of cough efficiency; we calculated this for sneezing in premature newborns. The values obtained while at rest and during spontaneous crying were compared. The values are tabulated in Table 7.2.

In the expulsive phase of sneezing, oesophageal pressure rose markedly. In this phase, the pressure reached rather high values (7 kPa) even in premature newborns. The volume of air expelled during this phase was 2.26 times greater of resting tidal volume, and the peak expiratory airflow was 6.63 times higher of quiet expiratory airflow. In the expulsive phase, total pulmonary resistance was

50.0 ± 0.7 kPa ´ l^{-1} ´ s and cough index was 60.9 ± 3.4 kPa ´ l^{-1} ´ s. Dynamic compliance was significantly lower ($p < 0.01$) in sneezing than in eupnoea.

The compliance of lungs decreased considerably, probably due to large and rapid lung volume changes. The evaluation of cough index has revealed that the index almost reaches the value 61 kPa ´ l^{-1} ´ s. Cough index, which is virtually a measure of high intrathoracic pressure required for quick and effective expiratory airflow, amounts to values 12.6–27.7 kPa ´ l^{-1} ´ s in adult humans[54] and 15.3 kPa ´ l^{-1} ´ s in cats.[45] Very high values of cough index indicate that the lumen of airways is small in premature newborns, and therefore the infants must use high transpulmonary pressure in order to eliminate noxious substances from the respiratory tract.

The evaluation of various parameters in the expulsive phase with and without an initial inspiration has revealed that expulsions preceded by deep initial inspirations had larger expiratory volumes and higher oesophageal pressures than expulsions without initial inspirations ($p < 0.01 – 0.001$). According to Burkart and Bucher,[57] a deep initial inspiration intensifies the consequent expulsions in sneezing and coughing through the increased activity of the SARs — pulmonary stretch receptors. In newborns, we found that expulsions were stronger when preceded by inspiratory efforts. This finding may indicate the importance of active Hering-Breuer inflation reflex in premature newborns.

Positive expiratory pressure during sneezing in premature newborns lasted 1.02 ± 0.05 s on average. The duration of compressive phase (from the beginning of the increase of oesophageal pressure above zero to the beginning of expiratory airflow) was 0.78 ± 0.05 s, which represents 76.5 per cent of the duration of the total pressure increase. As we can see also in Figure. 7.7, the expiratory effort lasted for a relatively long time, nevertheless, the expulsive phase was considerably shorter. Here, the closure of glottis contributes to the strengthening of the expulsive effect.

Crying is specifically seen in humans; and therefore, it cannot be studied in animals. During crying, the pattern of breathing changes considerably; (Table 7.2) respiratory rate in our study was significantly lower while crying than during quiet breathing. Inspiration was markedly shorter and expiration was prolonged, this produced marked changes in inspiration/expiration ratio. The ratio was 1 : 5.1 while crying, which is significantly less than that in eupnoea and this was due to a shorter inspiration as well due to the prolongation of expiration. During the inspiratory phase of crying, the oesophageal pressure decreased markedly and the airflow rose compared to values at rest and while sneezing ($p < 0.001$).

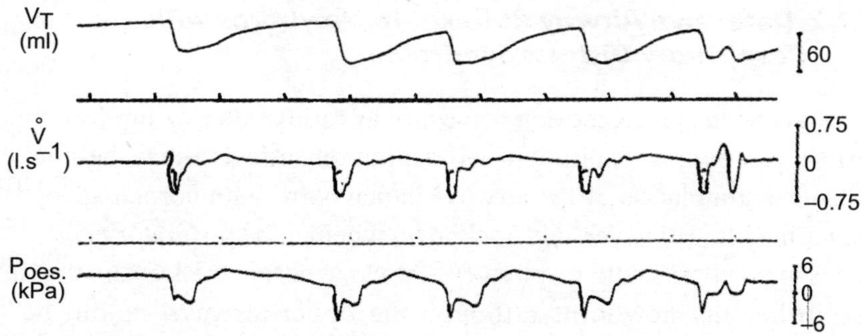

Fig. 7.10 Tidal volume (V_T), airflow (V) and oesophageal pressure (P_{oes}) in a premature newborn, while crying. (Reproduced from Ref. [56] with permission from Publisher).

During the expiratory phase of crying, the oesophageal pressure rose, although much less than during sneezing ($p < 0.001$). Expiratory flow increased 4.8 times of the value at rest, nevertheless it had a lower peak expiratory flow in sneezing ($p < 0.01$).

Mean tidal volume while crying was 43.1 ± 2.6 ml amounting to 20.1 ± 1.2 ml/kg body weight. It represents a 3.6 times greater volume of the eupnoeic tidal volume, being higher than in sneezing ($p < 0.001$). Maximum tidal volume while crying, was on average 72.1 ± 6.4 ml, which is 33.8 ± 3.0 ml/kg body weight. Ventilation, while crying was increased 3.6 times ($p < 0.001$) of values when quiet. Dynamic compliance in crying was similar to that in sneezing but was less than that in eupnoea ($p < 0.001$). Total pulmonary resistance in crying was significantly higher ($p < 0.001$) than in quiet breathing, but significantly lower than in sneeze reflex.

Each cry is preceded by a sudden short lasting decrease in intrathoracic pressure and quick transition from negative to positive values (Fig. 7.10). In mature newborns, positive values of intrathoracic pressure are about 3.3–4 kPa during crying.[58,60] In our premature newborns, positive pressures attained values of 3.7 ± 0.2 kPa. Expiratory phase in crying is protracted through a special mechanism similar to that in speaking[59] or grunting. The ability to modify expiration, represents a mature mechanism in newborns, and it is most likely caused by laryngeal closure.[58]

7.3.2.2 Defensive Airway Reflexes in Newborns with Respiratory Distress Syndrome

As we have seen before, the defensive airway reflexes (sneezing, coughing and reactions resembling expiration and aspiration reflexes) may be elicited by mechanical stimulation of the airways in newborns with normal adaptation to extrauterine life. However, it is not known whether the respiratory responses or reflexes in newborns with respiratory distress syndrome (RDS) are the same as those in healthy newborns although the upper airways should be often mechanically cleaned or sucked. Therefore, we have analysed the sensitivity and nature of respiratory reactions evoked by mechanical stimulation of the upper airways in newborns with RDS and compared the results with the responses of healthy newborns.[61]

We studied 16 infants with RDS whose mean gestational age was 33 (28–40) weeks and the mean birth weight was 1.8 (0.9–2.5) kg. The mean postnatal age at the time of investigation was 39 (8–72h). From a group of 16 newborns with RDS, six (37.5%) died within 48 hours of examination. Eleven newborns had scores of 4 to 7 using the scoring system of Downes et al[62] indicating mild RDS; of these two died. Five other newborns had severe respiratory distress (scores 8–10) and four of these died. The results were compared with values obtained from 16 age-matched newborns who had no disturbances during adaptation. The mean values of birth weight and the gestational and postnatal age in both groups did not differ significantly ($p > 0.05$).

Newborns with RDS had the following blood gas and acid-base balance values: PCO_2 : 6.35 ± 0.74 kPa, pH : 7.297 ± 0.030, BE : –5.2 ± 0.9 mVal. l^{-1}, BB : 44,55 ± 2.00 mVal. l^{-1}, standard HCO_3^- : 20.27 ± 0.67 mVal. l^{-1}, actual HCO_3^- : 22.52 ± 2.05 mVal. l^{-1}. The values of blood gases and acid-base balance were not measured in control newborns.

During the study, newborns with RDS and a few controls lay supine in incubators, and some newborns of the control group lay in cots with neutral environmental temperature. Newborns with RDS were not ventilated artificially nor had a naso-oropharyngotracheal intubation before or during examination. At the beginning of the investigation, the infants were asleep. During examination, they were awake but quiet. Pressure in the thoracic segment of the oesophagus was recorded with an electromanometer through a polyethylene catheter filled with saline. The catheter was introduced for feeding purposes. A transducer with a flat frequency response up to 25 Hz was fixed at the level of the tip of catheter. In newborns with expiratory grunting, a respirophonogram was taken using a contact microphone along with an ECG (lead II). The parameters were simultaneously recorded on a polygraph with a linear frequency response up to 130 Hz. From oesophageal pressure recordings lasting for at least a minute, we were able to evaluate the breathing frequency, the mean duration of inspiratory and expiratory efforts, the intensity of the maximum inspiratory and expiratory efforts, the total expiratory and inspiratory intensity of the attack (the sum of all individual inspiratory and expiratory efforts) and the mean intensity of the attack (intensity of the attack divided by the number of efforts).

The responses to mechanical stimulation of the nasal, oropharyngeal and laryngeal mucosa were studied. The stimulations were simulation of clearing and sucking of mucus from the upper airways. We also evaluated changes in intrathoracic (oesophageal) pressure during crying in newborns with RDS. The results are given as mean and standard error of mean (± SEM).

In newborns with RDS, the mean frequency of breathing was 71.5 ± 3.9/ min; inspiration lasted for 0.2 ± 0.03 s and expiration for 0.7 ± 0.07 s. The ratio T_I/T_E was 1 : 3. The amplitude of respiratory changes of the oesophageal pressure was 1.60 ± 0.23 kPa. In the control group of healthy newborns, the mean frequency of breathing was 44.0 ± 5.1/ min; with inspiration lasting for 0.45 ± 0.09 s and expiration for 1.2 ± 0.1 s. The ratio T_i/T_e was 1 : 2.5. The amplitude of oesophageal pressure change was 0.49 ± 0.04 kPa during eupnoea. These values were significantly different from those in the controls ($p<0.02$–$p<0.001$).

Mechanical stimulation of nasal mucosa produced expulsive efforts (sneezing) in 45 per cent of newborns with RDS (from 104 stimulations). The number of expulsions for one sneezing attack was 2.6 ± 0.3 (mean value from 123 expiratory efforts). An apnoeic reaction with a mean duration of 2.0 ± 0.2 s was elicited by 11 nasal stimulations; three stimulations provoked a decrease in frequency of breathing and two, produced hyperpnoea. There were no respiratory responses in the remaining 41 cases. In healthy newborns, mechanical stimulation of the nasal mucosa produced an expulsive reaction in 94.5 per cent of 36 stimulations. It is significantly more ($p < 0.001$) than that in newborns with RDS. The number of expiratory efforts in one sneezing attack was 4.5 ± 0.5 (mean value from 152 expiratory efforts). In two other cases (5.5%), hyperpnoea was seen. Values of these parameters can be seen in Tables 7.3 and 7.4. A typical record of an apnoeic reaction elicited by mechanical stimulation of the nasal mucosa in a newborn with RDS is shown in Figure. 7.11.

Table 7.3 Inspiratory parameters of sneezing, coughing, inspiratory reactions and crying in newborns. Ti effort — time duration of inspiratory effort (in seconds), IMIe – intensity of the maximum inspiratory effort, TIiA — total intensity of inspiratory attacks, MIiA — mean intensity of inspiratory attacks, H-healthy, statistical significance H vs RDS: ** p < 0.01, *** p< 0.01, **** p< 0.001. [From 61]

		Sneezing	*Coughing*	*Inspiratory reaction*	*Crying*
Ti effort (s)	H	0.51±0.05	0.43±0.04	0.59±0.09	
	RDS	0.52±0.03	0.67±0.07**	0.61±0.06	
IMIe (kPa)	H	1.05±0.12	3.35±0.65	3.42±0.42	2.29±0.26
	RDS	2.48±0.28****	4.23±0.67	3.87±0.36	1.40±0.50
TIiA (kPa)	H	2.97±0.42	9.77±2.52		
	RDS	6.33±0.90****	15.29±2.40		
MIiA	H	0.81±0.10	2.08±0.37		
	RDS	2.08±0.44****	4.54±0.29***		

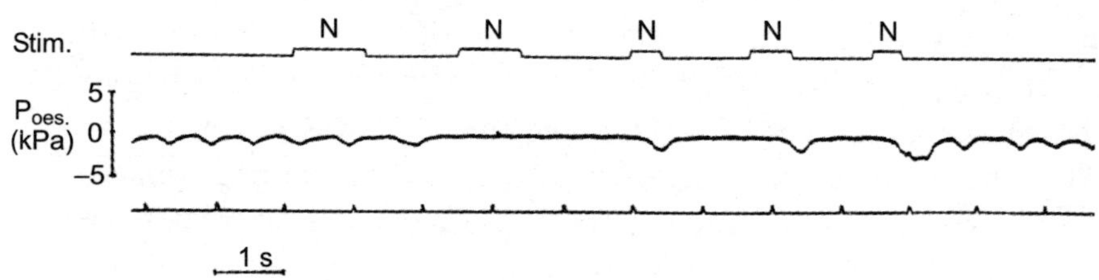

Fig. 7.11 Oesophageal pressure ($P_{oes.}$) in apnoeic reaction elicited by mechanical stimulation (Stim.) of nasal mucosa (N) in a premature newborn with respiratory distress syndrome. (Reproduced from Ref. [61] with permission from Publisher).

Mechanical stimulation of the oropharyngeal and laryngeal mucosa caused forced respiratory reactions in 48 per cent of the 83 stimulations in newborns with RDS. There were 13 cough attacks (16%) with 32 expulsive efforts (on an average 2.5 ± 0.4 in one attack), as well as 19 inspiratory (23 %) and 8 expiratory efforts (9%). Apnoeic reaction appeared in 13 cases (16%), with a mean duration of 2.4 ± 0.3 s. In the other 30 cases (36%), there was a decrease in respiratory frequency with or without a deepening of breaths accompanied by a slow increase in the expiratory positive pressure (e.g. as in vomiting). In healthy newborns, forced respiratory reactions were elicited from the oropharyngeal and laryngeal

Table 7.4 Expiratory parameters of sneezing, coughing, expiratory reaction and crying in newborns. Te effort — time duration of expiratory effort; IMEe - intensity of the maximum expiratory effort; TieA — total intensity of the expiratory attacks; MieA — mean intensity of the expiratory attacks; H — healthy newborns; RDS, those with respiratory distress syndrome. Statistical significance of H vs RDS: * $p < 0.05$ ** $p < 0.02$, *** $p < 0.01$, **** $p < 0.001$. [from 61]

		Sneezing	*Coughing*	*Exp.reaction*	*Crying*
Te effort (s)	H	0.97±0.04	0.69±0.07	0.157±0.035	
	RDS	0.86±0.04	1.16±0.10****	0.310±0.06*	
IMEe (kPa)	H	6.00±0.31	5.65±0.33	5.00±0.73	4.48±0.33
	RDS	4.59±0.24****	5.37±0.43	2.83±0.30**	2.73±0.28***
TIeA (kPa)	H	23.9±2.8	18.3±3.07		
	RDS	13.7±1.7***	16.9±3.05		
MIeA (kPa)	H	5.16±0.30	4.12±0.38		
	RDS	3.94±0.25***	4.93±0.51		

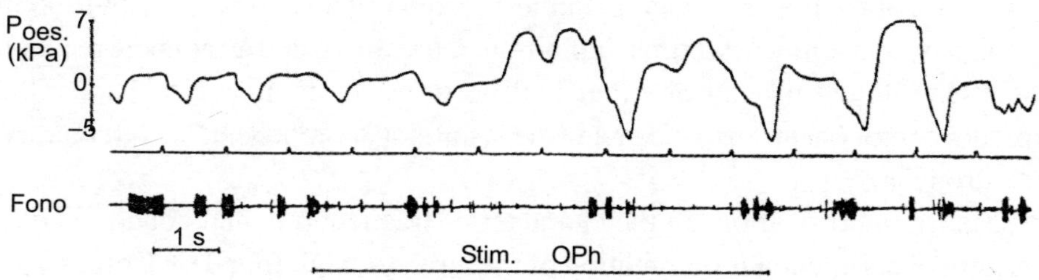

Fig. 7.12 Oesophageal pressure ($P_{oes.}$) and respirophonogram (Fono) in expulsive reactions elicited by mechanical stimulation of the oropharyngeal and laryngeal regions (Stim.OPh) in a newborn with respiratory distress syndrome (RDS) and expiratory grunting. (Reproduced from Ref. [61] with permission from Publisher).

regions in 74 per cent of 39 stimulations, and its occurrence was significantly greater ($p < 0.001$) than that in newborns with RDS. A depression of breathing followed by crying was produced in 26 per cent of the stimulations. The values of individual parameters of coughing, inspiratory and expiratory reactions in healthy newborns as well as in newborns with RDS are given in Tables 7.3 and 7.4. Expulsive reactions elicited by mechanical stimulation of the oropharyngeal and laryngeal regions in a newborn with RDS accompanied by expiratory grunting are shown in Figure 7.12.

Statistical comparison showed that the duration of inspiratory effort in coughing and the expiratory effort in coughing or expiratory responses were of longer duration in newborns with RDS. All parameters indicating the intensity of inspiratory effort in sneezing and the mean intensity of inspiratory cough attack were seen to be stronger in newborns with RDS. On the contrary, the expiratory-expulsive component of both sneezing and coughing was weaker in newborns with RDS. Mechanical stimulation of the upper airways elicited less expulsive respiratory reactions in the newborns with RDS compared to controls, and the depression of breathing was often seen instead of expulsive reactions (Fig. 7.13).

Crying in newborns with RDS: The maximum expiratory effort during crying was weaker in newborns with RDS (2.73 ± 0.28 kPa) than in controls (4.48 ± 0.33 kPa, $p < 0.001$). On the contrary, the maximum inspiratory effort during crying did not differ significantly ($p > 0.05$) in both groups (newborns with RDS: 1.40 ± 0.50 kPa, healthy newborns: 2.29 ± 0.26 kPa).

Our results showed that expulsive respiratory reactions to mechanical stimulation of the upper airways occur less frequently in newborns with RDS in comparison to healthy newborns. Inhibition of breathing and an apnoeic reaction was often elicited instead of expulsive reactions. In expulsive reactions, the expiratory component was weaker and the inspiratory component, on the contrary, was stronger.

Similar modifications in the character of tracheobronchial cough in adult cats with experimental inflammation of the airways were found by Korpas.[63] A marked increase in the inspiratory component of cough in experimental inflammation was considered to result from hypersecretion and subsequent mechanical stimulation in the airways. The action of subthreshold stimuli from the inflammatory mucosa and their summation with the mechanical stimuli could not be ruled out. In addition, large amounts of secretions in the airways can give rise to receptor adaptation, especially in children with bronchitis.[45] This mechanism may be involved in newborns with RDS, where hypersecretion is aggravated by oxygen therapy due to hypertrophy of mucus-producing goblet cells and depression of the mucociliary function.[64]

Immaturity of the reflex arc could also be responsible for modification of the defensive airway reflexes in newborns with RDS. Fleming et al.[18] found that in intubated newborns with RDS, who had signs of apnoea and transient tachypnoea, a direct stimulation of the bronchial mucosa with a fine catheter often produced a paradoxical response, i.e. an increased inspiratory effort or an

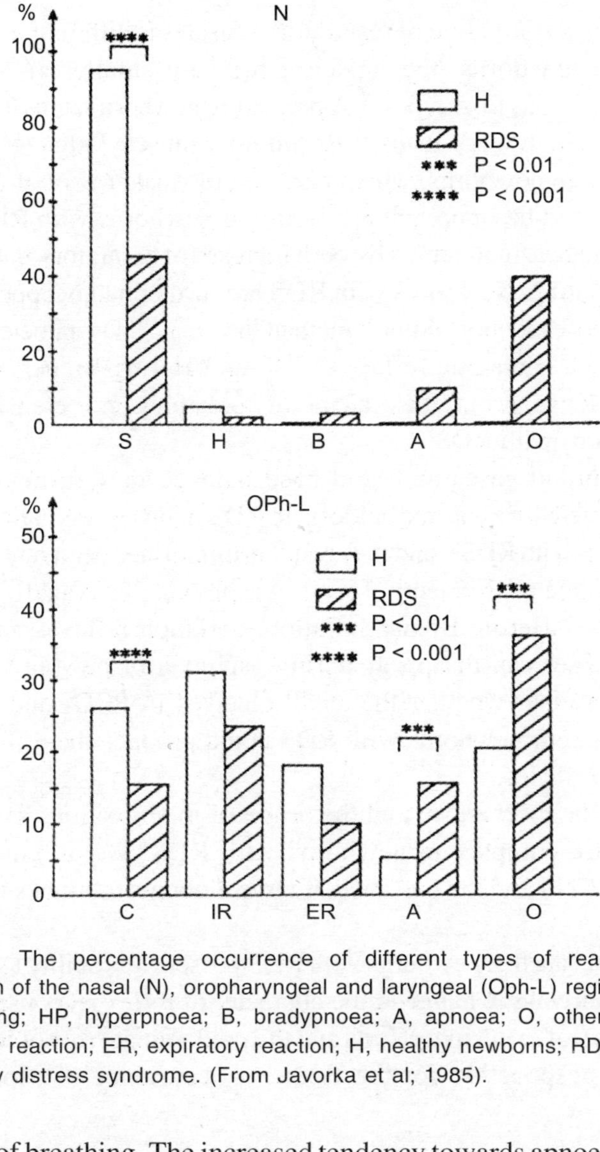

Fig. 7.13 The percentage occurrence of different types of reaction evoked by stimulation of the nasal (N), oropharyngeal and laryngeal (Oph-L) regions, respectively. S, sneezing; HP, hyperpnoea; B, bradypnoea; A, apnoea; O, others, C; cough; IR: inspiratory reaction; ER, expiratory reaction; H, healthy newborns; RDS, newborns with respiratory distress syndrome. (From Javorka et al; 1985).

inhibition of breathing. The increased tendency towards apnoea in response to a mechanical stimulation of the airways, also seen in our study, was possibly due to an incomplete myelination of the vagus nerve. Differences in respiratory reflexes between adults and newborns may further depend on the maturity of the receptors and or synaptic connections of peripheral nerve fibres to specific neurons.[20] Deficient dendritic arborisation and inadequate synaptic connections in newborns could play an important role in the origin of the differences.[65,66]

Histologically, the structure of respiratory muscles is different in newborns and in adults. In newborns, the muscle fibres are smaller and not fully differentiated into various fibre types.[65] A premature newborn seems to be poorly equipped to sustain high work-loads.[67] Respiratory muscle fatigue can quickly develop in premature newborns, which can lead to weaker expiratory efforts. The mechanism could be important especially in newborns with RDS, where alveolar gas exchange is maintained by both increase of expiratory muscle work and expiratory grunting. Newborns with RDS are further handicapped because their chest wall is soft and more compliant than the lungs.[64] Dyspnoeic breathing activates intercostal-to-phrenic reflexes[30,31,68] and Hering-Breuer reflexes in the newborns. All these specificities can modify breathing and defensive airway reflexes in newborns with RDS.

Changes in blood gases and acid-base balance may influence reflex responses. Progressive hypoxia and acidosis in RDS may depress cardiovascular reflexes in newborns with RDS[69] and may result in diminished heart rate variability and in fixed heart rate as frequently found in asphyxia.[70-72] Vagally mediated respiratory reflexes (Hering-Breuer inflation, deflation reflexes and Head´s paradoxical response) can disappear during asphyxia of newborn rabbits.[73] However, it is not clear whether the small changes in PCO_2 and acid-base balance of blood in our newborns with RDS could produce the differences in defensive airway reflexes.

It seems that the mechanism and the origin of modifications in defensive airway reflexes are complex in newborns with RDS. We assume that the immaturity of the CNS and the presence of large amounts of mucus in airways play a major role.

The results indicate that newborns with RDS possess less ability to eliminate irritants from the airways. Change in the character of reflex responses, mainly the poor elicitability of expulsive efforts and the predominant role of inspiratory efforts, could be responsible for the frequent occurrence of aspiration in premature newborns.

7.4 VENTILATION AND COUGHING IN CHILDREN

Maturation of the respiratory system including ossification of thoracic bones, growth of the airways specifically that of the alveoli, continues through childhood. The position of the larynx descends vertically in the first in 6 months of the postnatal life. The volume of dead space (VD), which in newborns is about 7–

8 ml, increases to 40 ml (in the age 6–8 years) and to 150 ml in adults. Cartilage support for the conducting airways increases rapidly in the first 2 months and thereafter, through childhood, more slowly. At the time of birth, there could be about 20 million terminal air sacs and alveoli, and by 8 years, the alveolar number increases to 300 millions. Alveolar diameter doubles in size during maturation and by 2 months of age, alveoli measures 150 to 180 microns. By adulthood, the alveolar diameter doubles in size.

The peripheral airways contribute the most to R_{aw} until 5 years of age after which the upper airway resistance predominates (seen in adults). Compliance of the lungs rises in absolute values, however, the specific CL (after recalculation from the lung volumes VC, FRC or TLC) does not depend on the size of the body.

Pecularities of the regulation of breathing in children including defensive airway reflexes are not well known. Frequency of breathing declines with early postnatal age. Abnormal maturation of the breathing control probably is associated sudden infant death syndrome (SIDS). Although the cause of the SIDS is multifactorial, where different endogenous and exogenous factors act simultaneously, imaturity of the regulation — chemical with regard to the biphasic response to hypoxia versus hypercapnia of breathing and/or neural, can play a crucial role in some cases.

The cause of apnoea or coughing could also be gastroesophageal reflux (GER). The reflux of the gastric content to oesophagus or up to the respiratory system (larynx, trachea) stimulates vagal receptors. Other causes of cough in children are respiratory infections, inflammation of the upper and lower airways, suppurative lung diseases (bronchiectasis), intrinsic and extrinsic foreign bodies, airway lesions, environmental factors (smoke and other pollutants) and sinusitis or postnasal drip.[74]

REFERENCES

1. Harned HS Jr. Respiration and the respiratory system. In: Stave U, editor. Perinatal Physiology. New York, London: Plenum Medical Book Company, 1978;p53–101.
2. Manning FA. Fetal breathing movements as a reflection of fetal status. Postgraduate Medicine 1977;61(4):116–22.
3. Bystrzycka E, Nail BS, Purves MJ. Central and peripheral neural respiratory activity in the mature sheep foetus and newborn lamb. Respiration Physiology 1975;25:199–215.
4. Maloney JE. The perinatal development of the respiratory system. Proceedings of the Australian Physiological Pharmacological Society 1978;9:7–14.

5. Rigatto HA. A critical analysis of the development of peripheral and central respiratory chemosensitivity during the neonatal period. Abstracts Wenner-Green Center Symposium, Stockholm 1978;21–3.
6. Rigatto H. Control of ventilation in the newborn. Annual Review of Physiology, 1984;46:661–74.
7. Avery ME, Chernick V, Dutton RE, Permutt S. Ventilatory response to inspired carbon dioxide in infants and adults. Journal of Applied Physiology, 1963;18:895–903
8. Cross KW, Klaus M, Tooley WH, Weisser K. The response of the new-born baby to inflation of the lungs. Journal of Physiology [London] 1960;151:551–65.
9. Javorka K, Tomori Z, Zavarska L. Effect of lung inflation on the respiratory frequency and heart rate of premature neonates. Physiologica Bohemoslovaca, 1982;31(2):1129–1359.
10. Olinsky A, Bryan MH, Bryan AC. Influence of lung inflation on respiratory control in neonates. Journal of Applied Physiology 1974;36:426–9.
11. Kirkpatrick SML, Olinsky A, Bryan MH, Bryan AC. Effect of premature delivery on the maturation of the Hering-Breuer inspiratory inhibitory reflex in human infants. Journal of Pediatrics [St. Louis] 1976;88(6):1010–4.
12. Thach BT, Frantz ID, Adler SM, Taeusch HW Jr. Maturation of reflexes influencing inspiratory duration in human infants. Journal of Applied Physiology 1978;45(2):203–11.
13. Widdicombe JG. Respiratory reflexes in man and other mammalian species. Clinical Science 1961;21:163–70
14. Koller EA, Ferrer P. Studies on the role of the lung deflation reflex. Respiration Physiology 1970;10:172–83.
15. Sellick J, Widdicombe JG. Vagal deflation and inflation reflexes mediated by lung irritant receptors. Quarterly Journal of Experimental Physiology 1970;55:153–63.
16. Dawes GS, Mott JC. Reflex respiratory activity in the newborn rabbit. Journal of Physiology [London] 1959;145:85–97.
17. Trippenbach T. Laryngeal, vagal and intercostal reflexes during the early postnatal period. Journal of Developmental Physiology 1981;3:133–59.
18. Fleming PJ, Bryan AC, Bryan MH. Functional immaturity of pulmonary irritant receptors and apnoea in newborn preterm infants. Pediatrics 1978;61:515–8.
19. Ponte J, Purves MJ. Types of afferent nervous activity which may be measured in the vagus nerve of the sheep foetus. Journal of Physiology [London] 1973;229:51–6.
20. Fisher JT, Mathew OP, Sant' Ambrogio FG, Sant' Ambrogio G. Reflex effects and receptor responses to upper airway pressure and flow stimuli in developing puppies. Journal of Applied Physiology 1985;58:228–64.
21. Jakus J, Tomori Z, Stransky A. Neuronal deteminants of breathing, coughing and related motor behaviours. Wist, 2004;333.
22. Thach BT, Taeusch HW Jr. Sighing in newborn human infants: role of inflation-augmenting reflex. Journal of Applied Physiology 1976;41(4):502–7
23. Thibeault DW, Wong MM, Auld PAM. Thoracic gas volume changes in premature infants. Pediatrics 1967;40:403.
24. Coleridge JC, Coleridge HM. Afferent vagal C fibre innervation of the lungs and airways and its functional significance. Reviews of Physiology Biochemistry and Pharmacology, 1984;99:1–110.
25. Widdicombe JG. Sensory neurophysiology of the cough reflex. Journal of Allergy and Clinical Immunology 1996;98(5):84–90.

26. Paintal AS, Anand A. Respiratory control mechanisms and sensations. Delhi, Vallabhbhai Patel Chest Institute, 1998;350.
27. Paintal AS. Mechanism of stimulation of type J pulmonary receptors. Journal of Physiology (London) 1969;203:511–32.
28. Kalia M. Visceral and somatic reflexes produced by J pulmonary receptors in newborn kittens. Journal of Applied Physiology 1976;41:1–6.
29. Schleman M, Gootman N, Gootman PM. Cardiovascular and respiratory responses to right atrial injections of phenyl diguanide in pentobarbital-anesthetized newborn piglets. Pediatric Research 1979;13:1271–4.
30. Remmers JE. Inhibition of inspiratory activity by intercostal muscle afferents. Respiration Physiology 1970;10:358–83.
31. Knill R, Bryan AC. An intercostal phrenic inhibitory reflex in human newborn infants. Journal of Applied Physiology 1976;40 (3):352–6.
32. Hagan R, Bryan AC, Bryan MH, Gulston G. Neonatal chest wall afferents and regulation of respiration. Journal of Applied Physiology 1977;42(3):362–7.
33. Rudolph AM, Heymann MA. Fetal and neonatal circulation and respiration. Annual Review of Physiology 1974;36:187–207.
34. Cosmi EV. Fetal homeostasis. In: Scarpelli EM, Auld PAM, editors. Pulmonary physiology of the fetus, newborn and child. Philadelphia: Lea Febiger 1975;pp369.
35. Scarpelli EM, Condorelli S, Cosmi EV. Cutaneous stimulation and generation of breathing in the fetus. Pediatric Research 1977;11:24–8.
36. Kattwinkel J, Nearman HS, Fanaroff AA, Katona PG, Kalus MH. Apnea of prematurity. Journal of Pediatrics [St. Louis] 1975;86(4):588–92.
37. Javorka K, Zavarska L. Okulokardialny reflex u nedonosenych deti. Ceskoslovenska Pediatrie, 1978;33(3):138–40.
38. Javorka K, Zavarska L, Tomori Z. Some cardiorespiratory reflexes in newborns. Bulletin Européan de Physiopathologie Respiratoire. Clinical Physiology. 1983;19:50.
39. Allen WF. Effect of various inhaled vapors on respiration and blood pressure in anesthetized, unanesthetized, sleeping and anosmic subjects. American Journal of Physiology 1929;88:620–32.
40. Haddad GG, Mellins RB. The role of airway receptors in the control of respiration in infants. A review. Journal of Pediatrics 1977;91(2):281–6.
41. French MD, Morgan BC, Guntheroth WG. Infant monkeys—a model for crib death. American Journal of Diseases of Children 1972;123:480.
42. Sarnat HB. Olfactory reflexes in the newborn infant. Journal of Pediatrics [St. Louis] 1978;92:624–6.
43. Allen LG, Howard G, Smith JB, McCublin JA, Weaver RL. Infant heart rate response to trigeminal airstream stimulation: determination of normal and deviant values. Pediatric Research 1979;13:184–7.
44. Javorka K, Tomori Z, Zavarska L. Protective and defensive airway reflexes in premature infants. Physiologica Bohemoslovaca, 1980;29:29–35.
45. Korpas J, Tomori Z. Cough and other respiratory reflexes. Basel, Munchen, Paris, London, New York, Sydney: Karger, 1979;356.
46. Korpas J, Kalocsayova G. The mechanoreception of airways in cats in the first postnatal periods.Physiologica Bohemoslovaca, 1973;22:365–73.
47. Williams ML, Galvis AG. Pulmonary complications in infants. Surgical Clinics of North America 1974;54:1137–54.

48. Brady JP, Tooley WH. Cardiovascular and respiratory reflexes in the newborn. Pediatric Clinics of North America 1966;13:801–21.
49. Dawes GS. Foetal and neonatal physiology. Chicago: Year Book Medical Publications 1968;247.
50. Miller HC, Proud GO, Behrle FC. Variations in the gag, cough and swalow reflexes as determined by direct laryngoscopy in newborn infants. Yale Journal of Biology and Medicine 1952;24:284.
51. Korpas J, Gajdos E. Mechanoreception of the respiratory tract in guinea-pigs. Physiologica Bohemoslovaca 1971;20:623–30.
52. Tomori Z. Pleural, tracheal and abdominal pressure variations in defensive and pathologic reflexes of the respiratory tract. Physiologica Bohemoslovaca 1965;14:84–95.
53. Ivanco I, Korpas J. K otazke laryngealneho a trachealneho kasla. Bratislavske lekarske listy, 1954;34:1391–6.
54. Cohen BM. Respiratory and cough mechanics in antitussive trials. Responsivity of objective indices to the treatment of acute upper respiratory tract infections. Respiration 1975;32:32–45.
55. Pedersen OF. A new way to describe the mechanics of the expiration. Bulletin Européen de Physiopathologie Respiratoire 1972;8:569–85.
56. Javorka K, Tomori Z, Zavarska L. Mechanics of breathing during sneezing and crying in premature newborns. European Journal of Respiratory Diseases 1982;63:442–448.
57. Burkart F, Bucher K. Zur Bedeutung des Vagus für Husten und Niesen. Med Exp 1960;3:297–302.
58. Bosma JF, Truby HM, Lind J. Cry motions of the newborn infant. Acta Paediatrica Scandinavica 1965;163(Suppl.):62–92.
59. Dinwiddie R, Pitcher-Wilmott R, Schwartz JG, Shaffer TH, Fox WW. Cardiopulmonary changes in the crying neonate. Pediatric Research 1979;13:900–3.
60. Langlois A, Baken RJ. Development of respiratory time-factors in infant cry. Developmental Medicine and Child Neurology 1976;18:732–7.
61. Javorka K,Tomori Z, Zavarska L. Upper airway reflexes in newborns with respiratory distress syndrome. Bulletin Européan de Physiopathologie Respiratoire. Clinical Physiology 1985;21:345–9.
62. Downes JJ, Arya S, Morrow G, Boggs TR Jr. Transient respiratory distress syndrome in the newborn. Archives of Disease in Childhood 1967;42:659–64.
63. Korpas J. Reflexes from the larynx and their modification in disease. Advances in Physiological Sciences 1980;10:485–93.
64. Lew CD, Ramos AD, Platzker ACG. Respiratory distress syndrome. Clinical Chest Medicine 1980;1:297–309.
65. Bruce EN. Control of breathing in the newborn. Annals of Biomedical Engineering 1981;9:425–37.
66. Schulte FJ, Albani M, Schnizer H, Bentele K. Neuronal control of neonatal respiration-sleep apnea and the sudden infant death syndrome. Neuropediatrics 1982;13:3–14.
67. Bryan AC. Maturation of neuromuscular function in infants. Abstracts Wenner-Gren Center Symp. 1978;66.
68. Martin RJ, Nearman HS, Katona PG, Klaus MH. The effect of a low continuous positive airway pressure on the reflex control of respiration in the preterm infant. Journal of Pediatrics 1977;90:976–81.

69. Kero P. Heart rate variation in infants with the respiratory distress syndrome. Acta Paediatrica Scandiavica 1974;250(Suppl.):70.
70. Javorka K, Zavarska L. K otazke regulacie frekvencie srdca u nedonosenych deti s RDS. Ceskoslovenska Pediatria 1978;33:536–9.
71. Adamsons K, Myers RE. Perinatal asphyxia: causes, detection and neurological sequelae. Pediatric Clinics of North America 1973;20:465–80.
72. Gregory GA. Resuscitation of the newborn. Anesthesiology 1975;43:225–37.
73. Godfrey S. The loss of respiratory reflexes during asphyxia of new-born rabbits. Journal of Physiology [London] 1966;184:78–80.
74. Chang AB. Causes, assessment and measurement of cough in children. In: Chung KF, Widdicombe JG, Boushey HA, editors. Cough: causes, mechanisms and therapy. Oxford: Blackwell Publishing Ltd. 2003;pp57–73.

8 Cardiovascular Effects of Coughing

K Javorka

8.1 INTRODUCTION

The respiratory system is closely associated with the cardiovascular system not only anatomically but also functionally, so that the two systems are sometimes taken as one entity, i.e. as the cardiorespiratory system.

Coughing is the most important defensive reflex of the airways and lungs. Vagal and glossopharyngeal nerves with endings in the epithelium of the airway mucosa[1-3] and others in the parenchyma, e.g. J-receptors[4,5] are involved in giving rise to cough and with the possibity of modulating autonomic nervous system (ANS) activities just before a cough attack. Coughing itself is accompanied by an increased activity of the central inspiratory and expiratory neurones in accordance with the cough phases[6] and this activation modifies the cardiovascular functions through the central mechanisms, because the brainstem mechanisms mediating respiratory and cardiovascular controls are known to be closely cooperating up to the integration level. Richter et al[7] proposed a common controller of the respiratory and cardiovascular functions—'cardiorespiratory network'. Contractions of the respiratory muscles involved in the cough mechanisms[8,9] and mechanical effects (pressure changes in different sites of the body, i.e. intra-thoracic and intra-abdominal and intravascular) evoke ventilatory changes as well as changes in blood gases during and after coughing. Hence, it is not surprising that coughing is accompanied by a huge complex of cardiovascular effects.

Cardiovascular responses to cough depend on different physiological factors including the origin (e.g. laryngopharyngeal, tracheobronchial), intensity and duration of the cough attack. Cough may be seen as a single effort or as short bursts, or it may be spasmodic, i.e. resembling Valsalva's manoeuvre.

In our studies on the cardiovascular effects of coughing in animals and humans, we have come to the conclusion that the basic mechanical, sensory and humoral mechanisms of cough and accompanying changes of the cardiovascular system are very similar, and thus information about this obtained from experimental animals can help us to understand the mechanisms of these changes in humans.

8.2 INTRATHORACIC AND INTRA-ABDOMINAL PRESSURES

A forceful contraction of the inspiratory muscles in preparation for the inspiratory phase followed by a similarly vigorous contraction of the expiratory muscles in expiratory phase are typically seen during coughing. The immediate and direct outcome of these efforts are changes in intrathoracic and intra-abdominal pressures. At this stage, the intrathoracic (and pleural) pressure falls by about 15 to 35 mmHg.

In the expiratory phase, the pleural pressure rises up to 200 mmHg in healthy subjects;[10] and in some, the intrathoracic pressure, during cough attacks, has been noted to reach extremely high levels, i.e. to about 300 mmHg.[11]

On the other hand, the intra-abdominal pressure rises during inspiratory phase by the descent of the diaphragm, and it increases further, in the active expiratory phase by contraction of the abdominal muscles. The high intra-abdominal pressure attained during cough is transmitted to the pelvic organs and then to the intra-abdominal vessels.

8.3 VENOUS RETURN CHANGES

Changes in intrathoracic and intra-abdominal pressures affect the venous return and blood flow significantly not only in the intrathoracic vessels but also those in the periphery (e.g. splanchnic and cerebral circulations).

During a quiet inspiration, the negative intrapleural pressure is transmitted to the great veins and to other elastic intrathoracic structures. The drop in pressure in thorax and in the great veins at the entrance of the right atrium (CVP) enhances venous return. The intra-abdominal pressure rises towards the end of inspiration together with a descent of diaphragm.

The rise in pressure squeezes blood towards the heart because backflow is prevented by venous valves in the leg veins.

As an effect, the respiratory pump is affected by forced manoeuvres—it is more efficient during deep inspiration and less with expiratory efforts (such as coughing). The changes in venous return during *deep inspiration* are explained by two theories, which at first sight appear to be contradictory. The first one is a well-known mechanism of the respiratory *thoraco-abdominal pump*. The second, which is best explained by the *collapse theory*, states that a vast decrease in intrathoracic pressure cannot enhance the venous return because the great veins collapse in their passage through diaphragm, and the blood flow is obstructed. It is very likely that the partial collapse of the extrathoracic veins occurs only during deep inspiration and the venous return through the inferior vena cava during partial collapse is higher than in a respiratory pause.[12]

This partial obstruction can have a significant physiological role, e.g. the reduction in blood inflow can protect against an excessive flow of blood into the right atrium. This mechanism can protect the right ventricle from being overloaded.

During active expiratory efforts, venous return from abdominal veins depends on a gradient between the intra-abdominal and intrathoracic pressure. Intra-abdominal pressure can exceed intrathoracic pressure only when lung volumes are small. In this situation, the expiratory effort is performed dominantly by abdominal muscles.[13]

8.4 CARDIAC FUNCTIONS DURING COUGHING

8.4.1 Heart Rate

Heart rate is under the regulatory influence of the ANS in which tonic discharges are modified by reflex mechanisms. Besides neural regulation, heart rate responds very sensitively to local temperature and pressure, distention of the right atrium (Bainbridge effect) and hormonal activities. Resting heart rate, i.e. beat-to-beat or RR intervals, fluctuates in relation to breathing and changes in blood pressure which itself is influenced by baroreflexes and other local factors. The effect of quiet breathing in humans can be seen on ECG records as respiratory sinus arrhythmia, an increase in heart rate at the end of inspiration and a decrease at the end of expiration. These oscillations are mediated mainly via the parasympathetic vagal innervation. During coughing, the respiratory sinus arrhythmia is enhanced in its extent and depends on the number and intensity of

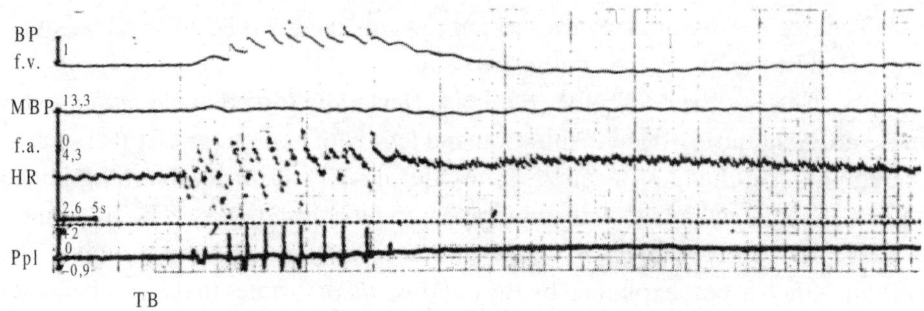

Fig. 8.1 A record of blood pressure changes obtained from the femoral vein (BP f.v.), mean blood pressure (through electronic averager), femoral artery (f.a.), heart rate (HR) and pleural pressure (Ppl) during and after a tracheobronchial cough (TB) evoked in an anaesthetised cat. (Modified from Ref. [15]).

cough efforts, fluctuations of negative / positive intrathoracic pressure and on blood pressure changes.

We studied heart rate variability during and after a cough attack in experimental animals[14,15] and in healthy volunteers.[16] In experiments on anaesthetized cats, at the beginning of a mechanically elicited cough, the positive intrathoracic pressure along with systemic arterial pressure changes, caused an enhancement of heart rate oscillations (Fig. 8.1) and a decrease in mean heart rate.

After a cough attack, there is a significant increase in heart rate (HR) along with a hypotensive effect. The HR reactions in cats without, and post-adrenergic block are shown in Figure 8.2. Beta blockade in contrast to alpha blockade inhibited the tachycardia response.

In human subjects, we found that the heart rate changes depend on the intensity of respiratory efforts. This was determined at different pulmonary volume levels at the beginning of the expiratory effort.[16] The subjects performed a single voluntary cough from functional residual capacity (FRC) and total lung capacity (TLC) levels. ECG was recorded and RR intervals were evaluated before and after cough. After a voluntary cough, the RR intervals became significantly shorter and at peak tachycardia heart rate increased noticeably between 4th and 5th RR interval. The increase in heart rate (coincident with the deep inspiration) was greater (Fig. 8.3) and longer lasting in cough from TLC, than from FRC (Fig. 8.3).

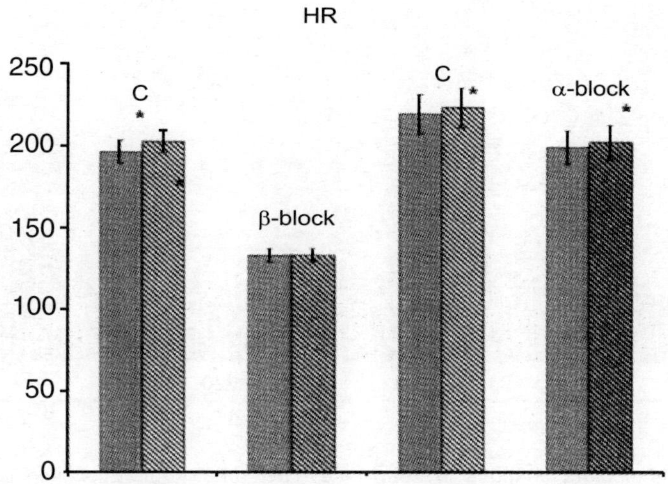

Fig. 8.2 Changes in heart rate (HR) in cats after coughing; heart rate before (grey column) and after coughing (striped columns) in untreated control animals (C) and after application of beta-(b-block) and alpha-(a-block) adrenergic blocking agents. * refers to the difference which is significant from initial values.

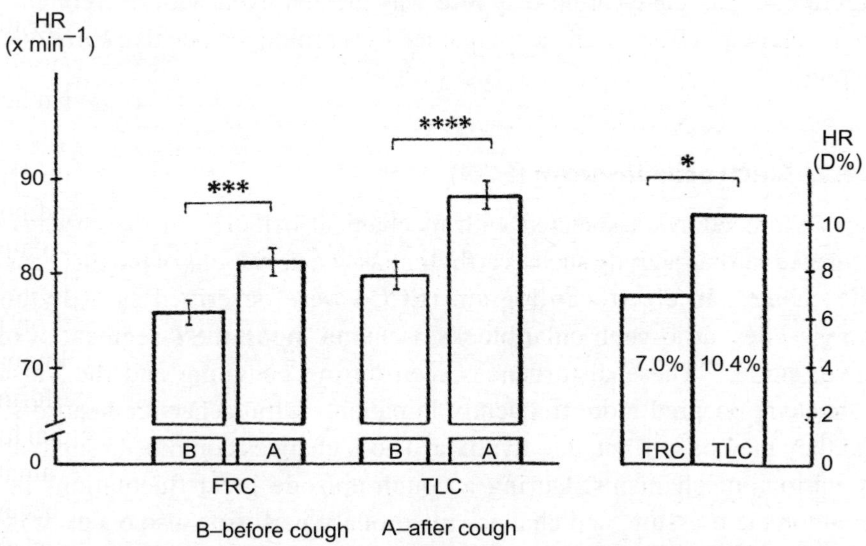

Fig. 8.3 Heart rate, HR (x min^{-1}) and per cent changes in HR (HR %) before (B) and after (A) one cough effort made from functional residual capacity (FRC) and total lung capacity) TLC levels. * $p < 0.05$. *** $p < 0.01$, **** $p < 0.001$/statistical significance of the difference between B and A values and FRC and TLC.

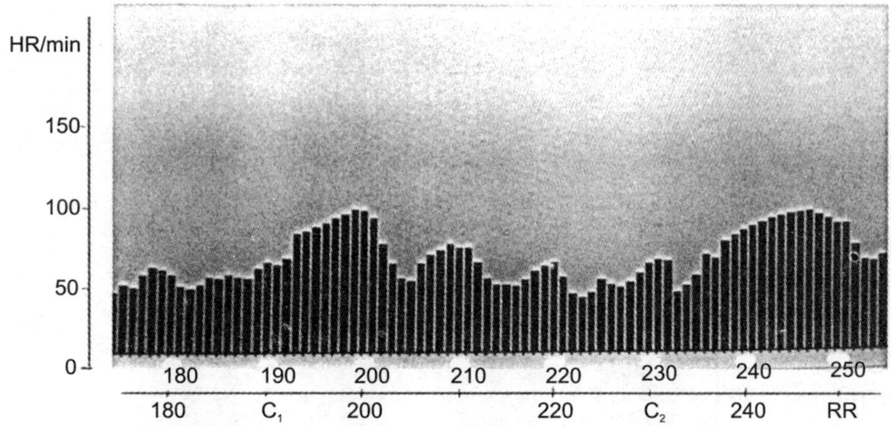

Fig. 8.4 Immediate changes in heart rate (HR) (beat-to-beat) evoked by a single voluntary cough (C_1) and by three cough efforts (C_2).

We studied the short-term variability of heart rate by means of a system known as VariaCor PF6 . The typical changes evoked immediately in resting heart rate by one or three cough bursts from the level of TLC are shown in Figure 8.4. The tachycardia response was present even with one cough, and three voluntary efforts were accompanied by a prolonged positive chronotropic response.[16]

8.4.2 Electrocardiogram (ECG)

Various procedures associated with mechanical irritation of the airways can influence cardiac activity such as arrhythmias and deviations of the ECG curves. The changes in electrocardiogram (ECG) were described as arrhythmia, extrasystoles, atrio ventricular blocks, ischemic signs of ST-segment or of T-wave, etc.[15-18] These disturbances seen during coughing and the Valsalva manoeuvre occured more frequently in patients with ischaemic heart disease and they may be attributed to hypoxia. These changes could be brought about by various mechanisms. During a cough episode great fluctuations in the intrathoracic pressure, and changes in coronary perfusion also occur. It is not clear whether these fluctuations are responsible for the arrhythmias.

In our experiments on anaesthetised cats, the attacks of coughing, sneezing and aspiration reflex were rarely seen (only in 5–15% of the instances) with changes in the ECG. In a majority of cases, no noteworthy changes in ECG occurred.

In our observations on healthy volunteers, coughing neither from FRC nor from TLC level was accompanied with pathological ECG changes.

8.4.3 Cardiac Output

Coughing can produce changes directly in stroke volume and in cardiac output. These variations may improve or worsen the pumping effect depending on venous return, blood flow through pulmonary circulation, or with intrathoracic pressure changes with phase of cardiac cycle. During a deep inspiration, end diastolic right ventricle volume (EDV) increases together with the enhancement of the respiratory pump effect on venous return. This leads to an increase in the right ventricle stroke volume followed by an increase in pulmonary artery blood flow. The greatest increase in the stroke volume was found at the end of a deep inspiration.[12]

A short-lasting high positive intrathoracic pressure as during the expiratory phase of coughing, acts on all structures inside the thorax. If the ventricles eject blood at the same time, the final effect is a result of summation of the pressures involved. Intrathoracic pressure is transmitted to the heart chambers and results in enhancing the force produced by the myocardium. However, this increase in the positive intrathoracic pressure also squeezes the intrathoracic vessels thereby increasing the afterload on the right ventricle and diminishing the overall effect.

The final result of the influence of an increase in positive intrathoracic pressure on cardiac functions, depends on the extent of its increase, the duration of expiratory phase, velocity of pressure changes as well as the timing of its change with reference to the phase of the cardiac cycle. If positive intrathoracic pressure is relatively stable (e.g. during artificial ventilation with positive-end expiratory pressure (PEEP) or in spontaneous breathing with continuous positive airway pressure (CPAP), its final effect is a decrease in the stroke volume and cardiac output (Scheme 8.1).[19]

However, if the increase in intrathoracic pressure is sudden and large and occurs at the beginning of the ejection phase of the cardiac cycle, it can improve stroke volume by 25 to 50 per cent as well as the pumping efficiency of the ventricles.[20,21] An influence of positive intrathoracic pressure on cardiovascular structures in the thorax can be seen not only during coughing, but also during high frequency intermittent positive pressure ventilation (HF IPPV) and jet ventilation (HFJV).

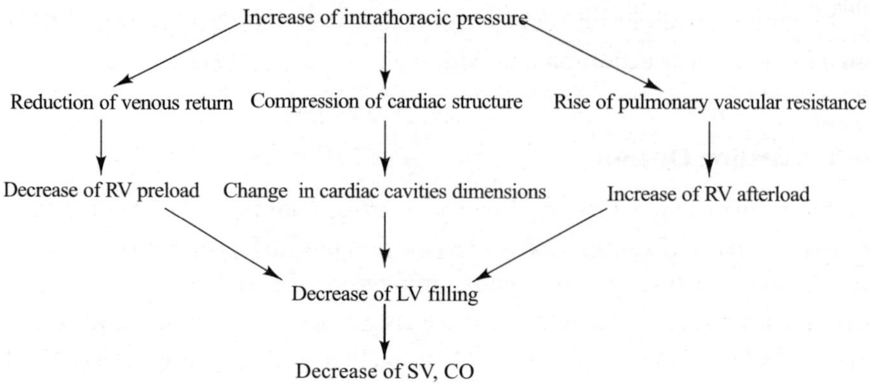

Scheme 8.1 Mechanisms and effects of constant positive intrathoracic pressure (e.g. during IPPV, combined with PEEP or with CPAP) on the cardiac pumping efficiency. RV—right ventricle, LV—left ventricle, SV— stroke volume; CO—cardiac output. (Modified from Gecelovaska V and Javorka K, 1996).[19]

The measurement of pericardial pressure in anesthetised dogs revealed a linear increment of pressure with elevation of intrathoracic pressure up to 15 cmH_2O during artificial ventilation.[22] The transmission of intrathoracic pressure occurs more readily through a thinner wall (e.g. the right ventricle). However, the right ventricle ejects blood to pulmonary circulation where the pressure is transmitted through the same mechanism, increasing both pressure and resistance in the pulmonary bed.[12,23] The effectiveness of the left ventricular pumping to the systemic bed is supported by the fact that the pressure in the extrathoracic part is normal or may even be less.[20,24] This effect was studied during high frequency jet ventilation (HFJV). If the positive intrathoracic pressure was synchronized (through ECG signal) at the end of diastole, or at early systole, the stroke volume increased.[25,26] This supporting effect of the HFJV synchronisation on cardiac output was enhanced in subjects with hypovolemia, hypotension and cardiac failure.[27]

8.5 CHANGES IN PERIPHERAL CIRCULATION

Coughing results in considerable oscillations in the peripheral blood pressure with an overall tendency towards causing hypotension. These changes are enhanced in a prolonged cough seizure, which if repeated many times, reduces venous return and central blood volume. The end diastolic volume, stroke volume and cardiac output of the left ventricle are thereby diminished. This is the reason

Table 8.1 Cardiovascular changes [HR—heart rate; BPsyst.—blood pressure systolic; BPdiast.—blood pressure diastolic; BPmean-mean blood pressure and mean blood flow (BF) in ml *x* min^{-1} per 100 g of the hindlimb evoked by mechanical stimulation of the tracheobronchial region in non-paralysed (spontaneous breathing) and paralysed anaesthetised cats. Mean values before (X_1), during stimulation (X_2) and after stimulation (X_3)—tracheobronchial coughing [only in non-paralysed cats]. Statistical significance of the difference in values (X_1) values: * $p< 0.05$, *** $p< 0.001$.

	Non-paralysed (spontaneous breathing)			Paralysed	
	X_1	X_2	X_3	X_1	X_2
HR (x min^{-1})	231.0	225.0*	241.2***	219.0	232.8***
BPsyst. (mmHg)	166	195***	143***	151	170***
BPdiast. (mmHg)	140	127***	119***	112	128***
BPmean (mmHg)	151	155*	125***	131	148***
BF				0.53	1.17***

why in a cough attack, when the expiratory efforts are dominant over inspiratory efforts there is a tendency to decrease the blood pressure and flow in aorta as well as in other peripheral arteries.

In our experiments on spontaneously breathing cats, a considerable inspiration-expiration oscillations of intrathoracic pressure were mechanically propagated, leading to marked oscillations of blood pressure in the systemic circulation. In the femoral artery, these were seen being accompanied by a sudden elevation of the systolic and a decrease of the diastolic blood pressure, but with mean blood pressure being raised (Table 8.1).

Typical changes in peripheral blood pressure registered by Finapres™ device (Ohmeda, USA) together with photoplethysmographic curves (ELCAT Germany) monitoring blood perfusion in fingers are shown in Figures 8.5 and 8.6. Each of the cough efforts is transmitted up to the finger circulation resulting in an increase in the parameters being monitored and this is seen in the expiratory phase of the cough.

Sudden changes in intrathoracic and intra-abdominal pressures are transmitted to the peripheral venous system, where they cause considerable and rapid changes in the venous blood pressure as it was seen in Figure 8.1. These rapid changes in blood pressure and flow in the veins and chambers of the heart may cause a release of venous thrombi leading to possible embolism. Mean blood pressure in venous peripheral system shows a tendency to increase as a consequence of an impairment of venous return and stagnation of blood in the veins.

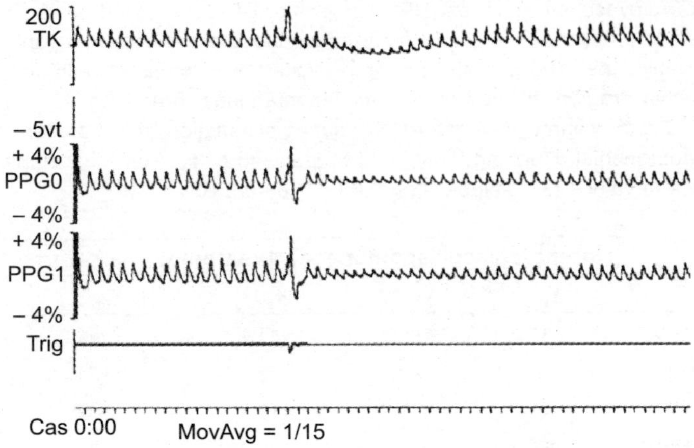

Fig. 8.5. Peripheral blood pressure (TK—upper trace) and photoplethysmographic curves (PPG0, PPG1) before, during (signal in Trig) and after one voluntary cough effort made from total lung capacity (TLC) level. Cas=time(s); mov Avg (signal processing).

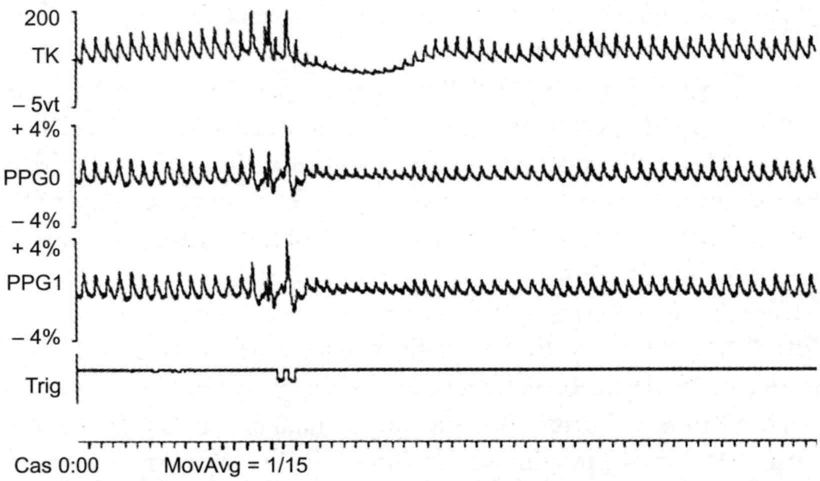

Fig. 8.6 Peripheral blood pressure (TK—upper trace) and photoplethysmographic curves (PPG0, PPG1) before, during (signal in Trig) and after three voluntary cough efforts made from total lung capacity (TLC) level.

Post-tussive reaction: After a cough attack, the peripheral systemic blood pressure decreases significantly; this hypotensive reaction is also seen in the acral circulation (Figs 8.5 and 8.6). Heart rate and blood flow in the abdominal aorta or femoral artery increase (Figs. 8.7, Table 8.1). The augmentation in blood flow can be due to mobilisation of accumulated blood in the venous system

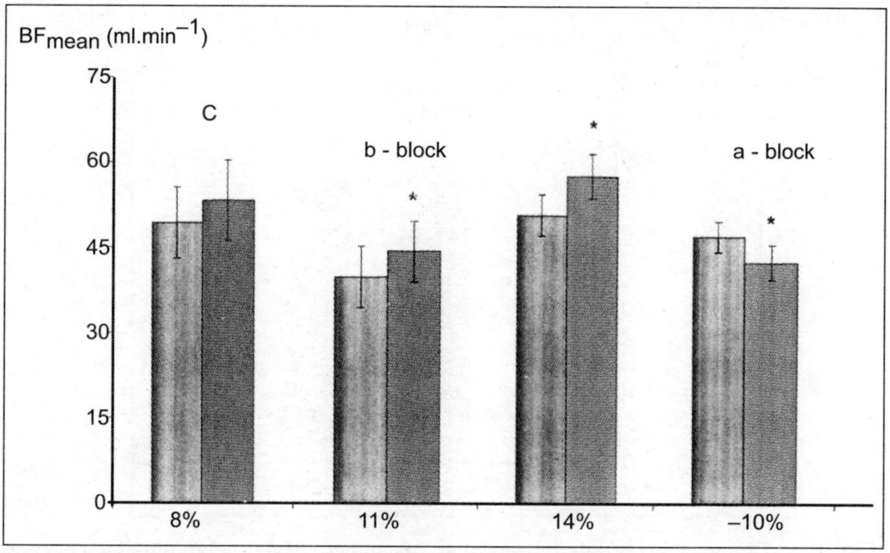

Fig. 8.7 Changes in mean aortic blood flow (BF mean) after (striped columns) coughing in cats in controls (C) and after application of beta - (b-block) and alpha - (a-block) adrenergic blocking agents. * -significant differences from initial values (grey columns). The post-tussive increase in blood flow was blocked by the alpha-blocker.

followed by changes in stroke volume and cardiac output. A decrease in the peripheral resistance also adds to the improvement of peripheral perfusion as also seen after coughing (Fig. 8.8).

The aim of peripheral hyperperfusion could be to improve the oxygen and nutrient delivery to tissues and organs which are likely to suffer during cough attack.

8.6 CEREBRAL CIRCULATION

Noteworthy changes in blood pressure and perfusion occur in the cerebral circulation during cough. Systolic blood pressure in the common and internal carotid arteries rises sharply during the expulsive phase of coughing, but diastolic pressure usually remains unchanged.[28] Despite this rise in systolic pressure, the cerebral blood inflow diminishes. The cause of this paradox lies in the intracranial pressure changes. The cerebral circulation has a special protective mechanism against excessive distension of cerebral vessels and rupture: the rise in intracranial pressure compresses the vessels from outside. It functions as an important

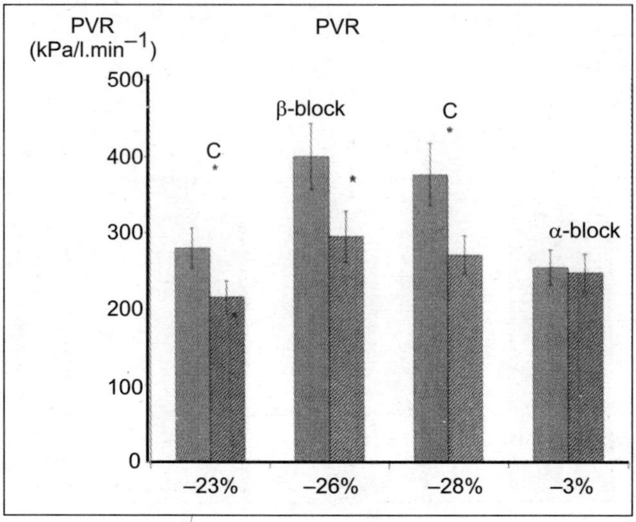

Fig. 8.8 Changes in peripheral vascular resistance (PVR) after (striped columns) coughing in cats under normal conditions (C) and after application of beta-(b-block) and alpha-(a-block) adrenergic blocking agents. It may be noted that the erstwhile post-tussive decrease in PVR after cough was inhibited by the alpha-blocker. * differences significant from initial values (grey columns).

mechanism against overdistention of the cerebral vessels thus preventing their rupture and cerebral apoplexy. This compression of the cerebral vessels during a cough prevents a rise in the transmural pressure to dangerous levels. However, small cerebral arteries, arterioles and capillaries may collapse with a great rise in intracranial pressure since the pressure inside them is at lower physiological levels. If a cough attack lasts for a long period, then the systolic and diastolic pressure in the carotid arteries begins to decline together with the cardiac output. Thus, cerebral perfusion may diminish and lead to cerebral hypoxia.

The fall in blood pressure and cerebral perfusion during a severe and prolonged cough attack may cause fainting, i.e. post-tussive or cough syncope.[29-32] Cough syncope can be seen mainly in middle-aged men in whom intrathoracic pressure can attain very high positive values. Susceptible subjects may have impaired vision at the height of a cough seizure and may lose temporary consciousness, i.e. for 1–2 s. Consciousness returns approximately in 10 s and the whole episode may last up to about 30 s. The attack can also be accompanied by clonic convulsions.

The main mechanism of cough syncope is thought to occur though changes in cerebral circulation. This occurs as a result of cardiovascular changes producing intermittent cerebrovascular insufficiency by means of a decrease in cerebral blood flow especially when it cannot be elevated to values necessary to meet the brain metabolic needs. The development of cough syncope may be contributed by several other factors such as peripheral vasodilation, collapse mechanism limiting venous return, reflex bradycardia, pulmonary vasoconstriction, decrease in cardiac output, and elevation of intracranial pressure.

Changes in arterial blood gas tensions during coughing may also play a role in the development of cough syncope. Coughing as a short hyperventilation can be accompanied by hypocapnia.[33] A fall in $PaCO_2$ has a constrictor effect on cerebral vessels and this cerebral vasoconstriction could be an important factor leading to the production of cough syncope.

In the post-tussive phase in rabbits, Murin[31] found that the cerebral inflow through carotid arteries was increased (on average from 9.2 to 12.0 ml/min), and this effect persisted for about 40 s.

8.7 PULMONARY CIRCULATION

During coughing, the pulmonary circulation, due to its location in the thorax, is affected by mechanical and other means. The systolic blood pressure in the pulmonary artery during preparation of a deep inspiration falls and in the expiratory phase it rises, but this depends on the prevailing intrathoracic pressure. The mean blood pressure in the pulmonary artery falls during coughing, especially when large inspiratory efforts are made. Pulmonary vascular resistance rises during coughing in cats not only in the expiratory phase but also in the inspiratory phase and is dependent on the lung volume.[12] This phenomenon can be explained by lengthening and narrowing of the pulmonary vessels. Though blood flow through pulmonary artery changes with the different phases of cough, its overall value shows a decrease.

During tracheobronchial coughing, when inspiratory efforts are not so deep the blood flow through the pulmonary artery in the expiratory phase increases.[12] Blood is diverted to the left atrium and left ventricle in the expiratory phase and central blood volume drops. In a prolonged cough attack, the resistance against inflow from the right ventricle increases and the return to the left atrium diminishes sharply.

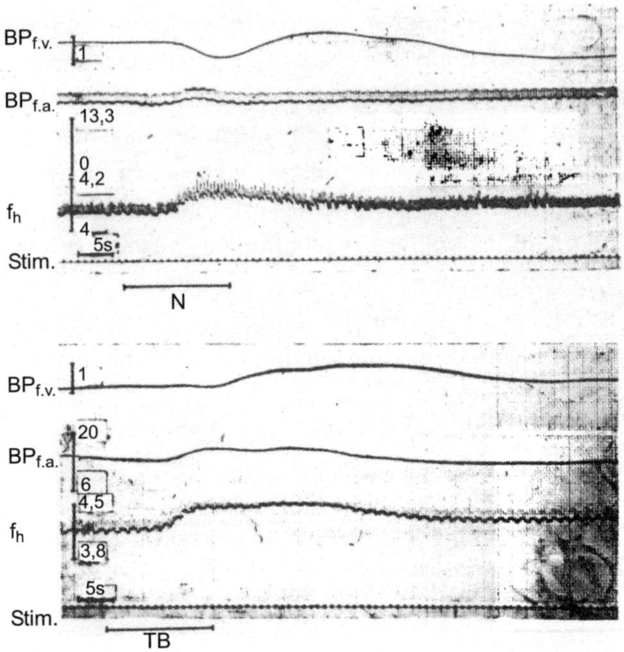

Fig. 8.9 Blood pressure in femoral vein ($BP_{f.v.}$), in femoral artery ($BP_{f.a.}$) and instantaneous heart rate (f_h) during and after mechanical stimulation (Stim.) of nasal (N) and tracheobronchial (TB) mucosa in anaesthetised, paralysed, artificially ventilated cat. (Modified from Ref. [15]).

8.8 MECHANISMS OF CARDIOVASCULAR CHANGES

Cardiovascular changes during coughing are produced by a combination of mechanical, reflex and chemical factors.

8.8.1 Mechanical Effects

Mechanical effects such as large fluctuations in intrathoracic, intra-abdominal and intracranial pressures evoked by respiratory muscle activity, are the dominant mechanisms of cardiovascular change at a glance. Seen during a cough attack a sudden increase or decrease in intrathoracic and intra-abdominal pressures can cause a reduction in venous return, changes in blood pressure and flow in different parts of circulation as well as that in the intracranial pressure. The pathway of how mechanical effects can produce cardiovascular changes has been described in the preceding section.

8.8.2 Reflex Effects

The reflex mechanisms are mediated by baroreflexes and generalised somatosympathetic reflex.

Baroreflexes: These are mainly involved in controlling blood pressure and flow in spontaneous breathing subjects, but they also produce their influence during cough which is seen as a vasodilation, by stimulation of high-pressure baroreceptors by sudden increases in arterial blood pressure during its expulsive phases. However, it was reported by Murin[31] that this post-tussive hypotensive effect can also be seen after denervation of the carotid sinuses and the aortic arch and that it was more prolonged than before. It seems that along with post-tussive baroreflex action there are other mechanisms (e.g. low-pressure intrathoracic baroreceptors) that contribute to these reflex changes.

The role of somatosympathetic reflexes has been studied in paralysed, artificially ventilated animals. Stimulation of the airways does not evoke ventilatory responses and mechanical effects in this experimental model, but primary reflex cardiovascular (and other) effects mediated through the ANS and humoral factors can be seen in a modified form. This model was used by Tomori and Widdicombe in 1969.[34] Mechanical stimulation of the airways evoked in paralysed and artificially ventilated cats produced marked tachycardia and hypertensive effects in the systemic arterial circulation.

In our experiments[14,15] on paralyzed and artificially ventilated animals, the stimulation of the airways evoked the above effect. In addition, it was also accompanied by vasoconstriction and thus a fall in blood pressure in the corresponding vein (Table 8.1, Fig. 8.9). This peripheral vasoconstriction lasted considerably longer than the reflex tachycardia and it was more marked when elicited by stimulation of the nasal mucosa in comparison to the lower airways.

In another group of anaesthetised cats, we studied the role of the sympathetic innervation on the circulatory changes produced by coughing. Figure 8.2 illustrates the block of post-tussive tachycardia by Trimepranol, a beta-adrenergic blocking agent in cats. From this, it is apparent that the beta-adrenergic system plays a significant role in the post-tussive tachycardia that is seen in cats. But whether or not a beta-block would inhibit this effect in humans has not been investigated, though it must be kept in mind that in contrast to most experimental animals; in them, the sinoatrial node is under dominant parasympathetic tone.

On the other hand, the block of alpha-adrenergic sympathetic innervation does not produce an increase in blood flow in the aorta (Fig. 8.7) and reduces the extent of fall in peripheral vascular resistance that is normally seen after cough (Fig. 8.8).

An important role of the sympathetic nervous system in post-tussive reactions (hypotension, bradycardia) was shown by Tomori and Widdicombe.[34] They found that discharge in cervical sympathetic nerves is diminished during the post-tussive phase.

In clinical practice, artificially ventilated patients often undergo procedures associated with mechanical stimulation of airways. There are reports of transient changes in the heart rate and short-lasting hypertension during laryngoscopy, intubation and suctioning of mucus from the airways.[35–37] General anaesthesia can significantly affect the cardiovascular functions and these largely depend on the type of anaesthetics used.[38]

8.8.3 Humaral Factors

Mechanical stimulation of the airways accompanied by ventilatory changes results in blood gas changes and an increase in secretion of some humoral substances.

Cough evoked experimentally in healthy cats represents hyperventilation. This causes a significant fall in $PaCO_2$ and a rise in PaO_2 and pHa after about 10 s from the onset of attack. Hypocapnia may trigger the development of a hypotensive reaction through a decrease in the vascular tone in the peripheral circulation. A special and strong effect of hypocapnia is in cerebral circulation were it evokes vasoconstriction. Russell et al[39] found that during endotracheal intubation in adult humans, the level of circulating catecholamines increases. It is likely that this would facilitate the sympathetic activity and contribute to vasoconstriction and tachycardia during mechanical stimulation of the airways as seen in artificially ventilated subjects.

Endothelial vasomotor substances: With cough, sudden changes in blood pressure (lateral and transmural) and blood flow occur. These actions can evoke changes in the synthesis and secretion of different endothelial vasomotor active substances; their role, however, has as yet not been studied.

8.9 PERSPECTIVES AND CLINICAL IMPLICATIONS

Besides the above-described cardiovascular effects of coughing, there could possibly be several others. To discover these, it is necessary that we utilise newer methods of investigation, e.g. continuous registration of blood pressure, peripheral and central perfusions, determination of different hormones and other substances. With these modern methods, one will be able to describe local changes in blood circulation and contribute to the understanding of pathological disorders like syncope, stroke or embolism during and after coughing.

At present, we have no idea about any other possible (positive) effects on the cardiovascular system, that coughing may have. It is very likely that coughing may, through enhancement of heart-rate variability, coordinate the activities of the respiratory and cardiovascular systems under different conditions. Enhanced respiratory sinus arrhythmia may help to maintain mean blood pressure and diminish energy expenditure by supressing unnecessary heartbeats during expiration[40] also in the special situation of coughing. Enhanced RSA may have a positive effect via harmonisation of the ventilation/perfusion match. Thus, the cardiovascular effects of coughing are not just passive consequences but may also have an important physiological role.

Petelenz and co-workers[41,42] have put forward a suggestion that voluntary cough could be utilised to produce cardiovascular changes for cardio-pulmonary-cerebral self-resuscitation (cough CPR). According to them, during a sudden arrhythmia subjects could be made to cough voluntarily and forcefully so as to maintain a sufficient blood flow to the brain. This idea is not entirely new. Criley et al[43] described successful resuscitation of patients undergoing coronary angiography from ventricular fibrillation by making them cough for up to one to three seconds. It seems the cough CPR can support circulation in certain cases where patients have abnormal heart rhythms and by coughing, compression of the heart by respiratory muscles ('internal heart massage') through intermittent and high-positive intrathoracic pressure, can help normalise them. This technique has been found to be useful in clinical situations, particularly during cardiac catheterisation under professional supervision.

8.10 CONCLUSION

The cardiovascular effects and mechanisms during coughing are complex processes, and research in this area/topic is of great importance. The clarification of different factors and their role in the development of cardiovascular effects during coughing will enable one not only to better understand the physiological mechanisms but also put forward simple preventive methods and treatment of their disorders.

REFERENCES

1. Widdicombe JG. Afferent receptors in the airways and cough. Respiration Physiology, 1998;114:5–15.
2. Widdicombe JG: Airway receptors. Respiration Physiology, 2001;125:3–15.
3. Mazzone SB. Sensory regulation of the cough reflex. Pulmonary Pharmacology Therapy, 2004;17:361–8.
4. Paintal AS. Vagal sensory receptors and their reflex effects.Physiological Reviews, 1973;53:159–226.
5. Dehghani GA, Sharif-Kazemi MB, Parvizi MR, Anand A., Paintal AS: A comparison of respiratory (J) sensations induced by intravenous lobeline injection and produced by exercise in subjects with coronary artery disease. Archives Iranian Medicine, 2005;8(1):36–44.
6. Jakus J., Tomori Z., Stransky A. Neuronal determinants of breathing, coughing and related motor behaviours. Martin, Wist, 2004;333.
7. Richter DW, Spyer KM, Gilbey MP, Lawson EE, Bainton CR, Wilhelm Z. On the existence of a common cardiorespiratory network. In: Koepchen HP, Huopaniemi T, editors. Cardiorespiratory and motor coordination. Berlin: Springer Verlag, 1991;pp118–30.
8. Sant´Ambrogio G, Widdicombe JG. Respiratory reflexes acting on the diaphragm and respiratory intercostal muscles of the rabbit. Journal of Physiology (London), 1965;180:766–9
9. Han JN., Gayan-Ramirez G., Dekhuijzen R., Decramer M.: Respiratory function of the rib cage muscles. European Respiratory Journal, 1993;6(5):722–8.
10. Langlands J. The dynamics of cough in health and in chronic bronchitis. Thorax 1967;22:88–96.
11. Sharpey-Schafer EP. Effects of coughing on intrathoracic pressure, arterial pressure and peripheral blood flow. Journal of Physiology (London), 1953;122:351–7.
12. Samseli A, Ivanco I, Murin M. Plucna cievna rezistencia pri pokojnom dychani a kasli u maciek. Ceskoslovenska Fysiologie, 1976;25:23–6.
13. Agostoni E, Rahn H. Abdominal and thoracic pressures at different lung volumes. Journal of Applied Physiology, 1960;15:1087–92.
14. Javorka K, Tomori Z. Kardiovaskularne efekty pri dra•dení hornych dychacich ciest. Ceskoslovenska Fysiologie, 1978;27:167–70.
15. Tomori Z, Javorka K. Cardiovascular effects due to the mechanical stimulation of the airways. Folia Medica Martiniana, 1981–1982;7–8:27–39.
16. Javorka K, Tomori Z, Kulišek V. Cardiovascular effects of coughing. Bulletin of European Physiopathology Respiratoire, 1987;23:64.
17. Urbach JR., Grauman JJ, Straus SH. Effects of inspiration, expiration, and apnoea upon pacemaking and block in atrial fibrillation. Circulation, 1970;42:261–70.
18. Salmi HJ, Takkanen J, Savolainen VP, Pyörälä K. Electrocardiographic changes during bronchoscopy. Annals of Clinical Research, 1972;4:89–94.
19. Gecelovska V, Javorka K. Cardiovascular and haemodynamic changes during artificial ventilation of the lungs. Bratislavske Lekarske Listy, 1996;97:260–6.
20. Pinsky MR, Summer WR, Wise RA, Permutt S, Bromberger-Barnea B. Augmentation of cardiac function by elevation of intrathoracic pressure. Journal of Applied Physiology, 1983;54:950–5.

21. Niemann JT, Rosborough JP, Niskanen RA, Alferness C, Criley J.M. Mechanical "cough" in cardiopulmonary resuscitation during cardiac arrest in dogs. American Journal of Cardiology, 1985;55:199–204.
22. Cabrera MR, Nakamura GE, Montague DA, Cole RP. Effect of airway pressure on pericardial pressure. American Review of Respiratory Diseases, 1989;140:659–67.
23. Ivanco I, Samseli A. Venozny navrat cez dolnu dutu zilu pri kasli a paroxyzmalnom inspiracnom usili. Ceskoslovenska. Fysiologie, 1970;19: 233–4.
24. Bradley TD, Holloway RM, McLaughlin PR, Roos BL, Walters J, Liu PP. Cardiac output response to continuous positive airway pressure in congestive heart failure. American Review of Respiratory Diseases, 1992;145:377–82.
25. Gotshall RW, Miles DS, Sexson WR, Spohn WA, Courtney SE. Oscillatory cardiopulmonary effects of high frequency jet ventilation. Respiration, 1986;49:283–91.
26. Matuschak GM, Pinsky MR, Klain M. Hemodynamic effects of synchronous high-frequency jet ventilation during acute hypovolemia. Journal of Applied Physiology, 1986;61:44–5.
27. Pinsky M.R. Ventricular support by synchronized jet ventilation. Applied Cardiopulmonary Pathophysiology, 1990;3:235–45.
28. Murin M, Ivanco I. Dynamika prietokovych zmien v mozgu pri pokojnom dychaní. Ceskoslovenska Fysiologie, 1975;24:443–6.
29. Hamilton WF, Woodbury RA, Harper HT. Arterial, cerebrospinal and venous pressures in man during cough and strain. American Journal of Physiology, 1944;141:42–50.
30. Sharpey-Schafer E.P. The mechanism of syncope after coughing. British Medical Journal, 1953;2:860–3.
31. Murin M. Sucasny stav nazorov na vznik kaslovej synkopy. Sbornik Prac (Kosice), 1970;13:151–9.
32. Korpas J, Tomori Z. Cough and other respiratory reflexes. Karger, 1979;pp356.
33. Tomori Z, Sedikova V, Javorka K. Changes in blood gas tensions and acid-base balance during respiratory reflexes. Physiologia Bohemoslovaca, 1973;22:305–14.
34. Tomori Z, Widdicombe JG. Muscular, bronchomotor and cardiovascular reflexes elicited by mechanical stimulation of the respiratory tract. Journal of Physiology (London), 1969;200:25–49.
35. Burman SO. Bronchoscopy and cardiorespiratory reflexes. Annals of Surgery, 1963;57:134–41.
36. Suzuki M, Kirchner JA. Laryngeal reflex pathways related to rate and rhythm of the heart. Annals (St.Louis) 1967;76:1–7.
37. Corbett JL, Kerr JH, Prys-Roberts C. Cardiovascular responses to aspiration of secretions from the respiratory tract in man. Journal of Physiology (London), 1969;201:51P–52P.
38. Lindgren L, Saarnivaara L. Cardiovascular responses to tracheal intubation in small children. British Journal of Anaesthesia, 1985;57:1183–7.
39. Russell WJ, Morris RG, Frewin DB, Drew SE. Changes in plasma catecholamine concentrations during endotracheal intubation. British Journal of Anaesthesia, 1981;53:837–40.
40. Hayano J, Yasumo F, Okada A, Mukai S, Fujinami T. Respiratory sinus arrhythmia: a phenomenon improving pulmonary gas exchange and circulatory efficiency. Circulation, 1996;94:842–7.

41. Petelenz T, Iwinski J, Chelbowczyk J, Czyk Z, Flak Z, Fiutowski L, Zaorski K, Petelenz T, Zeman S. Self-administered cough cardiopulmonary resuscitation (c-PR) in patients threated by MAS events of cardiovascular origin. Wiadomosci Lekarske 1998;51:326–36.
42. Petelenz T, Criley JM, Petelenz TJ. Cough cardiopulmonary resuscitation: a life-saving strategy for patients at high risk of sudden circulatory arrest. European Heart Journal, 2003;24:729P.
43. Criley JM, Blufuss JH, Kissel GL. Cough-induced cardiac compression. Self-administered form of cardiopulmonary resuscitation. JAMA—Journal of the American Medical Association, 1976;236:1246–50.

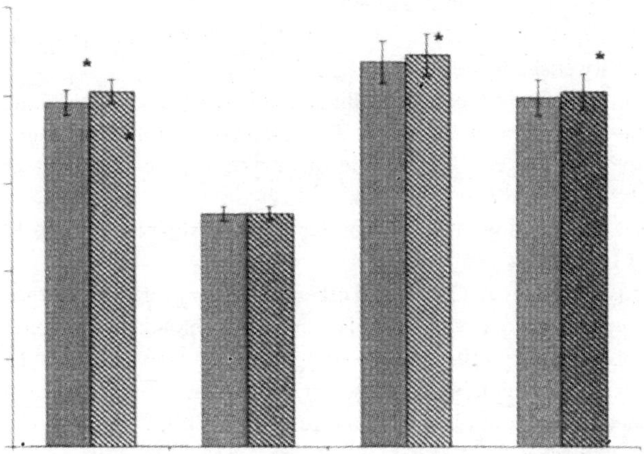

9 The Significance of Dry Cough

Ashima Anand, AS Paintal

9.1 INTRODUCTION

One of the better known functions of cough is to prevent entry of inhaled foreign material into the lungs by means of a forced expulsion. It is this reflex manoeuvre that prevents particles of food or water lodged inadvertently in the trachea, from travelling down any further. Cough, by this mechanism, is produced by stimulation of sensory receptors in the larynx and the tracheo bronchial tree (upper respiratory tract).[1,2] Other pulmonary receptors, such as the rapidly adapting pulmonary stretch receptors or "irritant" receptors, though activated by extraneous material such as irritant gases and cigarette smoke, do not actually give rise to cough in man as no cough arises when they are stimulated by their natural stimulus. This is concluded from the following demonstration. By forcefully and repeatedly deflating the lungs from functional residual capacity to about 120/min, a stimulation with which one would expect to produce an intense activity in these receptors (being a well-established stimulus in animals[3] does not however, produce a cough or even sensations of irritation in the throat. On the other hand, they produce a feeling of relief from breathlessness.[4,5]

Nevertheless, physicians have tacitly assumed that all kinds of cough arise from the pharynx and the upper airways by irritation or stimulation of the epithelium due to inflammation or the presence of accumulated secretions produced by bacterial or viral infections. This is not correct as it is also well known that cough is also produced at the alveolar level by the juxtapulmonary capillary (J) receptors.[6,7]

9.2 JUXTAPULMONARY CAPILLARY (J) RECEPTORS

The J receptors having been named so because they lie near the pulmonary capillaries in the lung parenchyma. This was at first evident from the short latencies with which the receptors were stimulated in response to right atrial or intravenous (IV) injections of appropriate chemicals or drugs. These are as short as 2.5 seconds in cats and dogs and 1 second in rats.[8-11] Further evidence was available with the presence of nerve endings surrounded by collagen tissue near the pulmonary capillaries in the electron micrographs of mouse,[12] rat[13] and human lung tissue.[14] They are innervated by vagal endings, 80 per cent of which are non-myelinated or C fibres (i.e., conduction velocities less than 2.5 m/second) and the remaining 20 per cent, by A-delta or myelinated fibres (conduction velocity above 2.5 m/s).[15-17] Thus, not all sensory endings innervating the J receptors are of the C-fibre type; and, therefore, it is inappropriate to refer sensory receptors with these characteristics as C fibres.

9.2.1 Stimuli and Reflex Effects of Receptors

In animals, stimulating the J receptors with chemicals gives rise to respiratory reflexes (tachypnoea, alternating with apnoea or vice-versa). In man similar reflexes are produced, when lobeline is injected intravenously and are also accompanied by irritating sensations in the throat and upper chest (Fig. 9.1). The J receptors are stimulated during interstitial congestion produced by pulmonary oedema.[10,18] In other words, the underlying stimulus is an increase in interstitial volume.[19] They are also significantly stimulated by an increase in blood flow through the lungs,[20] i.e., the cardiovascular response accompanying exercise.[21] Since the J receptors are stimulated during pulmonary congestion and even more intensely during pulmonary oedema, and as pulmonary capillary pressure rises during exercise, it was predicted that they might, therefore, terminate exercise. In anaesthetised animals stimulating the J receptors with chemicals, the monosynaptic reflexes; in awake freely moving ones, it dramatically stops the walking movements.[22-24]

Cough in response to injecting the alkaloid lobeline into humans intravenously, is well known.[25] It was assumed to have arisen by the stimulation of carotid chemoreceptors and the time of its appearance was used for determining the speed of circulation in a variety of patients with heart disease.[26-28] In 1995, Raj et al.[29] demonstrated that the only sensory receptor with a vagal innervation that could have produced this cough was the J receptor. This conclusion was

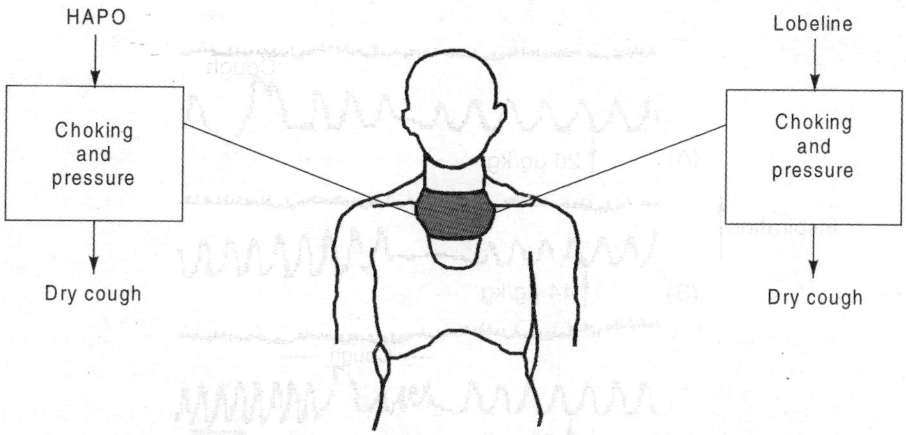

Fig. 9.1 Nature of J receptor-induced sensations and regions where they are felt after injections of lobeline or during high-altitude pulmonary oedema (HAPO). Darker shading indicates greater intensity of sensations. Intensification of sensations leads to dry cough.

arrived at by confirming that neither type of the pulmonary stretch receptors (SARs or RARs) could have contributed to the lobeline cough. That the lobeline cough was of pulmonary vagal origin was revealed by a study of bilateral lung transplant patients[30] into whom, injecting lobeline IV neither evoked respiratory reflexes including cough nor did they report the characteristic sensations in the upper chest. This was obvious in the case of patients who had received their transplants just about 2 weeks before the study (i.e. too early for re-innervation) and clearly ruled out the origin of lobeline-induced cough from carotid receptors.

9.3 DRY COUGH IN HIGH ALTITUDE PULMONARY OEDEMA

The knowledge that natural stimulation of J receptors leads to the genesis of cough in man was arrived at by comparing the effects of lobeline with those of high-altitude pulmonary oedema (HAPO).[31] Since in animals the J receptors are markedly stimulated during pulmonary oedema,[10,32] it is likely that they must also be stimulated in man during pulmonary oedema. Information available from soldiers indeed pointed out to this being the case. In a reinvestigation of the data obtained from healthy young soldiers who had HAPO, were afebrile and had no evidence of any respiratory infection; it was found that cough was reported by 96 per cent of them; and in 72 per cent of them, it was of the dry type (Fig. 9.1). It may be pointed out that the dry cough produced by natural stimulation of J

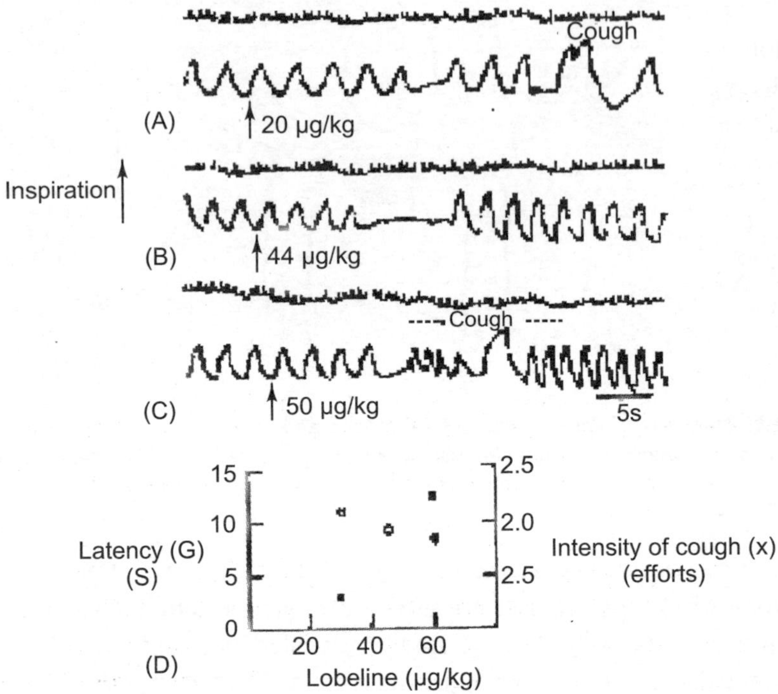

Fig. 9.2 Effect of injecting lobeline IV on the respiration of a spontaneously breathing comatose subject to increasing dose of lobeline. (A) With the least dose (26 μg/kg) a short-lasting apnoea appeared after a latency of 12 s and preceded the cough whose duration was 6 s and occurred with an intensity 1.3 'efforts'/s. Doubling this dose (C) decreased the latency of the respiratory response from 12 s to 8s and the intensity of the cough increased to 2.3 'efforts'/s (B) An intermediate dose (44 μg/kg) gave rise to a prolonged apnoea (8 s) after 9 s and was followed by an increase in control Rf from 26 to 34/s. Traces from top to bottom in each record are of ecg and pneumogram. (D) Illustrates the relationship of increasing doses of lobeline (A–C) to (i) the latency of appearance of the respiratory reflex (o) and (ii) to its intensity (x). (Reproduced from Ref. [7] with permission from Publisher]).

receptors (see above) is indistinguishable from the common cough produced by irritation of the upper respiratory tract during infection. The former, however, is accompanied by breathlessness and muscle weakness which is absent in the case of cough generated by pathophysiological conditions confined to the upper airways.

9.4 REFLEX ORIGIN OF COUGH FROM J RECEPTORS

Since lobeline also produces irritating sensations in the throat and chest which normally precede cough, investigators have been of the view that the 'coughing' especially with higher doses, which would have produced an intensification of these sensations, was a conscious attempt to get rid of them, i.e., much like clearing of the throat.

But the observation that in some subjects cough could be produced by small doses (threshold) of lobeline which would have produced only minimal-intensity sensations and not intense enough to got rid of, put in doubt the above conclusion. This controversy was resolved in a study published by Raj et al.[7] who studied unconscious individuals (comatose or anaesthetised) and found that lobeline produced the characteristic, distinct cough in all of them. Cough in response to intravenous lobeline persisted in all subjects into whom it was injected and also those under thiopental anaesthesia. Thus, this confirmed its origin as a reflex and one whose intensity increased with the stimulus, i.e. in this case, the dose of lobeline (Fig. 9.2). The above evidence has thus established that stimulation of J receptors does indeed give rise to a dry unproductive cough reflexely.

9.5 UNDERLYING STIMULUS FOR ALVEOLAR COUGH

It is well recognized that persistent, unproductive cough (dry) may be the only important clinical sign of left ventricular insufficienc, e.g., as in left ventricular failure, pulmonary hypertension and mitral stenosis.[33] It is accompanied by breathlessness and muscle weakness. It is also well known to be associated with acute mountain sickness and high-altitude pulmonary oedema.[31] Dry cough is not only a characteristic symptoms in human patients of left ventricular insufficiency but also in animals. It is reported in dogs with clear evidence of mitral stenosis[34] and in horses with congestive heart failure.[35]

In patients with left ventricular dysfunction (LVD), a natural stimulation of J receptors would be expected to occur due to transient interstitial oedema.[34] It is also likely that the level of stimulation would be enhanced during mild–moderate exercise by the increased cardiac output.[36] In the cat, increasing pulmonary blood flow by 133 per cent (i.e. to twice cardiac output) stimulated the normally silent J receptors to a level of 0.75 impulses/second (mean) which is sufficient to produce marked respiratory and somatic reflexes.[9,20] In a recent study, Dehghani et al[37] reported that moderate exercise in patients with left ventricular dysfunction produced not only lobeline-like irritating sensations (heat, burning) in their throat and upper chest, but also cough. In healthy subjects with no evidence of cardiac disease, comparable levels of exercise neither produced a cough nor a noteworthy appearance of lobeline-like sensations. However, the most notable observation in this study was that a majority of patients found a similarity between one or two lobeline sensations and those that are felt while exercising. While using target heart rate (THR) as a means of imposing equivalence in exercise, it was not surprising that this level (though similar), did not evoke noteworthy sensations in 50 per cent of healthy individuals, nor did more than 40 per cent of them, found more than one sensation to be alike. The underlying presence of natural stimuli of J receptors in LVD patients during exercise and the similarity of respiratory sensations and cough evoked by it, to those of lobeline IV suggests that they have a common origin i.e. the J receptors.

9.6 WHAT DOES DRY COUGH SPECIFY?

Dry cough with lobeline is known to be indicative of a greater level of J receptor stimulation.[28,29,37,38] Its presence thus, with modest level of exercise in patients, would also imply a greater level of J receptor stimulation. Although it is to be expected that J receptors would be stimulated in all individuals with exercise they may be stimulated to a greater degree and at a lower workload in the presence of left ventricular dysfunction. Thus, episodes of dry cough and sensations in the throat and upper chest in relation to exercise must not be overlooked as they indicate underlying pulmonary congestion. A close appraisal of these sensations and cough could be useful in identifying patients of latent or early heart disease. This would be important to keep in mind that when individuals hitherto undiagnosed for heart disease have a dry cough, or report experiencing sensations like heat, swelling or pressure in their throat and chest with exercise as moderate as climbing stairs or running short distances as for catching a bus or a train. It would be especially worthy of taking note if cough and these symptoms appear, every time the same level of exercise is undertaken.

REFERENCES

1. Sant'Ambrogio G. Afferent pathways of the cough reflex. Clinical Research in Physiology 1987;23(Suppl. 10):19s–23s.
2. Sant'Ambrogio G, Sant'Ambrogio FM. Role of laryngeal afferents in cough. Pulmonary Pharmacology, 1996:9;309–3114.

3. Widdicombe JG. Respiratory reflexes from the trachea and bronchi of the cat. Journal of Physiology 1954;123:55–74.
4. Fowler WS. Breaking point of breath-holding. Journal of Applied Physiology. 1954;6:539–45.
5. Flume PA, Eldridge FL, Edwards LJ, Houser LM. Relief of distress of breath holding: separate effects of expiration and inspiration. Respiration Physiology 1995;101:41–6.
6. Lazlo O. Respiratory Medicine. In: Read AE, Barrett DW, Langton HR, editors. Modem Medicine. Tunbridge Wells: Pitman Medical Publishing Co. Ltd., 1984;pp361–416.
7. Raj H, Bakshi OS, Tiwari RR, Anand A, Paintal AS. How does lobeline injected intravenously produce a cough? Respiratory Physiology & Neurobiology 2005;14579–90.
8. Coleridge JCG, Coleridge HM. Afferent vagal C-fiber innervation of the lungs and airways and its functional significance. Reviews in Physiology, Biochemistry & Pharmacology 1984;99:1–110.
9. Paintal AS.Impulses in vagal afferent fibres form specific pulmonary deflation receptors. The response of these receptors to phenyl digunaide, potato starch, 5-hydroxytryptamine and nicotine, and their role in respiratory and cardiovascular reflexes. Quarterly Journal of Experimental Physiology 1955;40:89–111.
10. Paintal AS.Mechanism of stimulation of type J pulmonary receptors. Journal of Physiology 1969;203:511–32.
11. Sapru HN, Willette RN, Krieger AJ. Stimulation of Pulmonary J receptors by an enkephalin-analog. Journal of Pharmacology & Experimental Therapeutics 1981;217:228–34.
12. Hung KS, Hertweck MS, Hardy JD, Loosli CG. Innervation of pulmonary alveoli of the mouse lung: an electron microscopic study. American Journal of Anatomy 1972;135:47–496.
13. Meyrick B, Reid L. Nerves in rat intra-acinar alveoli: an electron microscopic study. Respiration Physiology, 1971;11:367–77.
14. Fox B, Bull TB, Guz A. Innervation of alveolar walls in the human lung: an electron microscopic study. Journal of Anatomy 1981;131:683–92.
15. Coleridge HM, Coleridge JCG, Luck JC. Pulmonary afferent fibres of small diameter stimulated by capsaicin and by hyperinflation of the lungs. Journal of Physiology 1965;179:248–62.
16. Dixon M, Jackson DM, Richards JM. The action of sodium cromoglycate on "C" fibre endings in the dog lung. British Journal of Pharmacology, 1980;70:11–13.
17. Russell NWJ, Trenchard D. Non-myelinated vagal lung receptors in the rabbit. Journal of Physiology 1980;300:31.
18. Coleridge HM, Coleridge JCG. Afferent vagal C-fibres in the dog lung: their discharge during spontaneous breathing, and their stimulation by alloxan and pulmonary congestion. In: Paintal AS, Gill-Kumar P, editors. Krogh Centenary Symposium on Respiratory Adaptations, Capillary Exchange and Reflex Mechanisms. New Delhi: Vallabhbhai Patel Chest Institute, 1977;pp396–406.
19. Paintal AS. Vagal sensory receptors and their reflex effects. Physiological Reviews 1973;53:159–227.
20. Anand A, Paintal AS. Reflex effects following selective stimulation of the J receptors in the cat. Journal of Physiology 1980;299:553–72.
21. Astrand PO, Cuddy TE, Saltin B, Stenberg J. Cardiac output during submaximal and maximal work. Journal of Applied Physiology 1964;10:268–274.

22. Deshpande SS, Devanandan MS.1970. Reflex inhibition of monosynaptic reflexes by stimulation of type J pulmonary endings. Journal of Physiology 1970;206:345–57.
23. Kalia M, Koepchen H-P, Paintal AS. Somatomotor and autonomous effects of type J receptors in the awake freely moving and unrestrained cats. Pflugers Archives 1973;339(Suppl.):R80.
24. Wilette RN, Gatti P, Gertner SB, Sapru HN. Pulmonary afferent stimulants in the conscious rat: opioids and phenyldiguanide. Pharmacology Biochemistry of Behaviour 1982;17:19–23.
25. Robb GP, Weiss S. The velocity of pulmonary and peripheral venous blood flow and related aspects of circulation in cardiovascular disease. American Heart Journal 1934;9:742–763.
26. Berliner K. Use of alpha lobeline for measurement of velocity of blood flow. Reflex effects following selective stimulation of the J receptors in the cat. Journal of Physiology, 1940;299:553–72.
27. Bevan JA, Murray JF. Evidence for a ventilation modifying reflex from the pulmonary circulation in man. Proceedings of the Society for Biological Medicine 1963;114:393–6.
28. Stern S, Bruderman I, Braun K. 1966. Localization of lobeline-sensitive receptors in the pulmonary circulation in man. American Heart Journal 1966;71:651–5.
29. Raj H, Singh VK, Anand A, Paintal AS. Sensory origin of lobeline-induced sensations: a correlative study in man and cat. Journal of Physiology 1995;482:235–46.
30. Butler JE, Anand A, Crawford MR, Glanville AR, McKenzie DK, Paintal AS, Taylor JL, Gandevia SC. Journal of Physiology 2001;534:583–93.
31. Paintal AS. The visceral sensations-some basic mechanisms. Progress in Brain Research 1986;67:3–19.
32. Paintal AS. The mechanism of excitation of type J receptors and the J reflex. In: Porter R, editor. Breathing. Hering-Breuer Centenary Symposium. London: Churchill, 1970;pp59–71.
33. Braunwald EWB. The physical examination. In: Braunwald EWB,editor. Heart Disease: A Textbook of Cardiovascular Medicine. Philadelphia: WB Saunders Co., 1988.
34. Lehmkuhl LB,Ware WA, Bonagawa JD. Mitral stenosis in dogs. Journal of Veterinary and Internal Medicine 1994;8:2–17.
35. Davis JL, Gardner SY, Schwabenton B, Breuhaus BA. Congestive heart failure in horses: 14 cases (1984–2001). Journal of American Veterinary Medical Association 2002;220:1512–15.
36. Dehghani GA, Parvizi MB, Sharief-Kazemi M, Raj H, Anand A, Paintal AS. 2004. Presence of lobeline-like sensations in exercising patients with left ventricular dysfunction. Respiration Physiology & Neurobiology 2004;143:9–20.
37. Gandevia SC, Butler JE, Taylor IL, Crawford MR. Absence of viscerosomatic inhibition with injections of lobeline designed to activate human pulmonary C fibres. Journal of Physiology 1998;470:85–107.
38. Jain SK, Subramanian S, Julka DB, Guz A. Search for evidence of lung chemoreflexes in man: study of respiratory and circulatory effects of phenyldiguanide and lobeline. Clinical Science 1972;42:163–77.

10 Cough in Clinic

J Plutinsky

10.1 INTRODUCTION

Although cough is a non-specific symptom, yet it is one of the most common reasons for which patients visit physicians.[1] On the other hand, smokers whose cough sensitivity is diminished, do not think that cough is an expression of disease[2] and by the time they seek the physician's advice, it is seen accompanying advanced chronic obstructive pulmonary disease[3] or bronchogenic carcinoma.

Cough can be divided into two groups: acute and chronic. Acute cough lasts for less than 3 weeks and chronic, more than 3 weeks. Additionally, it is important to know whether the cough is dry (does not produce a large amount of sputum) or, productive.[4]

Characteristically, the sputum in productive cough is tinted with colour: white, white flecked with red (haemoptysis), red with coughed-up blood and yellow, green or greenish colour when purulent. Chronic cough is a frequent and serious medical problem; it is reported from all over the world and costs health-care a lot of money. For example, in the United States more than $ 1 billion are spent annually on non-prescription antitussive medications and treatment of other associated symptoms and in the United Kingdom, the costs go up to £ 94 million.[5,6]

The underlying pathology of cough is due to either inflammation or irritation. Inflammation of the airway mucosa or lung parenchyma, small and (or) large airway obstruction by some foreign body, hypertrophy of mucosa, infiltration of mucosa and obstruction of trachea or bronchus by tumour. Inflammation can be caused by viral or bacterial infections, mechanical, physical (radiation) or chemical irritation or as a result of allergic diseases (with a wide range of causal agents).

Irritation of lungs or airways can occur during deflation or re-expansion as in pneumothorax, and a mechanical irritation of lung parenchyma could occur, during thoracoscopy or thoracentesis or chest drainage.

10.2 PRINCIPAL APPROACH TO COUGH IN CLINICAL PRACTICE AND DIAGNOSTIC PROCEDURES

Since cough can arise due to a myriad reasons, the physician must take into account the patient's personal and work history, record of allergies and nicotine use. For differential diagnosis, the results of clinical examinations such as allergy testing, chest X-ray, fibreoptic bronchoscopy, high-resolution computer tomography (HRCT), laryngological examination, and radiograph of paranasal sinuses, are necessary to know. For an accurate diagnosis, it is also important to know if the patients with cough fall into the category of acute or chronic cough or a group that does not complain about its severity. Thereafter, we can use subjective and objective methods for its diagnosis.[7] In addition to the ones mentioned above, one has also to include, family allergies and medical history, use of ACE inhibitors (angiotensin converting enzyme inhibitors) a thorough physical examination; blood examination for the number of eosinophils and IgE; sputum test (bacteriological and cytological) and any indication of malignant disease. Furthermore, examinations of the lungs and nose with a fibreoptic bronchoscope and rhinoscope, respectively (in addition to checking mucous samples for eosinophilic inflammation) are recommended. Also, the following could be undertaken, carrying out assessment for allergies by skin-prick tests and pharmacological or metacholine bronchoprovocation investigations. It may also become necessary to do 24-hr oesophageal pH monitoring and spirometry which are all of indispensable for arriving at a conclusion about the origin of cough. Additionally, findings from fibreoptic gastroscopy and procedures like echocardiography and ergometry tests can assist the physician.[8]

10.2.1 Infection Aetiology of Cough

Haemophilus influenzae and *Streptococcus pneumoniae* are the most common agents in the acute exacerbation of chronic obstructive pulmonary disease, tracheitis and (or) tracheobronchitis. *H. influenzae* and *S. pneumoniae* with *Branhamella catarrhalis* are typical causative agents of pneumonia. Pneumonia is accompanied by dry cough and sometimes with rust-coloured sputum (streptococcal pneumonia), dyspnoea and fever. An acute cough precedes viral infections which may originate with an infection of respiratory syncytial viruses, rhinovirus, coronavirus, and adenovirus. These viral infections are typically seen during autumn or spring whereas those caused by influenza and para-influenza viruses are seen mostly in the months of February and March.

Infection with *Bordatella pertussis* (whooping cough) is a disease with a broad spectrum of clinical severity, ranging from a trivial cough to the classic picture of vomiting, whooping, and apnoea with paroxysmal coughing.[9] Seen mostly in children it can, however, infect adults who come in direct contact with those who are so infected.

Tuberculosis is another example of a bacterial infection in which chronic cough is seen. The cough is dry and patients have mild fever (37.0–37.6°C) in the evenings or at night and this is accompanied by loss of weight. However, in order to confirm tuberculosis, a microscopical and microbiological examination of the sputum along with a chest X-ray and tuberculin skin test are recommended. *Mycoplasma pneumoniae* and *Chlamydia pneumoniae* could also be causative agents for chronic cough.[10] The presence of chronic cough also indicates an upper or lower respiratory tract disease, rhinitis, tonsillitis, breathlessness, headache, joint pain and diarrhoea. It is important for the physician to be informed of the presence of a respiratory infection in the patient's family or a class or group of individuals that he or she associates with. Since bacteria are present as normal resident flora in the upper respiratory tract, the aetiological role of bacteria cultured from sputum samples is unclear and treatment with antibiotics is doubtful.[11] To be able to distinguish viral from bacterial infection is difficult, without carrying out specific tests for the two. Although microbiological investigation in acute bronchitis or acute exacerbation of chronic obstructive pulmonary disease in general practice is rarely carried out, yet it is recommended that it be done so with the assistance of speciality places.

10.3 COMMON DISEASES CAUSING COUGH

The management of acute and notably chronic cough is important in the process of diagnosis and therapy in clinical practice. When one uses such a diagnostic algorithm for identifying chronic cough which in past practice has yielded success, then in a majority of cases (88–100%) the cause of chronic cough can be accurately determined.[12] As the outset we must assume that multiple reasons contribute to it; in 79 per cent patients, French and coworkers[1] found more than two causes of chronic cough.

The correct diagnosis of the aetiology of cough is necessary if treatment is to succeed. The most common causes of chronic cough are postnasal drip syndrome, bronchial asthma, gastro-esophageal reflux disease, chronic bronchitis, eosinophilic bronchitis, bronchiectasis and in some cases the use of ACE inhibitors that are used for the treatment of ischaemic heart diseases or arterial hypertension. This group presents about 95 per cent of all causes of cough and 5 per cent are constributed by other diseases such as bronchogenic carcinoma, metastatic carcinomatosis, diffuse parenchymal lung diseases, tuberculosis, aspiration of foreign body. Acute cough can also result from thoracentesis.[5,12-14] On the other hand, gastro-oesophageal reflux-associated cough and postnasal drip-induced cough are very rare but cough variant asthma and atopic cough are major causes of isolated, chronic non-productive cough in Japan.[15]

Repeated diagnostic examinations can help towards a correct diagnosis, since it has been noted that at sometimes during the course of a cough, its cause could change. The newer diagnostic methods [high-resolution computer tomography (HRCT)] and approaches (combination of examinations) are helpful in finding new signs of 'older' causes of chronic cough.[12] The failure of differential diagnosis and unsuccessful treatment could occur in about 23 per cent of patients with chronic cough.[16]

10.3.1 Postnasal Drip Syndrome

The diagnosis of postnasal drip syndrome (PNDS) induced cough can be accurately arrived at by differential diagnosis, i.e. a combination of examinations carried out clinically and in the pathology laboratory as well as results of chest or paranasal X-rays and an estimate of the effectiveness of the treatment being used.

Patients with PNDS cough to clear postnasal drainage, i.e. they have a need to clear something 'foreign' stuck in their throat or in the oropharynx. There could also be a history of an upper respiratory tract infection,[5] but in some who do not have a cough, i.e. this clinical sign, a diagnosis of PNDS cannot be ruled out. PNDS can be established only after a clinical examination, laboratory tests and treatment. In some patients, the treatment is without effect; in them, an environment irritant-induced upper respiratory disease could be considered or gastro-oesophageal reflax diseases (GERD) that can mimic

PNDS.[12] A sinus X-ray examination can, however, confirm sinusitis and a suitable treatment should follow.

In those patients who have signs of seasonal problems, testing for allergies should be carried out to confirm the presence of seasonal (intermittent) allergic rhinitis or vasomotor rhinitis. Cough with allergic rhinitis caused by medication (nasal drops: oxymetazoline) or drug (cocaine) abuse is also well known and must be kept in mind while carrying out differential diagnosis.

10.3.2 Bronchial Asthma

Although chronic cough is just one of the symptoms of bronchial asthma, in the 'cough-variant asthma', it is the only symptom (besides an increase in airway hyper-responsiveness). Thiadens et al[17] examined 221 patients who had a cough lasting for at least two weeks and identified 39 per cent of them as having bronchial asthma. In another study, the frequency of cough-variant asthma was seen in 16 to 24 per cent of the cases examined.[17,18] A frequent feature of bronchial asthma is the presence of nocturnal cough[18] and other indications are breathlessness, attacks of dyspnoea with wheezing. Typically, these are reported in the morning and after exertion; during change of weather from warm to cold and during flowering time of trees and grasses (seasonal).

For the diagnosis of bronchial asthma, besides the personal medical history of the patient and that of the relatives, it is important to know the following: presence of atopic dermatitis in childhood, allergic rhinitis, positive allergy reports, positive skin-prick tests or peripheral blood eosinophilia, IgE, eosinophils in sputum[19] a hyper-responsiveness after exposure to metacholine or histamine,[20] reversible obstruction of airways. An airflow obstruction is variable and changes spontaneously or after treatment with an inhaled b_2-agonist.[5] In differential diagnosis we must exclude eosinophilic pneumonia, allergic bronchopulmonal aspergillosis.[22,23] Also to be ruled out is cardiac asthma, which typically presents with dyspnoea and cough, especially while lying down in the evenings and may also be accompanied by a swelling of the legs.

In performing a differential diagnosis of the cough-variant asthma, it is essential to carry out the histamine or metacholine provocation test.[19] The high sensitivity of this test in patients with cough-variant asthma may be produced by the high number of P-immunoreactive nerves in mucous airway.[23] A positive provocation test is typical not only in bronchial asthma but may also in other diseases such as in cystic fibrosis.

10.3.3 Gastro-esophageal Reflux Disease

Gastro-esophageal reflux disease (GERD) commonly leads to chronic cough;[13,20,24,25] it could be considered a possible cause of chronic cough especially when the patient has other symptoms of GERD such as heartburn and regurgitation[25] or when there is an absence of sinusitis, rhinitis or bronchial asthma.[26]Besides seeing it along with the classic symptoms (see above), it is also possible to see cough along with other symptoms of GERD such as epigastric or retrosternal discomfort and chest pain.[23] While diagnosing chronic cough as being GERD-related, it is useful to keep in mind that only 20 per cent of these patients have "classic" symptoms of GERD and another 30 per cent will be identified using endoscopic evidence (of reflux oesophagitis). Although laryngitis (oedema and redness) can result from reflux,[27] but one should be careful in connecting laryngitis with GERD as the latter can also occur in the absence of oesophagitis. Clinical examinations for the confirmation of GERD, include an endoscopic examination, 24-hour monitoring of pH, radiological examination of the oesophagus and reflux scintiscaning. A definite relationship between GERD and chronic cough is not always possible and to exclude PNDS, bronchial asthma would have to be excluded (normal chest X-ray). It is recommended that for a successful treatment of GERD,[26,28] a diagnosis be undertaken only when patients have the typical clinical symptoms of GERD.

Finally, we must consider that chronic cough is the result of a combination of other reasons (allergy, PNDS), particularly if treatment for GERD had failed to eliminate them.[28]

10.3.4 Eosinophilic Bronchitis

Eosinophilic bronchitis was first described in 1989 and was defined as an airway inflammation with chronic cough (an isolated symptom) with normal spirometry values and normal methacholine airway responsiveness.[29,30] The results of these tests are important to know for an accurate diagnosis and for distinguishing it from the cough-variant bronchial asthma or even chronic obstructive bronchitis. The pathogenesis of eosinophilic bronchitis is not clear.[12]

Fujimura and coworkers[15] use the term 'atopic cough' for a cough that is characteristically dry, and is accompanied by eosinophilic tracheobronchitis, hypersensitivity without bronchial hyper-responsiveness and an absence of eosinophils in the bronchoalveolar lavage.[15,31] These patients do not have symptoms of asthma, PNDS or GERD.[30] A typical finding is the presence of eosinophils in the sputum and better still, is histological proof of eosinophilic inflammation in the bronchial wall. According to some investigators the presence of eosinophils in bronchoalveolar lavage is more conclusive.[15] For this, a sample may be taken from the bifurcation of the upper apical and posterior bronchus on the right side during fibreoptic bronchoscopy.[19] The results from the provocation test of bronchial hyperresponsiveness are different from those carried out for bronchial asthma.

This atypical cough can be treated with topical steroids with good results; however, it is recommended that in those cases that it does not work, systemic steroids could be used.[12]

10.3.5 Chronic Bronchitis

Chronic cough is also a typical symptom of chronic obstructive pulmonary disease (COPD). Most of the patients with COPD are smokers or former smokers and may even have a family history of bronchitis. A history of smoking with lung function changes (spirometric) is important for diagnosis of COPD.[5]

The main symptoms besides cough are: production of mucoid sputum, dyspnoea, subjective fever, chills, and generalised malaise.[32] During acute exacerbation of COPD, the colour of the sputum or its amount may change and the dyspnoea could worsen. In addition, the patients can have others symptoms such as rhinitis, upper respiratory tract viral infections, signs of chronic respiratory insufficiency (snoring, change of sleeping time, confusion); in the later stages of the disease, heart failure could also occur.[33]

During differential diagnosis, the presence of a wheeze, resulting probably due to an exacerbation of COPD has also to be taken into account. An exacerbation of COPD can occur due to the presence of a bacterial infection—distinguished by the presence of purulent and copious amounts of sputum. If the production of purulent sputum is seen for a long time, then the underlying cause could be bronchiectasis (see following section).

In patients with chronic bronchitis, it is not unusual to see post-tussive syncope, especially after paroxysmal coughing.[35] It must also be borne in mind that dyspnoea without productive cough could be linked to underlying cardiac disease[35] and especially if there is a history of breathlessness and which is typically seen while lying down.

10.3.6 BRONCHIECTASIS

Bronchiectasis is the irreversible dilatation of a portion of the bronchial tree.[36] Recurrent respiratory infections remain the most common cause of bronchiectasis. Other aetiologies include cystic fibrosis, ciliary dyskinesia, recent pneumonia, tuberculosis, immunodeficiency disorders, and may be associated with rheumatoid arthritis.[37] Advanced radiological imaging techniques (HRCT) have improved the ability to detect bronchiectasis. It has made it possible to identify it in patients who are asymptomatic and in patients with other diagnoses, such as rheumatoid disease and obliterative bronchiolitis.[36] A destruction of bronchial wall by inflammatory process is the result of earlier insults (inhalation of chemicals, childhood infections) and dysfunction of the host-defence system.[5] These days the occurrence of bronchiectasis is quite rare.[38]

In a large number of patients, the clinical symptoms of bronchiectasis are present along with productive cough i.e. with expectoration of purulent sputum (sometimes copious); in 25 per cent of the cases, bronchiectasis accounts for haemoptysis and may even be the reason for recurrent haemoptysis.[37] Other accompanying signs of bronchiectasis are finger clubbing, amyloidosis, neuropathy and loss of weight when exacerbation of wheezing and rhonchi occur.[36] Its diagnosis can be determined by bronchography[5] and better still with HRCT examinations. Bronchiectasis is not related to any specific change in pulmonary functioning.[36]

10.3.7 ACE Inhibitor-induced Cough

Dry cough is a serious problem in non-smokers who use angiotensin-converting enzyme inhibitors (ACEI) for cardiac disease or for arterial hypertension. The incidence of cough as a side effect of ACE is about 15 to 60 per cent.[40,41] Cough occurs more frequently in women and in non-smokers and at a higher dosage but is not related to age, duration of treatment, or chronic respiratory disease.[41] This side effect of ACEI is typical for all types of ACEI that are in clinical use. Cough can either appear immediately (few hours) after start of treatment or after a few weeks or months.[5,42]

The pathogenesis of ACEI cough is unclear;[43] it has been suggested that it is related to an accumulation of bradykinins, tachykinins, substance P and neurokinin A, as this enzyme plays a key role in the degradation of these peptides.[44] Patients with ACEI cough have an increased sensitivity of the cough reflex;[5] it may also be associated with an increase in NO generation in bronchial epithelial cells.[43] That cough is due to the use of ACE-inhibitors can concluded, if after discontinuing them for four weeks, it disappears completely.[45]

10.3.8 Post-Infection Cough

If a cough is present for more than 8 weeks, then it could be the result of an earlier infection of the respiratory tract.[45] In this case one has to pay attention to the possible outbreak of epidemics, the number of times per year the patient has had a respiratory tract infection and in the case of children, the status of similar infections amongst their siblings or amongst their classmates and the time of the year, i.e., spring or autumn. All of this information is important for diagnosis. Cough is usually seen during an infection with microbes such as *Mycoplasma pneumoniae, Moraxella. catarrhalis, Chlamydia pneumoniae, Bordatella pertussis* respiratory syncytial and parainfluenza viruses *Moraxella catarrhalis* as a cause of chronic cough is frequently seen in children; in adults it may occur in the presence of other respiratory tract infections. *Moraxella catarrhalis* infection is confirmed from sputum or from a sample taken during bronchoscopy.

The chronic cough induced by *Bordatella pertussis* infection is seen in children who are incompletely immunised but has also been seen in those who have been well immunised.[5]

In order to confirm that the cough that is seen is due to an earlier infection, other more typical reasons have to be excluded at first. We can use clinical examinations, laboratory tests, bacteriological examination of sputum samples or samples acquired by bronchoscopy, laryngoscopy. X-ray of nasal sinuses (sinusitis) and of chest (pneumonia) are useful in this respect.

10.3.9 Bronchogenic Carcinoma

A history of cough and its character has a high diagnostic value; a change in the character of cough in persons who smoke or those who have discontinued to smoke could be assumed to occur as a result of bronchogenic carcinoma,[36,45] Though cough is a common symptom of lung carcinoma, but not every carcinoma of the lung is accompanied by cough.[5] For an accurate diagnosis, it is important to know the character of cough and its duration. Evidence of carcinoma is based on chest X-rays and examination by bronchoscopy.

It must be kept in mind that haemoptysis is common in patients with lung carcinoma. Bleeding occurs probably as a result of endotracheal or endobronchial growth of the carcinoma or due to necrosis of a lung tumour. A cough is seen more frequently in squamous cell or small cell carcinoma, and these have a tendency to be present in the central airways[5].By contrast adenocarcinoma is localized in the peripheral regions of the lungs where there is a low density of sensory receptors which could be stimulated to give rise to a cough.[5] Rarely does bronchoalveolar carcinoma, a subtype of adenocarcinoma, give rise to a cough. Patients have symptoms that include large quantities of mucoid sputum, breathlessness and their state of health declines fast. For its diagnosis, it is crucial to obtain a lung sample and this may be taken either by transbronchial biopsy, transparietal biopsy or via thoracotomy. A further confirmation is carried out by histological and cytological examination of the samples obtained.

The other specific kind of carcinoma which is accompanied by cough, is carcinomatosis of the lung. The carcinomatosis is the spread of carcinoma into the lung via blood or lymphatic vessels from the other parts of the body. The radiograph of the lung yields a picture of diffuse interstitial lung disease; its diagnosis is confirmed by lung biopsy and the prognosis is usually bad. Not only are chest X-rays and scans invaluable for diagnosis, but are also important for knowing the stage at which the carcinoma is and subsequently for its treatment.

10.3.10 Psychogenic Cough

Psychogenic cough is commonly seen in children and adolescents and occurs along with other respiratory problems such as dyspnoea, hyperventilation and vocal cord dysfunction; its presence too, assumes a psychosomatic nature.[47] Other simultaneously occurring features are various breathing sounds and tightness of throat.[48] Problems at school are one of the main underlying reason for these respiratory problems.[48,49]

Cough under such circumstances is sometimes difficult to distinguish from PNDS. Patients believe that they are rather ill and expect quick success from their medical treatment although their clinical examinations are negative for PNDS, GERD or bronchial asthma, and a differential diagnosis does not confirm other diseases that are accompanied by cough. Since its occurrence is common among adolescents and children, the physicians are advised to take into consideration, any problems that the child may have at school. This could require a consultation from the psychiatrists.

The prevalence of psychogenic cough is a little more common in girls than in the boys. In adults, after exclusion of other causes, a cough could also be considered as a sign of malingering.[5]

10.4 UNCOMMON CAUSE OF ACUTE COUGH: THORACENTESIS

In healthy subjects cough is produced by stimulation of vagal afferent endings located predominantly in the larynx, trachea and bronchi. This is considered as a part of the defence mechanism and a reflex act, which removes secretions from airways by means of mucociliary transportation.

Cough can occur by deep breathing and by irritation of the larynx and trachea. In experimental animals, it is more difficult to provoke cough by an irritation of the alveoli or the small airways. There are no explicit reports of provoking cough by direct stimulation or irritation of the pleura, either by mechanical or chemical means. However, we know from clinical practice that thoracentesis can be the cause of acute cough, seen either during or after it. This cough usually lasts from a few minutes to a few hours. At this point, it is not clear whether thoracentesis is the cause of cough or is accompanied by it. In our investigation, in which we were studying the origin of cough which related to thoracentesis, we found that the phenomenon of thoracentesis is not a complication, but a demonstration of re-expansion of the lung parenchyma which probably leads to a stimulation of the rapidly adapting pulmonary stretch receptors (RARs).

However, in 9 to 11 per cent of patients, cough is considered as a complication of thoracentesis and occurs as a consequence of the removal of pleural fluid that is seen alongside pneumothorax.[50]

10.4.1 Pathophysiology of Thoracentesis Cough

The visceral pleura is also innerved by branches of the vagus nerves, the sympathetic trunk and the parietal pleura is supplied by branches of the intercostal nerves.[51] According to Widdicombe,[52] a stimulation of C fibre nerve endings and rapidly adapting pulmonary stretch receptors during thoracentesis, could lead to cough that is seen in such patients.[53] It is also likely that under such circumstances, an irritation is produced by the inflammation processes, in the lung parenchyma[54] or by the (re)inflation of lung parenchyma after removal of pleural fluid. Although individual tolerance varies in patients, yet the re-expansion of the lung parenchyma after thoracoscopy produces a cough.

In our observation, no cough was elicited even at times when large amounts of fluid were removed with the chest open and the lungs not fully re-expanded, or when similar samples were taken out of the parietal and visceral pleura. But a cough arose when we compressed the lung with the thoracoscope. This means that not only does re-expansion, but also deflation (compression) can lead to cough but the unanswered question is, what is stimulated and how?

It is not clear whether, during these procedures, the RARs are compressed and stimulated or is it the shifting of the mediastinum and the carina, around which there is a great concentration of receptors, which on getting stimulated give rise to a cough. But one cannot suppose that cough is produced by a shift of the mediastinum or by stimulation of receptors in the area around the carina during thoracentesis. Patients have reported to us only chest pain, but no cough occurs when the mediastinum is shifted with our effort to re-expand the lung parenchyma at thoracoscopy.[55]

On the basis of our clinical findings, we can conclude that the direct stimulation of parietal and visceral pleura does not lead to cough. The role of other receptors, which could be stimulated by the underlying disease, for which the thoracoscopy was being carried out in the first place, are implicated and these therefore, cannot be excluded. A further study to identify the cause of cough seen in thoracentesis is needed.

10.5 COMPLICATIONS OF COUGH

Cough may be followed by complications resulting from high intrathoracic pressures that are reached during coughing. Moreover, the rapid motion of the diaphragm may also produce high pressure in the abdominal space which may affect the abdominal organs including blood vessels.

Thus cough itself could cause additional problems (complications) with respect to the respiratory, cardiovascular, central nervous, genitourinary and musculoskeletal systems. The following is a list of some of the common complications of cough.[5,36]

10.5.1 Respiratory

- Interstitial emphysema

- Risk of pneumomediastinum, pneumoperitoneum
- Pneumothorax (rupture of visceral pleura)
- Laryngeal trauma
- Tracheobronchial trauma (bronchial rupture)
- Intercostal lung herniation

10.5.2 Cardiovascular

- Dislodgement of venous or cardiac mural thrombi
- Displacement of right heart or central venous catheters
- Arterial hypotension
- Loss of consciousness
- Rupture of veins (nasal, anal)
- Malfunctioning of intravascular catheters
- Paroxysmal tachyarrhythmias
- Bradyarrhythmias

10.5.3 Neurologic

- Syncope (and death if syncope occurs while driving a vehicle)
- 'Benign' cough headache
- Cerebral air embolism (in patients on positive-air pressure ventilation)
- CSF fluid rhinorrhoea
- Acute cervical radiculopathy
- Malfunctioning ventriculoatrial shunts
- Seizures
- Stroke due to vertebral artery dissection
- Cough toothache

10.5.4 Gastrointestinal

- Rupture of oesophagus with mediastinitis
- Gastro-oesophageal reflux events
- Hydrothorax in peritoneal dialysis
- Malfunctioning of gastrostomy button
- Splenic rupture
- Inguinal hernia

10.5.5 Genitourinary

- Urinary incontinence
- Inversion of bladder through urethra

10.5.6 Musculoskeletal

- Elevation serum creatine phosphokinase
- Rupture of rectus abdominale muscles
- Rib fractures
- Injury of back

10.5.7 Miscellaneous

- Petechie and purpura
- Disruption of surgical wounds
- Lifestyle changes
- Self-consciousness, hoarseness, dizziness
- Fear of serious disease
- Decrease of quality of life
- Interference of speech and sleep

REFERENCES

1. French CL, Irwin RS, Curley FJ, Krikorian CJ. Impact of chronic cough on quality of life. Archives of Internal Medicine 1998;158:1657–61.
2. Dicpinigaitis PV. Cough reflex sensitivity in cigarette smokers. Chest 2003;123:685–8.
3. Schayck CP, Loozen JMC, Wagena E, et al. Detecting patients at a high risk of developing chronic obstructive pulmonary disease in general practice: cross sectional case finding study. British Medical Journal 2002;324:1370–83.
4. Davis CL. ABC of palliative care: breathlessness, cough, and other respiratory problems. British Medical Journal 1997;315:931–4.
5. Irwin RS, Boudet LPH, Cloutier MM, et al. Managing cough as a defense mechanism and as a symptom. A Consensus Panel Report of the American College of Chest Physicians. Chest 1998;114:113S–181S.
6. Schroeder K, Fahley T. Systematic review of randomised controlled trials of over the counter cough medicines for acute cough in adults. British Medical Journal 2002;324:329.
7. French CT, Irwin RS, Fletcher KE, Adams TM. Evaluation of a cough-specific quality-of-life questionnaire. Chest 2002;121:1123–31.
8. Palombini PC, Villanova CAC, Araújo E, Gastal OL, et al. A pathogenic triad in chronic cough: asthma, postnasal drip syndrome, and gastroesophageal reflux diseases. Chest 1999;116:279–84.

9. Jenkinson D. Natural course of 500 consecutive cases of whooping cough: a general practice population study. British Medical Journal 1995;310:299–302.
10. Miyashita N, Fukano H, Yoshida K, Niki Y, et al. *Chlamydia pneumoniae* infection in adult patients with persistent cough. Journal of Medical Microbiology 2003;52:265–9.
11. Fahey T, Stocks N, Thomas T. Quantitative systematic review of randomised controlled trials comparing antibiotic with placebo for acute cough in adults. British Medical Journal 1998;316:906–10.
12. Irwin RS, Madison JM. The persistently troublesome cough. American Journal of Respiratory and Critical Care Medicine 2002;165:1469–74.
13. Ogilvie CM. Clinical features: symptoms and signs in respiratory disease. In: Brewis RAL, Corrin B, Geddes DM, Gibson GJ, editors. Respiratory Medicine. 2nd edn. London: W.B. Saunders Company Ltd., 1995;pp247–49.
14. Glaspole I, Conron M, du Bois RM. Clinical features of parenchymal lung disease. In: Olivieri D, du Bois RM, editors. Interstitial Lung Diseases. European Respiratory Monograph 2000;14:p3.
15. Fujimura M, H Ogawa H, NishizawaY, Nishi K. Comparison of atopic cough with cough variant asthma: is atopic cough a precursor of asthma? Thorax 2003;58:14–18.
16. Irwin RS, Curley FJ, French CL. Chronic cough: the spectrum and frequency of causes, key components of the diagnostic evaluation, and outcome of specific therapy. American Review of Respiratory Disease. 1990;141:640–7.
17. Thiadens HA, de Bock GH, Dekker FW, et al. Identifying asthma and chronic obstructive pulmonary disease in patients with persistent cough presenting to general practitioners' descriptive study. British Medical Journal 1998;316:1286–90.
18. Irwin RS, Curley FJ, French CL. Chronic cough: the spectrum and frequency of causes, key components of the diagnostic evaluation, and outcome of specific therapy. American Review of Respiratory Disease 1990;141:640–7.
19. Sistek D, Tschopp J-M, Schindler C, Briutsche M, et al. Clinical diagnosis of current asthma: predictive value of respiratory symptoms in the SAPALDIA study. European Respiratory Journal 2001;17:214–9.
20. Carney IK, Gibson PG, Murree-Allen K, Saltos N, et al. A systematic evaluation of mechanisms in chronic cough. American Journal of Respiratory and Critical Care Medicine, 1997;156:211–6.
21. Pratter MR, Bartter T, Akers S, Dubois J. An algorithmic approach to chronic cough. Annals of Internal Medicine 1993;119:977–83.
22. Kurup VP, Banerjee B, Greenberger PA, Fink JN. Allergic bronchopulmonary aspergillosis: challenges in diagnosis. Medscape General Medicine 1999;1:3.
23. Plutinsky J, Ockovska V, Plutinska J, Polanova M. Familiar occurrence of allergic bronchopulmonary aspergillosis. Studia Pneumologica et Phtiseologica 1995;55:446–54.
24. Lee SY, Kim MK, Shin C, Shim JJ, et al. Substance P-immunoreactive nerves in Endobronchial biopsies in cough-variant asthma and classic asthma. Respiration 2003;70:49–53.
25. George RB, Payne DK. The respiratory history and physical examination. In: George RB, Light RW, Matthay MA, Matthay RA, editors. Chest Medicine: Essentials of Pulmonary and Critical Care Medicine. Philadelphia: Lippincott Williams & Wilkins 2000;pp59–67.
26. Irwin RS, Zawacki JK, Wilson MM, French CT, Callery P. Chronic cough due to gastroesophageal reflux disease: failure to resolve despite total/near-total elimination of esophageal acid. Chest 2002;121:1132–040.

27. Kiljander TO, Salomaa ERM, Hietanen EK, Terho EO. Chronic cough and gastro- oesophageal reflux: a double-blind placebo-controlled study with omeprazole European Respiratory Journal 2000;16:633–8.
28. Wong RKH, Hanson DG, Waring PJ, Shaw G. ENT manifestations of gastroesophageal reflux. American Journal of Gastroenterology 2000;95:S15–S22.
29. Poe RH, Kallay MC. Chronic cough and gastroesophageal reflux disease: experience with specific therapy for diagnosis and treatment. Chest 2003;123:679–84.
30. Gibson PG, Dolovich J, Denburg J, et al. Chronic cough: eosinophilic bronchitis without asthma. Lancet 1989;1:1346–7.
31. Joo JH, Park SJ, Park SW, Lee JH, et al. Clinical features of eosinophilic bronchitis. Korean Journal of Internal Medicine 2002;17:31–7.
32. Brightling CE, Ward R, Goh KL, Wardlaw AJ, et al. Eosinophilic bronchitis is an important cause of chronic cough. American Journal Respiratory and Critical Care Medicine 1999;160: 406–10.
33. Anzueto A. Contemporary diagnosis and management of bronchitis. 2nd edn. Newtown: Handbooks in Health Care Co., 1999;7.
34. Barnes P, Godfrey S. Chronic obstructive pulmonary disease. London: Martin Dunitz Ltd., 1997;2–10.
35. Taylor B, Green MS. Evaluating and Managing Syncope Clinical Review 2000;10:55–64.
36. Barnes PJ. Managing Chronic Obstructive Pulmonary Diseases. Singapore: Science Press Ltd., 1999;21–3.
37. Fraser RS, Müller NL, Colman N, Paré PD. Diagnosis of Diseases of the Chest. 4th edn. Philadelphia: W.B. Saunders Company 1999;2265–78.
38. Mansharamani NG, Koziel H. Chronic lung sepsis. Lung abscess, bronchiectasis, and empyema. Current Opinion of Pulmonary Medicine 2003;9:181–5.
39. Currie GP, McKay J. Chronic cough. British Medical Journal 2003;326:261.
40. Saruta T, Arakawa K, Iimura O, et al. Difference in the incidence of cough induced by angiotensin converting enzyme inhibitors: a comparative study using imidapril hydrochloride and enalapril maleate. Hypertension Research. 1999;22:197–202.
41. Lacourciere Y. The Incidence of Cough: A comparison of lisinopril, placebo and telmisartan: a novel angiotensin II antagonist. Telmisartan Cough Study Group International Journal of Clinical Practice 1999;53:99–103.
42. Rodgers JE, Patterson JH. Angiotensin II-receptor blockers: Clinical relevance and therapeutic role. American Journal of Health-System Pharmacy 2001;58:671–83.
43. Seedat YK, Ismail, Randeree IGH. Antihypertensive effect and tolerability of perindopril in Indian hypertensive and Type 2 diabetic patients 1-year randomised, double-blind, parallel study vs atenolol. Clinical Drug Investigation 1998;16:229–40.
44. Lee S-CH, Park SW, Kim D-K, et al. Iron supplementation inhibits cough associated with ACE inhibitors. Hypertension 2001;38:166–72.
45. McGarvey LPA, Savage DA, Phil D, Feeney SA, et al. Is there an association between angiotensin-converting enzyme gene variants and chronic nonproductive cough? Chest 2000;118:1091–4.
46. Irwin RS, Madison JM. The diagnosis and treatment of cough. New England: Journal Medicine 2000;343:1715–21.
47. Strebel P, Nordin J, Edwards K, et al. Population-based incidence of pertussis among adolescents and adults, Minnesota, 1995–1996. Journal of Infection Disease 2001;183:1353–9.

48. Homnock DN, Pratt HD. Respiratory diseases with a psychosomatic component in adolescents. Adolescent Medicine 2000;11:547–65.
49. Niggeman B. Functional symptoms confused with allergic disorders in children and adolescents. Pediatric Allergy and Immunology 2002;13:312–8.
50. Bhatia MS, Chandra R, Vaid L. Psychogenic cough: a profile of 32 cases. International Journal of Psychiatry Medicine 2002;32:353–60.
51. Collins TB, Sahn A. Thoracentesis. Clinical value, complications, technical problems, and patient experience. Chest 1987;91:817–22.
52. Harley R. Anatomy of the pleura. Seminar of Respiratory Medicine 1987;9:1–6.
53. Widdicombe JG. Neurophysiology of the cough reflex. European Respiratory Journal 1995;8:1193–202.
54. Plutinsky J. Cough and thoracentesis. European Respiratory Journal 1999;14:225S–226S.
55. Plutinsky J. Cough and chest diseases. European Respiratory Journal 2001;18:87S.

11 Cough Sensitivity Testing

RENATA PECOVA, M TATAR

11.1 INTRODUCTION

Over the last 20 years, cough sensitivity-testing has become an integral part of studying this reflex in clinical medicine. Currently, cough provocation investigations are being undertaken for studying epidemiological issues regarding the influence of age and gender on cough and in the prognosis of patients with chronic cough and monitoring its course with regard to therapy. It is also being used clinically to study the pathogenesis and therapeutics of chronic cough.[1]

Extensive studies were undertaken to test the cough sensitivity of patients with various respiratory diseases to capsaicin and to compare it with that of patients, with pathological findings in the nasal cavity and skin. These were undertaken to see if the responses of airway afferent nerve endings mediating cough in some patients were any different, from those who also had allergic rhinitis, atopic dermatitis and gastro-oesophageal reflux, but who did not complain of having a cough and other respiratory symptoms. With this additional information, one could either consider airway reactivity as a marker of 'subclinical' pathological processes in the nose, skin or gastrointestinal tract or assume that central sensitisation of the cough generated by afferent impulses from the upper airway, skin or gastrointestinal tract, occur.

11.2 COUGH SENSITIVITY

Inhalation cough challenge has become an accepted method of investigating antitussive agents.[2] Enhanced sensitivity of airway nerves that mediate cough is important in the pathomechanism of nonproductive cough, and successful treatment is associated with a reduction in cough sensitivity.[3]

Enhanced cough sensitivity is a hallmark of many airway diseases, and it reflects plasticity in the neural circuits regulating this defensive reflex. Increased afferent nerve fibre excitability produces changes in afferent nerve fibre anatomy, and facilitatory interactions between the sensory nerve fibres subtypes may produce increased cough sensitivity. This may reduce the stimulation of sensory nerve fibres or produce an inhibition of synaptic transmission in the brainstem, thereby providing new sites of action of pharmaceutical agents used for relief from cough. The contributions of other mechanisms in cough sensitivity, including complex alterations in central processing or changes in stimulus perception, have yet to be defined, and these when described could provide other useful targets for future therapeutic strategies.[4]

11.3 INHALATION COUGH CHALLENGE

Inhalation cough challenge has been used for many years in the investigation of the cough reflex.[5] It is mainly carried out by the single dose or the dose-response method. The single-dose inhalation challenge consists of administering only one dose of the tussive agent. This method is used for screening large populations to find the reproducible dose for cough.[6] and is used widely in the investigation of the properties and duration of antitussive action of pharmacological agents.[7,8] Owing to a smaller number of inhalations required, this method has been associated with a lower propensity for tachyphylaxis which had confounded previous dose-response inhalation cough testing with agents such as citric acid, distilled water and capsaicin.[2,9]

The dose-response method involves inhalation of incremental doses of the tussive agent under investigation and is alternated with inhalation of placebo. Depending on the length of inhalation, this method can be further subdivided into single breath or fixed-time inhalation challenges (usually between 15 and 60 seconds).[10] The fixed-time 1-minute inhalation method has been used to test both capsaicin[9,11] and citric acid.[12] However, as this type of cough challenge involves a long inhalation period, it has been associated with difficulties in the delivery of accurate amount of tussigenic agents.[10] Nevertheless, the single-breath method has acquired a much broader usage. There are also some variations of this method. A less reliable approach involving simple inspiratory manoeuvres such as vital capacity-volume inhalation, is also used sometimes.[13]

Thus, easier and more accurate methods that use a single-breath, dosimeter-controlled nebuliser for delivering tussigenic agents have acquired a wider usage.[10] This method is used particularly for testing the influence of gender[14] and gastro-oesophageal reflux on the genesis of cough.[15] The single-breath method is preferred for assessing the cough sensitivity to citric acid[16] and capsaicin.[17] However, the most relevant usage of this method has been in the investigation of antitussive effects of pharmacological agents.[18]

A large number of chemical substances are currently used for the induction of cough in humans and three different kinds of substances used frequently are—capsaicin and vanilloid-related substance, citric acid or related organic acids, and low chloride solutions. A wide variety of cough challenge methodologies are available now, and allow the investigator to select the best one suited for the investigation. However, there is also a need to use a standardised method so as to be able to compare data from different laboratories.[10]

11.4 ASSESSMENT OF COUGH SENSITIVITY

At first, the measurement of the cough threshold to capsaicin (the pungent extract of red pepper that stimulates the vanilloid receptors-TRPV1 (formerly VR1), is a ligand-gated ion channel that is expressed by a large percentage of mammalian nociceptive C-fibre nerves.[19] TRPV1 is required for activation of sensory nerves by using vanilloids such as capsaicin for the measurement of cough threshold. According to the method of Fujimura et al[20] the subject at first inhales an aerosol of physiological saline (control solution), followed by progressively increasing doses of capsaicin. Two litres of aerosol are inhaled every 60 seconds through the mouth while wearing a nose clip (Pari Werck™, Germany). Aerosols containing larger doses are inhaled until two or more coughs are elicited. The mean diameter of the capsaicin particles is kept at 1.2 micrometres. The number of capsaicin-induced coughs that arise are counted and the lowest concentration of capsaicin eliciting two or more coughs, is considered as an index of airway cough sensitivity.

The capsaicin cough challenge test is a simple and reproducible laboratory method for the assessment of cough in a wide variety of respiratory diseases.[21]

Inhaled capsaicin has been postulated to induce cough via release of tachykinins. Tachykinins are rendered inactive by neutral endopeptidase (NEP).

It has been shown that NEP activity is decreased in bronchoalveolar lavage fluid from patients with lung cancer.[22]

11.4.1 Cough Sensitivity in Patients Suffering from Respiratory Diseases

Cough is diagnosed as chronic, if it persists for more than 8 weeks, and it may signify the seriousness of underlying disease. According to Higenbottam's classification[23] a persistent cough is that which occurs along with upper respiratory tract infections, but it usually disappears after about 6 to 10 days. Bronchial hyper-responsiveness that accompanies chronic cough is considered a consequence of increased sensitivity of the reflex mechanism involving coughing. The chief factors that influence the cough reflex in disease are the location of sensory receptors in the airways whose afferents are to be stimulated, the effect of airway calibre and the effect of respiratory tract infections if already present.[23] The cough reflex response to capsaicin is enhanced during well-known lung diseases such as bronchogenic carcinoma, interstitial pulmonary processes, and bronchopneumonia. In order to evaluate the sensitivity of the cough reflex to capsaicin, particularly in patients with these diseases who had chronic cough, but who had normal chest radiograms and no recent respiratory infection or a personal history of allergic diseases, were studied.

The difference in the cough sensitivity to capsaicin found amongst patients with interstitial pulmonary processes, chronic bronchitis, chronic cough, and control group was significant. The changes in cough sensitivity in patients with bronchopneumonia and bronchogenic carcinoma were not noteworthy, although those with chronic cough and bronchogenic carcinoma, were note worthy[24] (Fig. 11.1).

In interstitial lung disease, there is evidence of an increased sensitivity to inhaled capsaicin in producing cough. This effect is not as a result of the lungs' reduced capacity or the chest being strapped or evidence of enhanced capsaicin responsiveness.[17] The mechanisms that sensitise proximal cough receptors in interstitial pulmonary disease affecting the parenchyma and bronchioles are unknown. It is possible that sensitisation of the cough reflex could occur through inflammation of proximal airways.[25] A likely possibility is that the pulmonary C-fibres, which can inhibit reflex cough, could have been damaged by the inflammatory processes in the lung parenchyma,[26] leading to greater levels of central influences which render the reflex more sensitive.

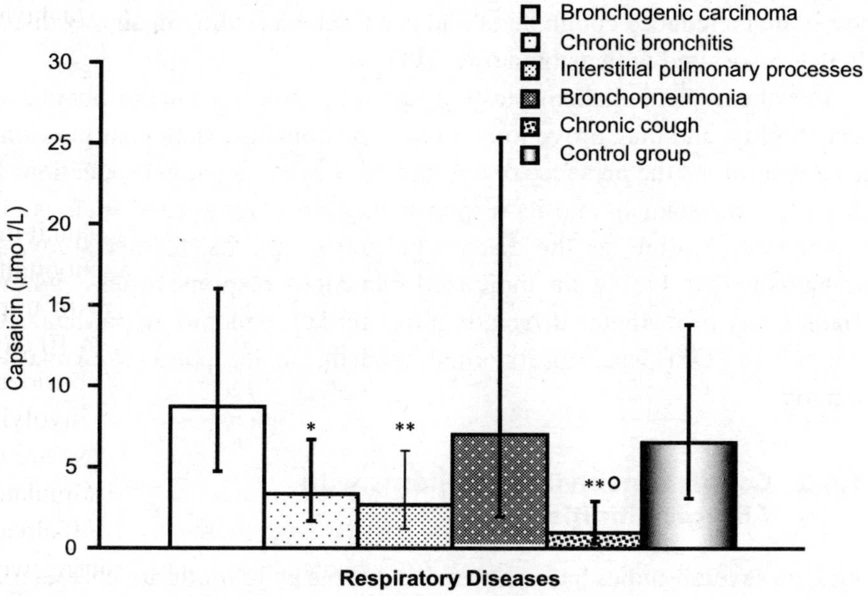

Fig. 11.1 Cough sensitivity to capsaicin in patients with respiratory disease. Subjects control group; 0 seg * $p<0.05$, ** $p<0.001$, o$p<0.05$ * Control group of subjects; o patient group. (Reproduced from Ref. [24] with permission from publisher).

Cough sensitivity to capsaicin in patients with bronchopneumonia was not found to have been significantly changed as compared to that in the control group. A substantial number of patients with recurrent pneumonia do not have any other obvious underlying reasons, but they may exhibit certain characteristics as a consequence of infection. For example, in patients with recurrent pneumonia, the cough threshold is significantly higher than in controls.[27]

On the other hand, Fujimura et al[28] indicated that cough threshold to inhaled capsaicin or tartaric acid was not enhanced during acute *Mycoplasma pneumoniae* with lymphocyte-predominant bronchitis. Cough sensitivity to capsaicin in patients with chronic bronchitis was increased significantly as compared to that in normals.

A lowered citric acid cough threshold (increased cough sensitivity) in patients with chronic obstructive pulmonary disease (COPD), which could be due to the effect of cigarette smoke on citric acid sensitive receptors in larynx and upper airways has been reported by Wong and Morice.[16] Doherty et al[17] showed that a reduced cough threshold is a frequent finding in airway disease, whether associated with asthma or COPD.

Use of capsaicin-challenge testing gives objective information about cough susceptibility, and may prove to be more discriminating than just questioning the patients about the presence or absence of cough or sputum production. The role of this mechanism and its responsiveness to other agents, such as citric acid or low chlorine, as the disease progresses merits, further study. The mechanisms producing an increased capsaicin responsiveness, whether inflammatory or mediator-driven, requires further exploration, particularly in patients with COPD where an abnormal cough threshold, appears to be relatively common.

11.4.2 Cough Sensitivity in Patients with Allergic Rhinitis

Although several studies have shown that asthma and rhinitis are characterized by a similar inflammatory process, pathophysiological interactions between upper and lower airways are not entirely understood.[29,30] It is, however, clear that the condition of the upper airways definitely influences the lower airways. In patients with allergic rhinitis but without bronchial hyper-reactivity, signs of allergic inflammation of the lower airways have been found in induced sputum, bronchoalveolar lavage, and bronchial biopsy specimens.[31,32] Nasal-bronchial reflex, altered breathing patterns pulmonary aspiration of nasal contents, and increased levels of inflammatory factors in blood may give rise to lower airway dysfunction in patients with rhinitis.[33,34]

In general, neuroregulation of nose and lower airways are similar, but there are significant differences in the effector tissues at these two sites.[35] The interrelationship between upper and lower airway manifestations of allergy remains incompletely investigated. Little is known about the critical factors that determine sensitivity of the cough reflex in subjects with allergic rhinitis.

The most common cause of chronic cough in non-smokers, in all age groups, is post nasal drip syndrome (PNDS) and is seen in a number of upper respiratory tract conditions;[36] with the cough reflex appearing to have a normal sensitivity in them.[37] Since PNDS generally occurs as a result of different types of nasal infections, allergic rhinitis or sinusitis, an evaluation of the cough reflex sensitivity in pollen-sensitive patients with allergic rhinitis, was evaluated by

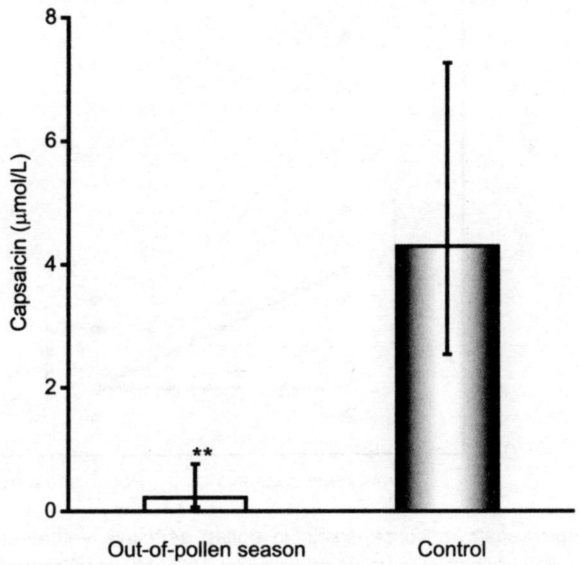

Fig. 11.2 Cough sensitivity to capsaicin in pollen sensitive volunteers during out-of-pollen season. (*** $p<0.001$). (Reproduced from Ref. [38] with permission from publisher).

us. This was carried out in persons exhibiting sensitivity to grass pollen during both, when it was in seasons and when not.

Capsaicin cough sensitivity in patients with allergic rhinitis in out-of-pollen season and in healthy controls was significantly increased[38] (Fig. 11.2).

Cough sensitivity to capsaicin found in the patients with allergic rhinitis which were examined out-of-pollen season and in pollen season was significantly higher[38] (Fig. 11.3). Cough sensitivity is significantly increased in pollen-sensitive subjects suffering from seasonal allergic rhinitis; nevertheless it is evaluated in, out-of or during pollen season.

Nasal inflammation has been well demonstrated in allergic rhinitis with different kinds of stimuli being capable of producing inflammation of nasal mucosa. During inflammatory responses, newly generated inflammatory mediators may be released from resident cells in the nasal mucosa (mast cells, goblet cells, lymphocytes, macrophages).[39] Mediators such as leukotrienes, prostaglandins and platelet-activating factor will increase vascular permeability with local tissue oedema, secretion of mucus and glandular proteins (rhinorrhoea). Nasal secretions may be aspirated into the lower airways in

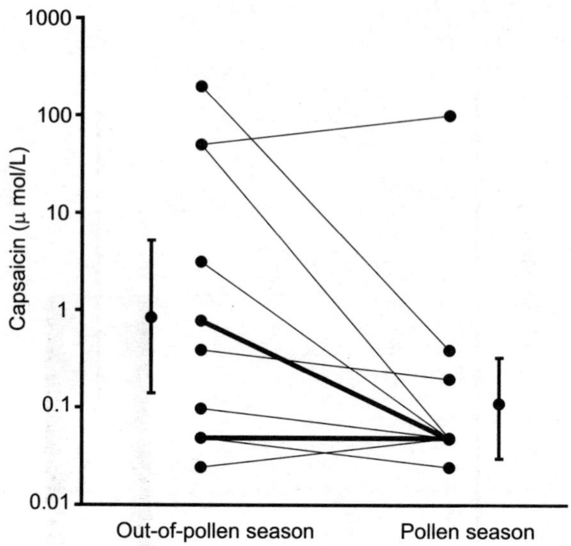

Fig. 11.3 Cough sensitivity to capsaicin in pollen sensitive volunteers out-of-pollen season and in pollen season. (Reproduced from Ref. [38] with permission from publisher).

patients with upper airway diseases. Thus a hypothesis which links nasal disease with increased airway responsiveness could be: a postnasal drip of mucus mediators or chemotactic factors into the lower airways, either reactivity or causing airway inflammation.[40]

Braunstahl et al[34] found an allergic inflammatory response, similar to asthma, in the lower airways of patients with rhinitis but without bronchial hyper-reactivity after segmental bronchial provocation. Interestingly, the allergic response was also not restricted to the allergen-challenged bronchial segment, but was more widespread: eosinophilia occurred in some parts of the lung and seen the in peripheral blood. They found increased inflammatory cell numbers in the nasal mucosa after segmental bronchial provocation, together with signs and symptoms of allergic rhinitis, indicating that the nose is involved in this systemic effect. They also observed a clear difference in the time course and the degree of clinical and immunopathologic findings in the nose and bronchi of allergic subjects after local allergen challenge.

Although allergic rhinitis and asthma are disorders that commonly occur together, very little is known about inflammatory features in bronchial airways of subjects with allergic rhinitis and no evidence of asthma. Bronchoalveolar lavage and bronchial biopsy studies have shown that subjects with allergic rhinitis may exhibit inflammatory changes in the airways.[41]

It is well established that stimulation of the nasal mucosa in animals precipitates reflex bronchospasm.[42] Circumstantial evidence supports the hypothesis that similar reflexes initiated in the nose during allergic rhinitis might exacerbate lower airway disease.[43] The severity of asthma symptoms correlates with the symptoms of allergic rhinitis. Moreover, treating allergic rhinitis can reduce the symptoms of asthma, whereas inducing allergic inflammation in the nose worsens it. Attempts to associate the consequences of allergic rhinitis on the lower airways with altered neural reflexes have yielded conflicting results. Given that the necessary anatomical substrate for producing such reflexes exist, and there is clear evidence for reflex bronchospasm initiated from nose, it is reasonable to assume that afferent hyperexcitability in nose will worsen the symptoms and physiology of asthma through neuronal mechanisms.[44]

The nervous system plays an essential role in regulating nasal function. Dysfunction of the nerves innervating the nose is likely in contributing to the pathogenesis of rhinitis.[44] Recent studies indicate that neuronal activation can precipitate inflammation of the human nasal mucosa through axonal reflexes.[45] These observations highlight the integral role played by the nervous system in rhinitis. Allergic inflammation can initiate hyper-reflexia in the nose, which might exacerbate pre-existing conditions such as asthma.[44]

Capsaicin cough sensitivity in allergic asthmatic patients increases during birch pollen season. Sensory reactivity in allergic asthmatic patients may be increased during prolonged allergen exposure during the pollen season. This finding suggests that allergic inflammation in the lower and/or upper airways may trigger neurogenic mechanisms of significant clinical importance.[46] There was no difference in capsaicin sensitivity between patients sensitive to or insensitive to methacholine who underwent a bronchial methacholine test, primarily because of suspected asthma.[47]

Cough sensitivity is influenced by allergic processes localised outside the lower airways; cough sensitivity is increased in patients with atopic dermatitis and other respiratory symptoms. There is no significant change in cough sensitivity between healthy subjects and patients suffering from psoriasis vulgaris who have no complaint of cough or other respiratory symptoms.

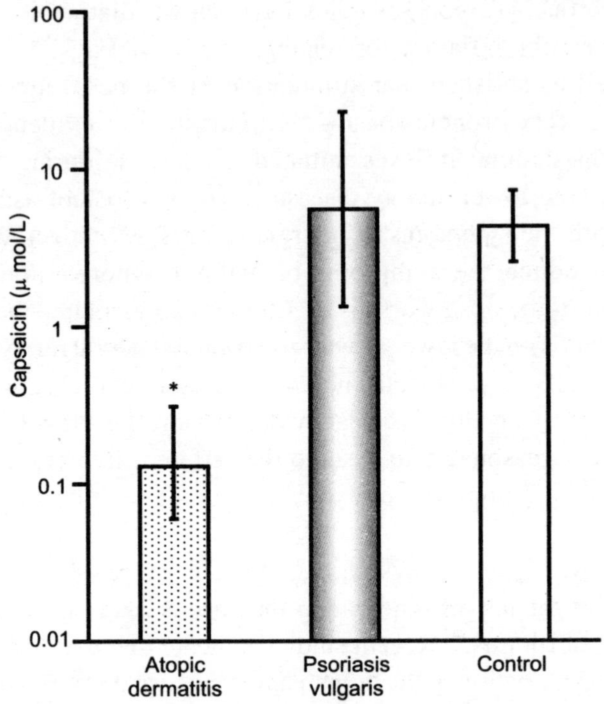

Fig. 11.4 Capsaicin cough sensitivity in patients with atopic dermatitis and psoriasis vulgaris as compared to control group (*p<0.001). (Reproduced from Ref. [48] with permission from publisher).

It is likely that atopic dermatitis as a clinical manifestation of skin atopic processes could be accompanied by ´subclinical´ inflammation of the airways.[48]

Cough sensitivity in patients suffering from allergic rhinitis is significantly increased during the pollen-season, nevertheless patients are treated with antihistamines. These findings are supported by increased cough intensity seen in experiments conscious guinea pigs with ovalbumine-induced allergic rhinitis.[49]

In our study, the difference in sensitivity of C2 (capsaicin dose causing 2 or more coughs) between the sexes was significant. There is an influence of gender that is seen on cough reflex sensitivity.[50,51]

11.4.3 Determining Cough Sensitivity in Patients with Atopic Dermatitis

Allergic sensitivity may be experienced all over the body; clinically, it is most pronounced only in the organ with most intensive inflammatory processes.Thus, it may be seen as allergic rhinitis or as atopic dermatitis. Atopic dermatitis is a chronic skin disorder frequently associated with elevated serum IgE levels.[52,53] When bronchial hyper-responsiveness was estimated in children who had atopic dermatitis, but no past history of bronchial asthma, about 32 to 82 per cent, exhibited a positive response.[54,55]

In a study aimed to investigate cough sensitivity to capsaicin, of patients suffering from atopic dermatitis but without any respiratory symptoms (e.g. cough, nasal discharge). The following study was carried out. The sensitivity of airway afferent nerve-endings mediating cough of healthy subjects was compared to that of patients suffering from psoriasis vulgaris who had some respiratory symptoms.[53,56] Capsaicin cough sensitivity was increased in patients with atopic dermatitis compared with healthy subjects and patients with psoriasis. Capsaicin cough sensitivity in patients with psoriasis was not significantly changed compared to healthy subjects[48] (Fig. 11.4).

One would also have to consider the role of allergic inflammatory processes of the skin due to atopy, in influencing sensitivity of the airway nerve endings mediating cough. Thus, cough sensitivity was significantly increased in patients with atopic dermatitis but who did have a cough or other respiratory symptoms as compared to healthy controls.

Cough reflex can be modulated by the irritation of sensory nerve endings outside of the lower respiratory tract. In experimental studies, stimulation of cardiac[57] and abdominal receptors[58] modulates the intensity of mechanically induced cough. Atopic dermatitis patients typically have marked pruritus—the factor that could exert a reflex influence on cough sensitivity by the irritation of skin sensitive nerve-endings. We found that cough sensitivity in patients with psoriasis vulgaris who also have marked pruritus does not change compared to that in healthy subjects. These data suggest that irritation of sensitive nerve endings in the skin does not play an important role in the regulation of cough sensitivity.

Disturbances of lower airway function in atopic dermatitis patients except that of bronchial hyper-responsiveness, have not been fully defined as yet. The percentage of cases that showed bronchial hyper-responsiveness was 32 to 82 per cent in atopic dermatitis in children who had never suffered from bronchial

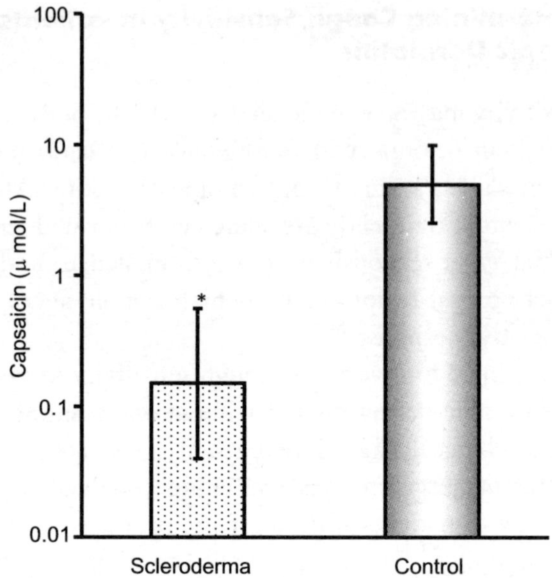

Fig. 11.5 Capsaicin cough sensitivity in patients with localised scleroderma as compared to control group (* p<0.001). (Reproduced from Ref. [60] with permission from publisher).

asthma.[54,55] We suppose that pathological processes in the airways which is a mechanism linking bronchial hyper-responsiveness could help to explain increased cough sensitivity. Whatever the mechanisms linking the airway eosinophilia and bronchial hyper-responsiveness to adenosine-5'monophosphate, there is no doubt that subclinical inflammatory changes within the lower airways are present in subjects with allergic rhinitis (even in the absence of clinical asthma).[41] Allergic rhinitis without clinical symptoms from lower airways was accompanied by increased cough sensitivity.[38]

It is suggested that atopy is not a determinant of airway cough sensitivity in healthy, nonasthmatic subjects; airway cough reflex to inhaled capsaicin were not associated with atopy in nonasthmatic young females.[20] Neither was an increased cough sensitivity seen in conscious guinea pigs sensitised to ovalbumine.[59]

11.4.4 Cough Sensitivity in Patients with Localised Scleroderma

The cough reflex measured using capsaicin is markedly increased in patients with cryptogenic fibrosing alveolitis. Cryptogenic fibrosing alveolitis is a disabling form of interstitial pulmonary fibrosis.[17] There is an increased cough reflex in patients with interstitial lung disease and this may represent sensitisation of airway sensory nerves.[24,25]

Capsaicin cough sensitivity in patients suffering from localised scleroderma without respiratory symptoms (i.e. cough or dyspnoea) was increased compared to that in healthy subjects (Fig. 11. 5).[60] The pathological process in scleroderma is localised not only in the skin but also in the respiratory system that may be involved in progressive systemic sclerosis. Scleroderma is a disease that causes alteration and fibrosis of connective tissue in skin and internal organs including lung.[61]

Localised scleroderma was used as a model of pathological autoimmune process clinically manifested in the skin and a capsaicin cough test can show a functional change in airway afferent nerve endings expressed as a cough in its presence.

11.5 CONCLUSION

Our data suggest that the capsaicin cough test can show functional changes of airway afferent nerve endings leading to cough during allergic atopic process with clinical inflammatory symptomatology in nose and skin. Although very little is known about allergic atopic processes spreading to the airways and its detection by capsaicin cough test, yet it merits further investigation, especially for testing the hypothesis that functional change of nerve endings could be a marker for a subclinical form of pathological process in the airways.

REFERENCES

1. Fuller RW. Cough sensitivity: the use of provocation tests. In: Chung F, Widdicombe J, Boushey H, editors. Cough: Causes, Mechanisms and Therapy. 1st edn. Oxford: Blackwell Publishing; 2003;pp49–55.
2. Morice AH, Higgins KS, Yeo WW. Adaptation of cough reflex with different types of stimulation. European Respiratory Journal 1992;5:841–7.
3. O´Connell F, Thomas VE, Pride NB, Fuller RW. Capsaicin cough sensitivity decreases with successful treatment of chronic cough. American Journal of Respiratory and Critical Care Medicine 1994;150:374–80.
4. Mazzone SB, Canning BJ. Plasticity of the cough reflex. The European Respiratory Review 2002;12(85):236–42.
5. Bickerman HA, Barach AL, Itkin S, Drimmer F. Experimental production of cough in human subjects induced by citric acid aerosols. Preliminary studies on the evaluation of antitussive agents. The American Journal of the Medical Sciences 1954;228:156–63.

6. Thompson RR, Wright C, Morice AH. Female gender and enhanced citric acid induced cough response. Thorax 1999;54:A75.
7. Wright CE, Thompson R, Meller S, Morice AH. Prolonged inhibition of the cough reflex by dextromethorphan: comparison with its metabolite dextrorphan. Thorax 1999;54:A75.
8. Grattan TJ, Marshall AE, Higgins KS, Morice AJH. The effect of inhaled and oral dextromethorphan on citric acid induced cough in man. British Journal of Clinical Pharmacology 1995;39:261–3.
9. Midgren B, Hansson L, Karlsson JA, Simonsson BG, Persson CGA. Capsaicin-induced cough in humans. American Review of Respiratory Disease 1992;146:347–51.
10. Morice AH. Inhalation cough challenge in the investigation of the cough reflex and antitussives. Pulmonary Pharmacology 1996;9:281–4.
11. Collier JG, Fuller RW. Capsaicin inhalation in man and the effects of sodium cromoglycate. British Journal of Pharmacology 1984;81:113–7.
12. Aauffarth B, de Monchy JG, van der Mark TW, Postma DS, Koeter GH. Citric acid cough threshold and airway responsiveness in asthmatic patients and smokers with chronic airflow obstruction. Thorax 1991;46:638–42.
13. Pounsford JC, Saunders KB. Diurnal variation and adaptation of the cough response to citric acid in normal subjects. Thorax 1985;40:657–61.
14. Dicpinigaitis PV, Rauf K. The influence of gender on cough reflex sensitivity. Chest 1998;113:1319–21.
15. Ferrari M, Olivieri M, Sembenini C, Benini L, Zuccali V, Bardell E, Bovo P, Cavallini G, Vantini I, Lo Cascio V. Tussive effect of capsaicin in patients with gastroesophageal reflux without cough. American Journal of Respiratory and Critical Care Medicine 1995;151:557–61.
16. Wong CH, Morice AH. Cough threshold in patients with chronic obstructive pulmonary disease. Thorax 1999;54:62–4.
17. Doherty MJ, Mister, R, Persson MG, Calverley PM. Capsaicin responsiveness and cough in asthma and chronic obstructive pulmonary diseease. Thorax 2000;55:643–9.
18. Morice AH, Marshall AE, Higgins KS, Grattan TJ. Effect of inhaled menthol on citric acid induced cough in normal subjects. Thorax 1994;49:1024–6.
19. Caterina MJ, Julius D. The vanilloid receptor: a molecular gateway to the pain pathway. Annual Review of Neuroscience 2001;24:487–517.
20. Fujimura M, Kasahara K, Yasui M, Myou S, Ishiura Y, Kamio Y, Hashimoto T, Matsuda T. Atopy in cough sensitivity to capsaicin and bronchial responsiveness in young females. European Respiratory Journal 1998;11:1060–3.
21. Choudry NB, Fuller RW. Sensitivity of the cough reflex in patients with chronic cough. European Respiratory Journal 1992;5:296–300.
22. Kita T, Fujimura M, Nishi K, Abo M, Ueda A, Yasui M, Kasahara K, Nakao S. Cough receptor sensitivity to capsaicin in patients with lung cancer. European Respiratory Journal 2001;18(Suppl.33):104s.
23. Higenbottam T. Chronic cough and the cough reflex in common lung diseases. Pulmonary Pharmacology & Therapeutics 2002;15:241–7.
24. Pèèová R, Tatár M, Rozborilová E, Buchancová J. Cough sensitivity in patients with respiratory diseases (in Slovak). Studia Pneumologica et Phtiseologica 1999;59:115–9.
25. Lalloo UG, Lim S, DuBois R, Barnes PJ, Chung KF. Increased sensitivity of the cough reflex in progressive systemic sclerosis patients with interstitial lung diseases. European Respiratory Journal 1998;11:702–5.

26. Tatar M, Webber SF, Widdicombe JG. Lung C-fibre receptor activation and defensive reflexes in anaesthetized cats. Journal of Physiology 1988;402:411–20.
27. Niimi A, Matsumoto H, Ueda T, Takemura M, Suzuki K, Tanaka E, Chin K, Mishima M, Amitani R. Impaired cough reflex in patients with recurrent pneumonia. Thorax 2003;58(7):645–6.
28. Fujimura M, Myou S, Matsuda M, Amemiya T, Kamio Y, Iwasa K, Ishiura Y, Yasui M, Tagami A, Matsuda T. Cough receptor sensitivity to capsaicin and tartaric acid in patients with *Mycoplasma pneumoniae*. Lung 1998;176(4):281–8.
29. Chanez P, Vignola AM, Vic P, Guddo F, Bonsignore G, Godard P. Comparison between nasal and bronchial inflammation in asthmatic and control subjects. American Journal of Respiratory and Critical Care Medicine 1999;159:588–95.
30. Bradley BL, Azzawi M, Jacobson M, Assoufi B, Collins JV, Irani AM, Schwartz LB, Durham SR, Jeffery PK, Kay AB. Eosinophils, T-lymphocytes, mast cells, neutrophils, and macrophages in bronchial biopsy specimens from atopic subjects with asthma: comparison with biopsy specimens from atopic subjects without asthma and normal control subjects and relationship to bronchial hyper-responsiveness. Journal of Allergy and Clinical Immunology 1991;88:661–74.
31. Foresi A, Leone C, Pelucchi A, Mastropasqua B, Chetta A, D´Ippolito R, Marazzini L, Olivieri D, Giovanni SS. Eosinophils, mast cells, and basophils in induced sputum from patients with seasonal allergic rhinitis and perennial asthma: relationship to methacholine responsiveness. Journal of Allergy and Clinical Immunology 1997;100:58–64.
32. Sedgwick JB, Calhoun WJ, Gleich GJ, Kita H, Abrams JS, Schwartz LB, Volovitz B, Ben-Yaakov M, Busse WW. Immediate and late airway response of allergic rhinitis patients to segmental antigen challenge: characterization of eosinophil and mast cell mediators. American Review of Respiratory Disease 1991;144:1274–81.
33. Corren J. Allergic rhinitis and asthma: how important is the link? Journal of Allergy and Clinical Immunology 1997;99:S781–786.
34. Braunstahl GJ, Kleinjan A, Overbeek SE, Prins JB, Hoogsteden HC, Fokkens WJ. Segmental bronchial provocation induces nasal inflammation in allergic rhinitis patients. American Journal of Respiratory and Critical Care Medicine 2000;161:2051–7.
35. Widdicombe JG. Neuroregulation of the nose and bronchi. Clinical and Experimental Allergy 1996;26:32–5.
36. Fuller RW, Jackson DM. Physiology and treatment of cough. Thorax 1990;45:425–30.
37. Irwin RS, Boulet LP, Cloutier MM, Fuller R, Gold PM, Hoffstein V, Ing AJ, McCool FD, O´Byrne P, Poe RH, Prakash UBS, Pratter MR, Rubin BK. Managing cough as a defense mechanism and as a symptom–a consensus panel report of the American College of Chest Physicians. Chest 1998;114:133S–181S.
38. Pecova R, Vrlik M, Tatar M. Cough sensitivity in allergic rhinitis. Journal of Physiology and Pharmacology 2005;56(Suppl 4):171–8.
39. Andersson M, Svensson C, Andersson P, Pipkorn U. Objective monitoring of the allergic inflammatory response of the nasal mucosa in patients with hay fever during natural allergen challenge. American Review of Respiratory Disease 1989;139:911–4.
40. Aubier M, Levy J, Clerici Ch, Neukirch F, Herman D. Different effects of nasal and bronchial glucocorticosteroid administration on bronchial hyperresponsiveness in patients with allergic rhinitis. American Review of Respiratory Disease 1992;146:122–6.
41. Polosa R, Ciamarra I, Mangano G, Prosperini G, Pistorio MP, Vancheri C, Crimi N. Bronchial hyperresponsiveness and airway inflammation markers in nonasthmatics with allergic rhinitis. European Respiratory Journal 2000;15:30–5.

42. Sant´Ambrogio G, Tsubone H, Sant´Ambrogio FB. Sensory information from the upper airway: role in the control of breathing. Respiration Physiology 1995;102:1–16.
43. Togias A. Mechanisms of nose-lung interaction. Allergy 1999;54(Suppl 57):94–105.
44. Canning BJ. Neurology of allergic inflammation and rhinitis. Current Allergy and Asthma Reports 2002;2:210–5.
45. Baraniuk JN, Ali M, Yuta A, Fang S-Y, Naranch K. Hypertonic saline nasal provocation stimulates nociceptive nerves, substance P release, and glandular mucous exocytosis in normal humans. American Journal of Respiratory and Critical Care Medicine 1999;160:655–62.
46. Weinfeld D, Ternesten-Hasseus E, Lowhagen O, Millqvist E. Capsaicin cough sensitivity in allergic asthmatic patients increases during the birch pollen season. Annals of Allergy, Asthma and Immunology 2002;89:419–24.
47. Ternesten-Hasseus E, Farbrot A, Lowhagen O, Millqvist E. Sensitivity to methacholine and capsaicin in patients with unclear respiratory symptoms. Allergy 2002;57:501–7.
48. Pecova R, Frlickova Z, Pec J, Tatar M. Cough sensitivity in atopic dermatitis. Pulmonary Pharmacology and Therapeutics 2003;16:203–6.
49. Tatar M, Karcolova D, Pecova R, Kollarik M, Plevkova J, Brozmanova M. Experimental modulation of the cough reflex. European Respiratory Review 2002;85:264–9.
50. Dicpinigaitis PV, Rauf K. The influence of gender on cough reflex sensitivity. Chest 1998;113:1319–21.
51. Kastelik JA, Thompson RH, Aziz I, Ojoo JC, Redington AE, Morice AH. Sex-related differences in cough reflex sensitivity in patients with chronic cough. American Journal of Respiratory and Critical Care Medicine 2002;166:961–4.
52. Leung DYM, Rhodes AR, Geha RS, Schneider L, Ring J. Atopic dermatitis (atopic eczema). In: Fitzpatrick TB, Eisen AZ, Wolff K, Freedberg IM, Austen KF, editors. Dermatology in General Medicine. New York: McGraw Hill, 1993;1534–56.
53. Braun-Falco O, Plewig G, Wolff HH, Burgdorf WH. Dermatology. Berlin Heidelberg, Springer-Verlag, 1996;585–613.
54. Miyabayashi Y. Bronchial hyperresponsiveness in atopic dermatitis. Acta Paediatrica Japonica 1997;39:205–9.
55. Salob SP, Laverty A, Atherton DJ. Bronchial hyperresponsiveness in children with atopic dermatitis. Pediatrics 1993;91:13–16.
56. Christophers E, Sterry W. Psoriasis. In: Fitzpatrick TB, Eisen AZ, Wolff K, Freedberg IM, Austen KF. Dermatology in General Medicine. New york: McGraw Hill, 1993, 490–511.
57. Tatar M, Nagyova B, Widdicombe JG. Veratrine-induced reflexes and cough. Respiratory Medicine 1991;85:51–5.
58. Tatar M, Nagyova B. Abdominal capsaicin-sensitive receptor activation and mechanically-induced cough in anaesthetised cats. Prague: Regional Meeting IUPS, 1991;98s.
59. Tatar M, Karcolova D. Role of repeated allergen challenge on cough reflex in awake guinea-pigs with experimental rhinitis. European Respiratory Journal 1999;Suppl 14:223–4.
60. Pecova R, Frlickova Z, Pec J, Tatar M. Cough sensitivity in localized sclerodermia with no clinical symptoms from lower airways. Journal of Physiology and Pharmacology 2003;54(Suppl. I): S25–S8.
61. Habif TP. Clinical Dermatology: A Color Guide to Diagnosis and Therapy. St. Louis, Missouri: C.V. Mosby Company, 1990;p756.

12 Pharmacotherapy of Cough

G Nosalova, S Franova, J Mokry, M Sutovska

12.1 INTRODUCTION

Cough represents one of the important ways of transmitting infections besides being a reflex for keeping the respiratory tract clean.[1] Coughing prevents the airways from being blocked and prevents mucus from getting into the lungs and the bronchi. In healthy persons, cough may be seen in a situation where the mucociliar apparatus and alveolar macrophages are unable to clean the airways, as during accidental dropping of food particles into the airways or by the inhalation of irritant gases.[2]

Cough, as is well known, is an affliction for which people visit physicians most frequently.[3] Cough is considered a pathological reflex from the moment it starts to burden the patient's organs. Pathological cough (especially the chronic form) has significant impact on patient's physical activity or psychosocial domain. Coughing patients, often suffer from insomnia, exhaustion, nausea and vomiting, or urinary incontinence. In many, it could lead to a need for changing their jobs or refraining from participating in important social activities.[4] The intrathoracic pressure changes during cough (inspiration –13 kPa and expiration +30 kPa) can cause costal fractures, cough syncope, pneumothorax, pneumomediastinum and even herniation. In patients with coronary lesions, even anginal pain can be initiated. Antitussive drugs such as codeine and dextromethorphan are among the most commonly used prescription and over-the-counter (OTC) drugs.[5] The widespread use of antitussive medications for the treatment of cough, associated with upper respiratory tract infection together with therapy of chronic cough generates millions of dollars for the pharmaceutical industry.[6] These facts

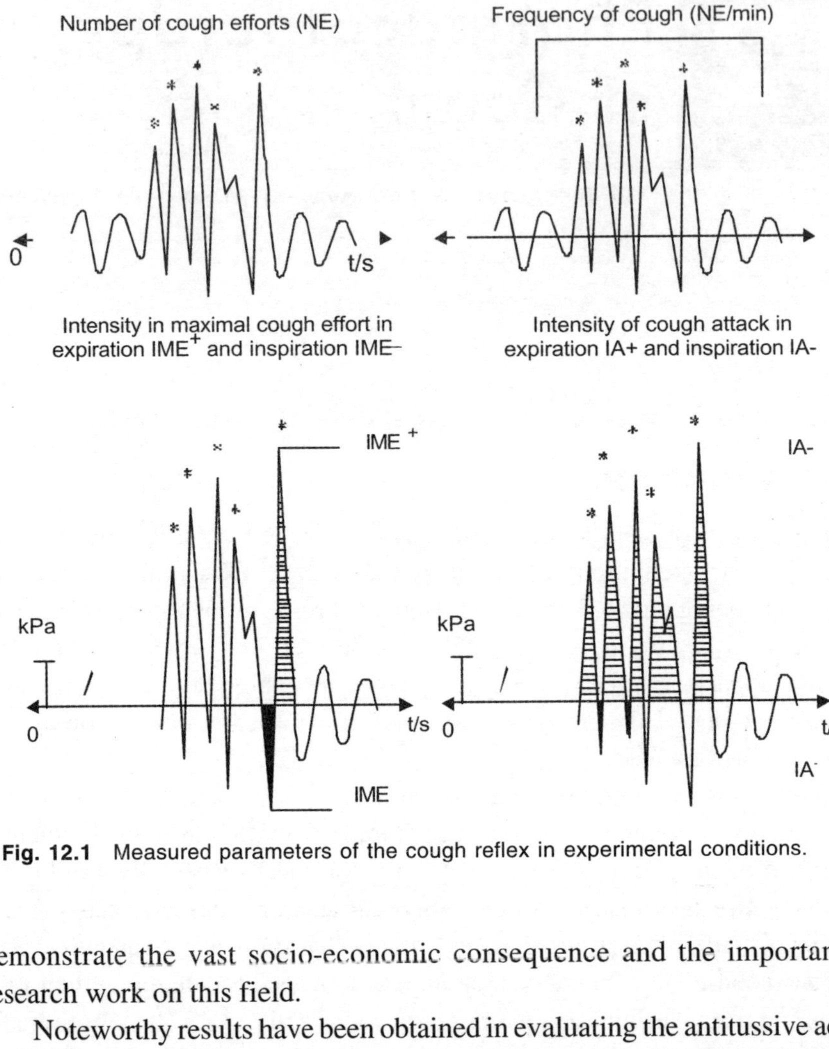

Fig. 12.1 Measured parameters of the cough reflex in experimental conditions.

demonstrate the vast socio-economic consequence and the importance of research work on this field.

Noteworthy results have been obtained in evaluating the antitussive activity of various substances based on objective methods for cough reflex evaluation,[7,8] which include studies on conscious animals and therefore without any influence of anaesthetics. A big advantage of this evaluation is the possibility of assessing the efficacy of agents in suppression of cough from laryngopharyngeal and tracheobronchial mucus areas separately (Table 12.1). Furthermore, there is a possibility to assess the antitussive activity according to the number of cough efforts, frequency, intensity of cough attack, and intensity of maximal cough effort in expiration or in inspiration (Fig. 12.1).

Table 12.1 Differing influence of drugs with antitussive activity on cough arising from laryngopharyngeal (LPh) and tracheobronchial (TB) areas of the airways

Higher efficacy in Lph area	*Higher efficacy in TB area*
Procaine	Tramadol
Azipranone	Tilidin
Glaucine	Pentazocine
Butamirate citrate	
Dropropizine	L-propoxyphene
Isoprenaline	Dextromethorphan
Guaifenesin	Clobutinol
Diazepam	Gabalid

12.2 PHARMACOLOGICAL MANAGEMENT OF COUGH

Agents used in pharmacotherapy of cough are divided into two main categories:

1. Drugs that selectively inhibit or moderate the cough reflex are called antitussive agents.
2. Agents that can make cough reflex more effective are called protussive drugs.

A 'lessening' of the cough could be considered as a reduction in the number of cough efforts, a decrease in its duration or of its intensity.[9] Pharmacologically, it is important to know that cough as a reflex can be modulated by agents acting at various levels of reflex arc, i.e. at the level of the receptors, afferent nerves, cough centre, efferent nerves and effectors, as well as by alteration of bronchial secretions. Some of the agents can exert an influence at several levels with a predominance at any one of them.

According to their source, cough-suppressive substances can either be natural or synthetic agents. The most common division of antitussive drugs, is according to their place of action, namely centrally acting agents, and agents with peripheral action.[10,11] (Fig 12.2). Nevertheless, many of the drugs have both, a central and a peripheral action. Table 12.2 shows a classification of these agents according to their particular action.

The terms 'specific and non-specific therapy of cough' relate to whether the therapy is aimed at the elimination of the underlying disease or only to its symptoms. Specific antitussive therapy helps the elimination of aetiological agents or pathophysiological mechanisms. Some examples are; stopping to smoke by patients with chronic bronchitis, elimination of postnasal discharge in allergic rhinitis and chronic sinusitis, and killing of bacilli in tuberculosis.[12,13] Identifying

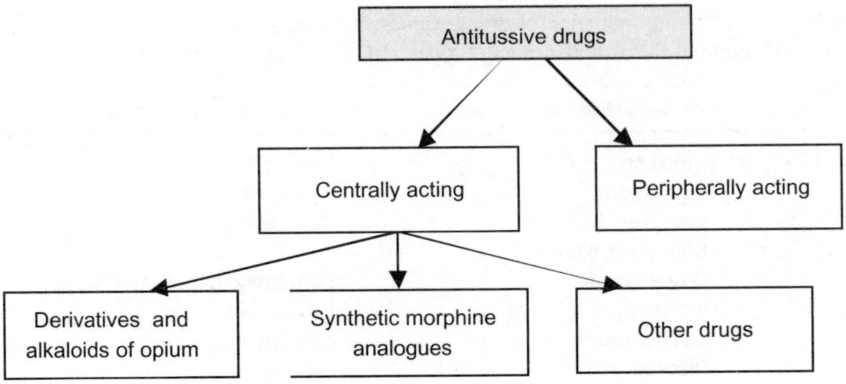

Fig. 12.2 Classification of drugs with antitussive activity.

the correct reason for cough is essential for the efficacy of specific antitussive therapy in 97 per cent of the cases. Non-specific antitussive therapy is focussed more on the removal of disease symptoms than on its aetiology or pathophysiological mechanism. It is indicated in cases when no specific therapy is possible as the cause evoking the cough is not known. Non-specific antitussive agents work in either of the following three ways:

A. Modulation of central coordination of cough reflex—either by increasing the irritation threshold or by depressing the activity of the central structures of cough reflex control in the medulla oblongata or the cortical areas of the central nervous system (CNS).[14,15]

B. Modulation of peripheral coordination of cough reflex—either by decreasing the sensitivity of peripheral reflexive zones or by interrupting the conduction of nerve impulses in afferent or efferent nerve fibres of the cough reflex arc.[16-18]

C. Changing bronchial secretion.[19,20]

12.2.1 Drugs Modulating Central Coordination of Cough Reflex

There is clear evidence that airway sensory afferents, irrespective of whether they are myelinated or non-myelinated, terminate within the brainstem in dorsal medulla NMDA, i.e. in nucleus tractus solitarius.[21,22] The fact that opiate receptors, receptors, and 5-HT receptors are able to modulate transmission through nucleus tractus solitarius is well known. This region is anatomically adjacent to the area postrema, where the blood-brain barrier (BBB) is weak or

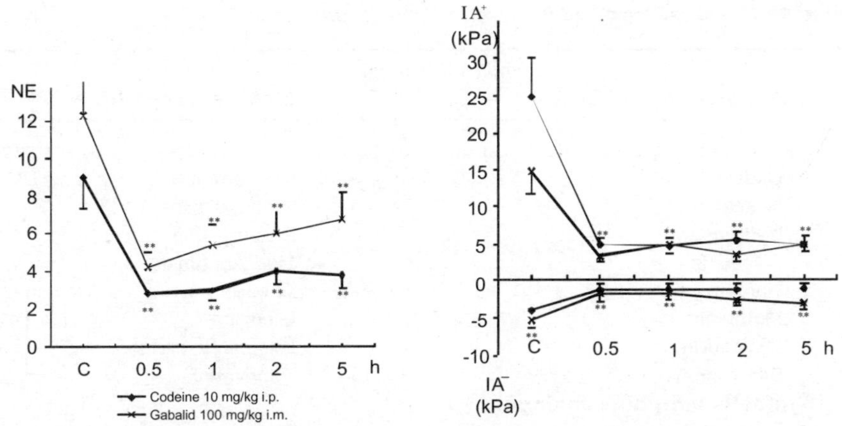

Fig. 12.3 Comparison of antitussive effect of gabalid with cough-suppressing activity of codeine from tracheobronchial area of the airways; before drug administration (C – control) and during 5 hours after administration. Evaluated cough parameters: number of cough efforts (NE), intensity of cough attacks in expiration (IA^+) and inspiration (IA^-).

absent, so that, these antitussive drugs given peripherally could be acting at the sensory side of the system. Other areas such as nucleus ambiguus and the dorsal vagal nuclei also contain these types of receptors and could be considered as additional sites of action. Activation of NMDA receptors and opiate and serotonergic systems can modify the central respiratory network.

In spite of a large body of work carried out by experimentalists, all the neurochemical processes participating in the mechanism of action of antitussive agents are still not known. Hedner et al[23-25] highlighted an important role of gamma-aminobutyric acid (GABA) in tonic modulation of respiratory activity. As breathing and cough centres are closely associated, we decided to verify the ability of GABA-ergic substance to influence cough reflex. We obtained original priority results,[26,27] which support the statement that GABA-ergic substances are able to suppress cough (Fig. 12.3) and that these mechanisms can participate in the action of other cough-suppressing agents.

Centrally acting antitussive drugs are classified as follows (Table 12.2):

- Derivatives and alkaloids of opium
- Synthetic morphine analogues
- Other drugs.

Derivatives and Alkaloids of Opium

In the past, derivatives and alkaloids of opium were the only drugs the physicians

Table 12.2 Classification of antitussive acting drugs

	Antitussive drugs	
	Higher efficacy in Lph area	*Higher efficacy in TB area*
A.	**Derivatives and alkaloids of opium**	
	Codeine	Benzonatate
	Noscapin	Prenoxdiazine
	Hydrocodon	Dropropizine
	Folcodine	Medazonamide
	Narcein	Azipranone
	Morphine	Glaucine
	Oxycodon	Butamirate citrate
	Ethylmorphine	Papaverine
B.	**Synthetic morphine analogues**	
	Dextromethorphan	Ganglioplegics
		Local anesthetics
C.	**Other drugs**	
	Clobutinol	Mucoactive substances
	Anxiolytics (diazepam, guaifenesin)	Demulcerative substances
	Hypnotics (pentobarbital)	
	Neuroleptics (chlorpromazine)	
	Antihistamines (clemastine, cimetidine)	
	Opioid analgesics	
	GABA-ergic substances (gabalid)	

used for cough suppression. The antitussive activity of these agents was associated with their ability to decrease the sensitivity of the cough centre to nerve impulses coming from airway receptors[28] and inhibition of expiratory motor drive and reduction of cough number.[29] The chief cough suppressive agent from the opioid family was codeine (3-methylmorphine, $C_{18}H_{21}NO_3$).

Oral as well as parenteral application of codeine in different doses[5,10,15] (mg/kg body weight) suppressed cough significantly[30] Cough-suppressive activity of codeine was not significantly influenced in pathological conditions, such as inflammation of the airways provoked by application of croton oil or by *Staphylococcus aureus* infection was not influenced by the suppressive activity of codeine[31] (Fig. 12.4).

It is well known that codeine, an alkaloid of opium has analgesic properties. The effect of this agonist, mediated mainly through interaction with μ-opioid receptors (via activation of μ_1 type of receptor[32-34] was studied for its role in antitussive action. It was found that codeine inhibited cough reflex in doses

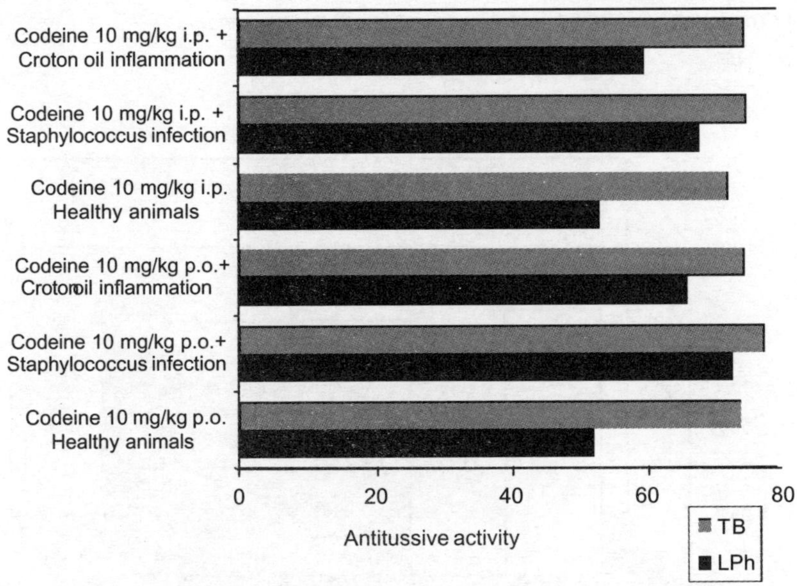

Fig. 12.4 Antitussive effect of codeine on cough elicited from laryngophar-yngeal (LPh) and tracheobronchial (TB) areas of the airways when administered intraperitoneally (10 mg/kg) or perorally (10 mg/kg) during control (physiological) and under pathological conditions (inflammation of the airways with croton oil and Staphylococcus aureus airways infection).

Table 12.3 Relationship between dose and analgesic activity of codeine

Dose of codeine	*Analgesic activity*
2.5 mg/kg	20%
5.0 mg/kg	20%
10.0 mg/kg	40%
20.0 mg/kg	70%

lower than those, that are necessary for analgesic activity (Table 12.3). Thus, 5 mg/kg codeine, which has only 20 per cent of its analgesic activity, significantly reduced the parameters of cough.[35] Results from our laboratory suggest that codeine can suppress cough in subanalgesic doses; which, in other words, means that antitussive activity of codeine is mediated through other types of opioid receptors.

Numerous data indicate cough suppression by stimulation of k-receptors as well as s-receptors.[36,37] This has been supported by the finding that, a

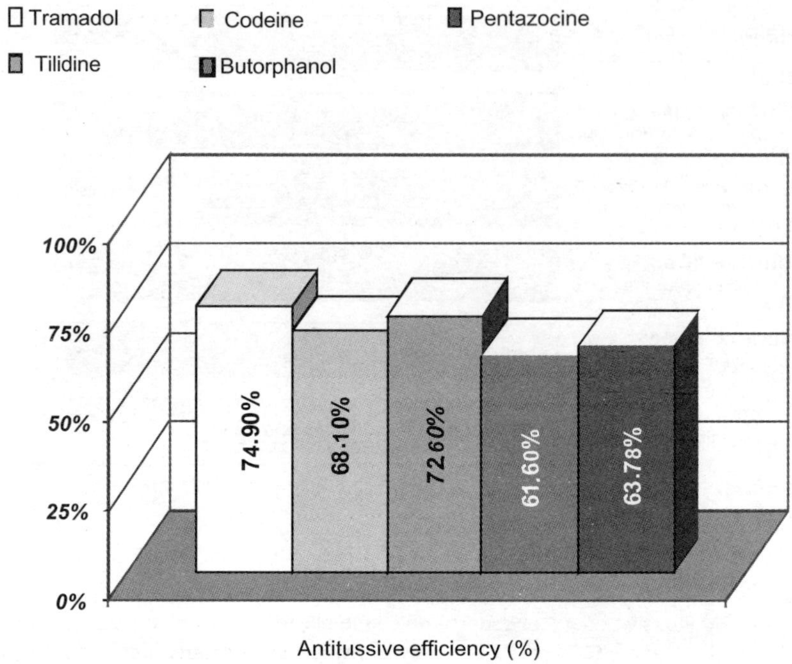

Fig. 12.5 Antitussive effect of opioid analgesics (tramadol, codeine, tilidine, butorphanol, pentazocins) on cough induced by mechanical stimulation of the airways.

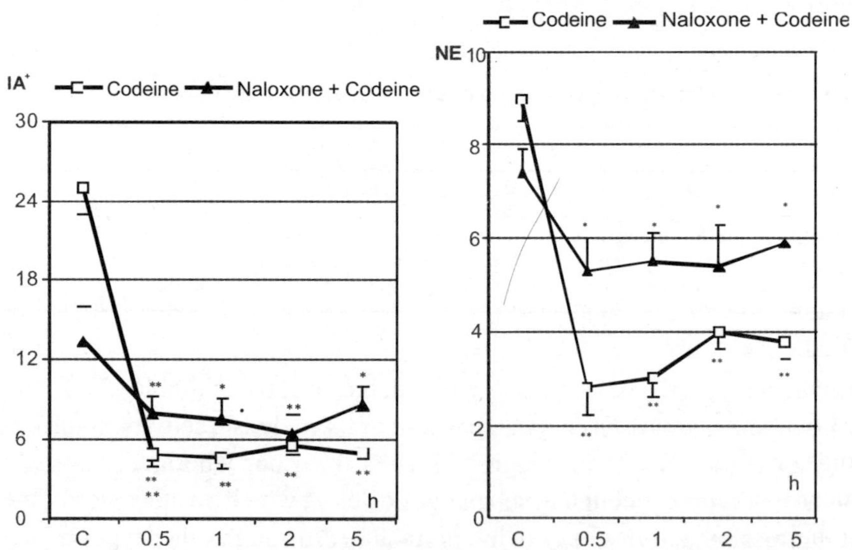

Fig. 12.6 Changes in antitussive activity of codeine (10 mg/kg i.p.) induced by pretreatment with naloxone (10 mg/kg i.p.); before drug administration (C–control) and during 5 hours after administration. Cough parameters studied: number of cough efforts (NE) and intensity of cough attacks in expiration (IA$^+$) from tracheobronchial area of the airways.

significant decrease in the parameters of cough, after application of substances influencing different types of opiate receptors, was seen[38] (Fig. 12.5).

This fact was also supported by our experiments with naloxone (antagonist of μ-opioid receptors). A pretreatment with naloxone, before codeine administration, did not significantly suppress the antitussive activity of codeine (Fig.12.6). These results also confirm that there are other important types of opioid receptors that could be responsible for a complete antitussive activity.

In early 1990s, it was hypothesised that an antitussive effect could be observed by the modification of endogenous opioid nervous system via d-opioid receptors. Therefore, it was suggested that d-opioid receptors are a potential target for the development of antitussive agents. Saitoh et al[39] confirmed this fact. Although the involvement of d-receptors in cough has been described,[32,40-42] some receptors, especially of d_1 type, are controversial. Kamei[41,42] showed antitussive effect of d_1 antagonists, contrary to Kotzer's finding,[43] who pointed out the dose-dependent ability of different agonists of μ, k, and d receptors to reduce cough. The mechanism of cough-suppressant effect of d agonists seems to be independent from μ and k receptors. The function of the e-type opiate receptors is still not clear. The new classification of opioid receptors by the International Union of Pharmacology Subcommitee on Opioid Receptors (IUPSOR) recommended designating d receptors as OP1, k receptors as OP2 and μ receptors as OP3.[44,45]

The function of ORL_1 (opioid-like receptors) is related to the inhibition of adenylatecyclase activity, sensory nerve activity in airways and may be an excellent target for new antitussive treatment.[46,47]

In peripheral tissues, including lungs, there occur probably the same types of opiate receptors as those in CNS. This is clear from those studies that verified the cough-depressant properties of 'type-specific' opiate receptor modulators, after administering them locally.[48] The potency and rapid onset of the action of inhaled codeine suggest that it exerts its effects without being metabolised to morphine.[37]

Precise mechanisms of action of opiates are incomplete. We know that opioids interact with stereospecific and saturable binding sites in CNS and other tissues, with highest concentration in limbic system, thalamus, striatum, hypothalamus, midbrain and spinal cord.[49-51] Their effects may result from mimicing the actions of enkephalins, beta-endorphins and other exogenous ligands, which have been found to occupy the same binding sites.[52] These actions appear to alter the rate of release of neurotransmitters. Opioids and exogenous peptides

Table 12.4 Effect of haloperidol pretreatment on the antitussive activity of codeine.

Treatment	*Antitussive activity (%)*
Codeine 10.0 mg/kg i.p.	68.6%
Haloperidol 0.1 mg/kg i.p. 15 minutes before codeine	69.8%
Haloperidol 0.1 mg/kg i.p. 30 minutes before codeinem	61.9%

inhibit the release of acetylcholine, norepinephrine, and substance P in the nerves, as well as influence the release of dopamine.[53-55]

From these, it appears that the opioid receptors are not the only ones that mediate antitussive activity.

The question was: which of the other types of receptors take part in antitussive activity of agents? Numerous data describe a close relationship between opiate and serotoninergic systems in nociception as well as cough regulations.[56-58] We found that pretreatment with 5-HT_2 receptor antagonist ketanserine reduced cough-depressant activity of codeine only by 10 per cent and tramadol by 20 per cent.[38] These observations are similar to those seen by others[59,60] (Fig.12.7). The fact that monoamines are involved in the mechanism of action of opiates is an accepted fact. Reserpine produces depression of brain levels of norepi-nephrine, dopamine and serotonine.[56] Nosalova[61] verified the results of Kamei[56] and showed that reserpine application before it diminished the property of codeine to reduce cough parameters (Fig 12.8). From this, it is clear that the level of monoamines is important for a full antitussive activity of agents. Now, the question was, which type of monoamines (except serotonines whose properties are well known) play the most important role in these processes? Is it dopamine? We found that the ability of codeine to reduce the cough parameters was unchanged after pretreatment with haloperidol[38] (Table 12.4). Some authors indicated the ability of dopaminergic agonists to modulate cough reflex through inhibition of vagal depolarisation.[62,63]

Cellular Mechanisms of Action

Opioid receptors belong to the family of G-protein-coupled receptors that inhibit adenylatecyclase, leading to reduction of intracellular cAMP levels.[44] Codeine is a pure agonist on μ-receptors (+++), ძ-receptors (+) and k-receptors (+). All three receptor subtypes decrease the levels of cAMP and affect ion channels directly through coupling G protein with these channels.

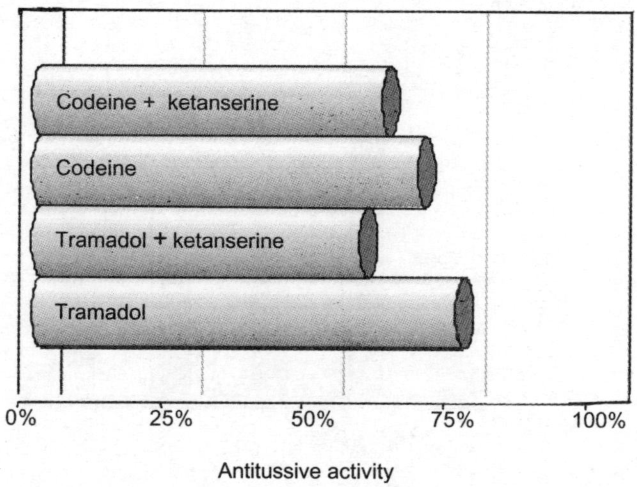

Fig. 12.7 Changes in antitussive factivity of codeine (10 mg/kg i.p.) and tramadol (10 mg/kg ip) induced by pretreatment (15 minute earlier) with ketanserine (1.0 mg/kg i.p).

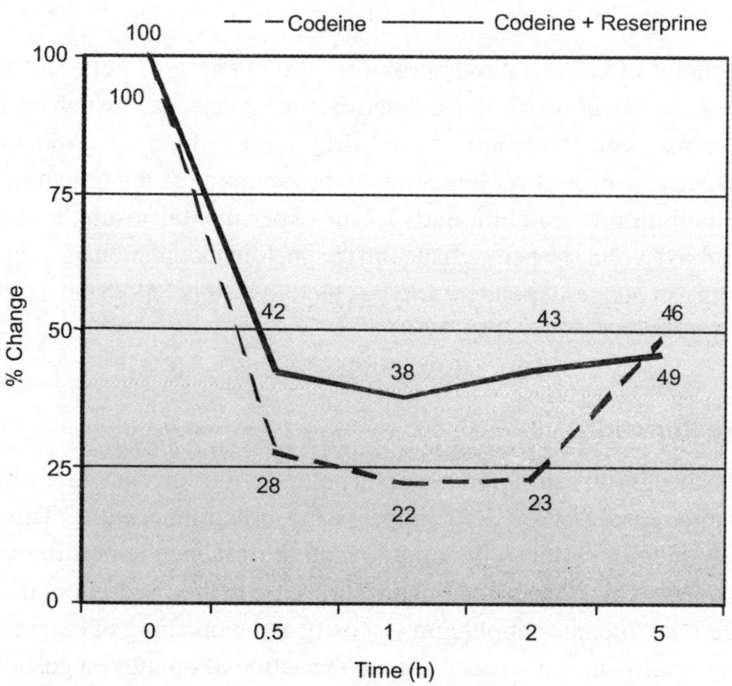

Fig. 12.8 Effect of reserpine pretreatment (2.5 mg/kg i.p. 24 hours before codeine) on the antitussive activity of codeine.

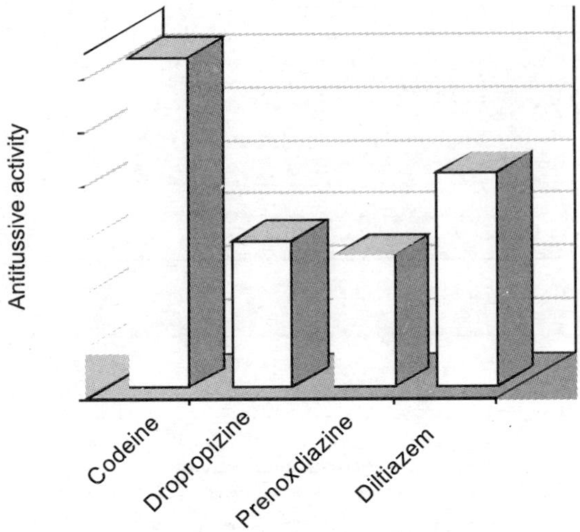

Fig. 12.9 Comparison of the antitussive activity of diltiazem (30 mg/kg) with the cough-suppressing effect of codeine (10 mg/kg i.p.), prenoxdia-zine (50 mg/kg i.p.) and dropropizine (30 mg/kg i.p.) on experimentally induced cough.

The latter effect of opioids promotes the opening of potassium channels and inhibits the opening of voltage-gated calcium channels,[64] which are important for reducing both neuronal excitability (since the increased potassium conductance causes hyperpolarisation of the membrane) and transmitter release (due to inhibition of calcium entry). Our experimental results confirmed the participation of voltage-operated calcium channels in modulation of cough reflex.[65] Diltiazem, as voltage-dependent L-type calcium channel blocker, showed a high cough-suppressing ability (Fig. 12.9).

Adverse Reactions

Although this group can suppress cough potently, the current worldwide trend is to limit their use as they also suppress the breathing centre. This effect is especially seen in children. Its other negative influence is on diminishing the activity of bronchial glands leading to a decrease in their secretion, inhibition of ciliary activity, increase of phlegm viscosity and worsening of expectoration.

Constipation may also occur due to the action of opiates on gastrointestinal tract. Codeine increases muscle tone and decreases gastric motility, especially in elders. An adverse effect of codeine is that it induces drug dependence. A long-term use of opiate antitussives is not recommended except for palliative purposes in patients with lung cancer.

Synthetic Morphine Analogues

Dextromethorphan is a dextroisomer of opiate levomethorphan, and it has no analgesic or sedative properties. This drug is a commonly used antitussive in the USA.[45] Dextromethorphan is the most important member in the group of synthetic morphine derivatives (Rhinotussal, Romilar), with no suppressive effect on breathing centre. Our results suggest that dextromethorphan possesses an excellent antitussive activity.[66] It is a substance with NMDA agonistic activity coupled with activation of sigma opioid receptors.[67,68] Its main metabolite is dextrorphan. Braga[67] showed a comparable antitussive activity of metabolite dextrorphan with the basic agent. Its adverse effects, occurring in less than 1 per cent of patients, include drowsiness, dizziness nausea, and abdominal disorders. Respiratory depression may occur in case of overdose. No constipation was observed. Since all opiates and opiate analogues can release histamine leading to bronchospasm, both codeine and dextromethorphan are relatively contraindicated in patients with bronchial asthma or chronic obstructive pulmonary disease.[69] A well-known advantage of this drug is that it does not cause dependence although its psycho-mimetic effects that have been pointed out, are via s-receptor activation.[70] Recent data suggest that it may be a clinically useful neuronal nicotinic receptor antagonist, that possibly aids persons addicted to smoking.[71] Dextromethorphan is contraindicated in persons taking monoamine oxidase inhibitors (MAOIs). The mechanism of this reaction has not been established. The obvious advantage of these drugs is that they do not cause dependence and that their psycho mimetic effects are produced via stimulation of s-receptors.

Other Drugs

Clobutinol (Silomat, KAT 256) is a drug with a central cough-suppressing effect (Table 12.5). Clobutinol has no addictive properties of codeine, nor does it suppress, but can stimulate the breathing centre. The agent has no analgesic activity. It is suitable for therapy of cough caused by haemoptysis during endoscopial procedures in the respiratory system during severe pertussis. Many centrally acting agents showed cough-suppressive efficacy apart from other pharmacological activities.

Table 12.5 Antitussive activity of non-opioid drugs with central cough-suppressing effect

Substance	*Dose*	*Antitussive activity (%)*
Clobutinol	20.0 mg/kg i.p.	36.1
Diazepam	0.3 mg/kg i.p.	32.4
Guaifenesin	5.0 mg/kg p.o.	33.6
Pentobarbital	15.0 mg/kg i.v.	16.6
Chlorpromazine	5.0 mg/kg i.p.	44.2
Clemastine	0.1 mg/kg i.p.	27.4

Anxiolytics

Diazepam is a modulator of $GABA_A$ receptors that function via interaction with specific binding sites. It activates chloride channels, hyperpolarises neurocyte membrane and reduces cellular reactivity.[68] Increased gabaergic transmission is the main mechanism of action of this drug. We observed (Table 12.5) an interesting antitussive activity of diazepam in doses of 0.05 mg/kg body weight intraperitonelly. This effect was especially related to the reduction of number of cough efforts and intensity of cough attacks. Both antitussive and sedative effects might be useful in the treatment of psychogenic cough.

Diazepam is not recommended for respiratory tract infection with hypersecretion of mucus, especially in paediatric practice. Cough-suppressing effect in this situation would have a negative influence on the therapeutic process.

Control of cough is of paramount importance for the quality of bronchoscopy, as this facilitates viewing the bronchial tree and obtaining good biopsy samples. Moreover, excessive cough can increase the risk of complication or prevent the performance of invasive procedures during bronchoscopic examination. The current guidelines of British Thoracic Society do not recommend the combined use of benzodiazepine or opiate during flexible bronchoscopy for suppressing cough. Stolz et al[72] in a randomised, placebo-controlled, double-blind study showed that the combination of midazolam and hydrocodone markedly reduced cough during flexible bronchoscopy without causing significant desaturation. This combination improves operating conditions due to its antitussive effect.

Guaifenesin has been used as an expectorant over the last 25 years. It was thought to act through stimulation of the vagal afferent nerves in gastric mucosa. These nerves stimulate the secretion of fluids from the bronchial glands, thereby decreasing the viscosity of or liquefying the mucus and facilitating expectoration. It was reported to possess muscle relaxant (via inhibition of

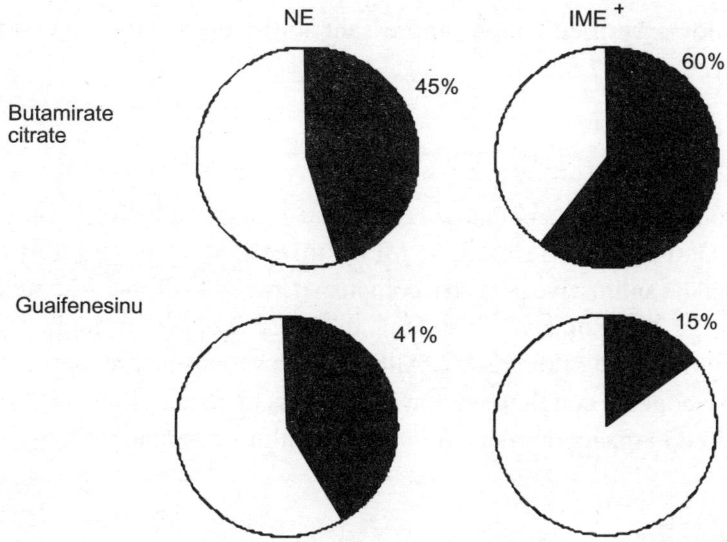

Fig. 12.10 Comparison of antitussive activity of butamirate citrate and guaifenesin seen as an influence on number of cough efforts (NE) and intensity of maximal cough effort (IME⁺).

polysynaptic spinal reflexes) and anxiolytic activities without analgesic efficacy. However, data about its cough-depressant property are controversial. Nosalova et al[73] and Parvez et al[74] reported that this agent had antitussive activity (Table 12.5). Guaifenesin decreased all parameters of cough except intensity of maximal cough effort (Fig. 12.10). These results supported the fact that guaifenesin does not reduce the efficacy of expectoration. We suppose that guaifenesin reaches cough-suppressive activity through interaction with gabaergic receptor system.

Guaifenesin interferes in tests for detecting certain cancers and could, therefore, mask their diagnosis. Such patients are to be advised to refrain from taking guaifenesin for three days prior to the testing.[75] Guaifenesin also reduces plasma level of uric acid.[76]

Hypnotics

Pentobarbital interacts with a different binding site at the same receptor as diazepam. Yamada et al[77] showed that pentobarbital evokes respiratory depression through interaction with gabaergic system localised in medulla oblongata. The same effect can occur in antitussive action of this agent. Korpas and Nosalova[1] verified cough suppressant ability of this drug in experimental conditions (Table 12.5).

Neuroleptics

Chlorpromazine is a phenothiazine derivative used primarily for its antipsychotic, sedative and antiemetic effects. Many investigators have published data evaluating the antitussive property both in experimental (Table 12.5) and clinical conditions.[78-81] Hosokawa[82] found that this agent is able to influence cough at a higher control level of the reflex. Although we suppose a great potency of this drug in psycogenic cough treatment is due to its main activities, yet care should be exercised in the recommendation of phenothiazine analogues.

Antihistamines

H_1 receptors are related to the pathophysiology of cough during allergic disorders such as eosinophilic bronchitis, and, therefore H_1 antihistamines might be a good choice for these patients.[83] The older known antihistamines block both histamine H_1 receptors and muscarinic receptors and can cross the blood-brain barrier (BBB). Their effectiveness may be exerted primarily due to the interactions of neuropharmacological histaminic and muscarinic receptors. Newer generation of antihistamines blocks mainly H_1 receptors that are relatively lipophobic and do not affect cough reflex sensitivity in healthy conditions.[84] Since the cough is an entirely vagally mediated phenomenon, the antitussive effects of the older and newer generations of antihistamines are explained by their relative anticholinergic activity and not by H_1 antagonism alone.[85,86] Antitussive effect of H_1 antihistamines might also be partly due to the inhibition of substance P (SP) release from sensory nerves.[87] Some antihistamines (chlorpheniramine) given together with opiate agonists are able to increase their antitussive effect.[88] Cough suppressive property of H_1 antagonist clemastine have been tested during our experimental studies.[89] We showed a reduction in cough parameters from both parts a airways after application of a dose of 0.1 mg/kg body weight intraperitoneally (Table 12.5).

H_2 receptors function is still being debated; their stimulation in the stomach leads to an increase of gastric secretion; and therefore H_2 antihistamines are used in treatment of gastric ulcerations for long time periods. Williams et al[90] published information describing a bronchodilating activity after stimulation of

H_2 receptors. Cimetidine stimulates gabaergic release and probably this mechanism participates in modulation of cough found during our experiments[91,92] Cimetidine typically reduced the number of cough efforts and intensity of cough attack from both parts of the airways. Bolser[93] showed that there is no influence of H_2 blocking drugs on capsaicin-induced cough in guinea pigs, this might be due to species (experimental animals) difference.

Opioid Analgesics

Opioid analgesics are another group of substances with great potency to inhibit an experimental cough. This property was verified during our experimental work, and our results[38] are similar to other published data[57,94] (Fig. 12.5). The antitussive activity of tested opioid analgesics is related to their affinity to various types of opioid receptors.

12.2.2 Drugs Modulating Peripheral Coordination of Cough Reflex

From pharmacological point of view, it is important to know that agents modulating cough reflex via interaction with peripheral structures are able to relax the smooth muscle of the airways or can have local anaesthetic or anti-inflammatory activity, and could possibly change the quality and quantity of mucus. These pharmacodynamic properties are associated with their ability to inhibit cholinergic and μ-adrenergic receptor activity or non-cholinergic-non-adrenergic (NANC) system to decrease release of tachykinins (SP, neurokinin A or NKA) and the synthesis of prostaglandins and leukotrienes.

Larynx and Pharynx : Laryngopharyngeal Type of Cough

Knowing what structures participate in the genesis of this defense mechanism is important for antitussive therapy, because the mechanism of both peripherally and centrally acting antitussive drugs may depend on the identity of afferent pathways involved.

Larynx, being the sentinel of the lungs, possesses abundant sensory innervations, which can produce violent coughing. Afferent activity may be elicited from the larynx by mechanical or chemical irritants. Most of the sensory traffic from larynx is conveyed in the superior laryngeal nerves.[95,96] Three types of

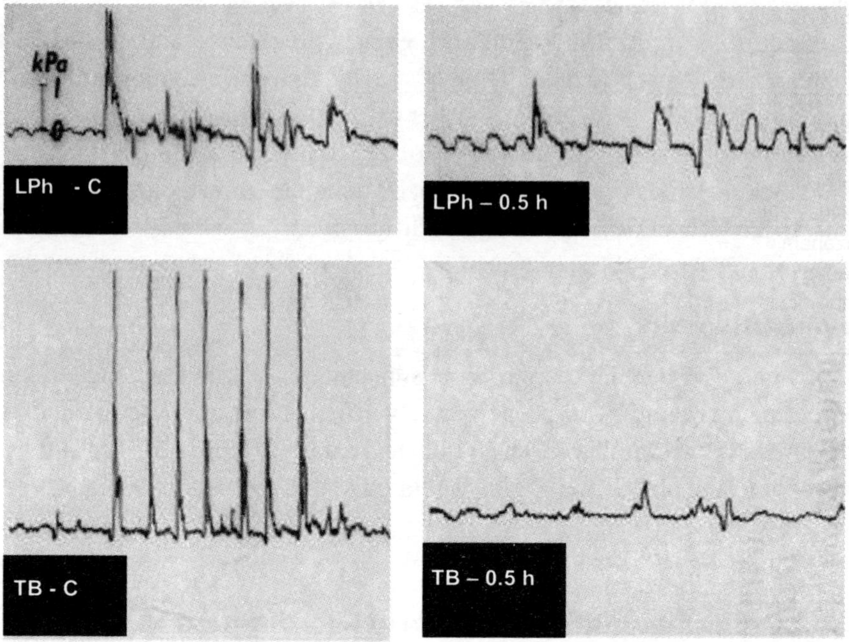

Fig. 12.11 Record of cough induced experimentally from laryngophary-ngeal (LPh) and its tracheobronchial (TB) area before application of antitussive drug (C) and half an hour after its application (0.5 h).

receptors, i.e. pressure, drive and cold take part in a clear respiratory modulation. Pressure receptors respond to changes in translaryngeal pressure; drive receptors are stimulated by passive or active motion of larynx; cold or flow receptors respond to a decrease in laryngeal temperature. Although respiratory-modulated receptors play an important role in the function of the upper airways, they are not generally viewed as a primary factor in the elicitation of cough reflex.

There are two types of receptors localised in the laryngeal mucosa that are part of the cough reflex. They are as follows.

Rapidly adapting stretch receptors (RARs) Cough reflex is probably caused by the stimulation of these irregularly firing receptors. They are usually silent in quiet breathing and activated by mechanical or chemical irritant stimuli (e.g. cigarette smoke, distilled water, CO_2). Since they are blocked promptly by topical anaesthetics, they are considered as having a superficial location.[97]

Our results suggest that application of nebulised procaine (Table 12.6) leads to a decrease in the mechanically evoked cough reflex.[98] Other investigators showed that an inhalation of procaine, lidocaine and bupivacaine inhibits this

Table 12.6 Antitussive efficiency of drugs modulating the cough reflex peripherally

Substance	*Dose*	*Antitussive activity (%)*
Procaine	10.0 mg/kg	39.2
Butamirate citrate	5.0 mg/kg i.p.	57.3
Dropropizine	100.0 mg/kg i.p.	27.3
Prenoxdiazine	30.0 mg/kg i.p.	24.7
Medazonamid	10.0 mg/kg i.p.	21.4
Azipranon (R.U. 20201) inhaled	200.0 mg/kg	46.9
Enprophylline	10.0 mg/kg i.p.	31.6
Propentophylline	10.0 mg/kg i.p.	36.4

reflex when elicited both by mechanical and chemical stimulations. The anatomical localisation of cough receptors in airways enables the use of local anaesthetics, which could be ideal from the pharmacological point of view. But these are not selective enough for use. Inhalation of anaesthetising aerosols leads to desensitisation of cough receptors as well as other segments of mucous membranes (in mouth, upper and lower parts of respiratory system), and increases the risk of aspiration.[99,100] The application of nebulised local anaesthetics (lidocaine or bupivacaine) gives short-term relief for severe cough but causes undesirable inhibition of important upper airway reflexes, and therefore cannot be recommended. In the clinic, local anaesthetics are used for the elimination of cough before diagnostic procedures such as laryngoscopy, bronchoscopy and intubations.

In the mechanism of action of some cough-suppressing agents with peripheral action,[1] a local anaesthetic activity takes part (benzonatate, dropropizine and azipranon). These drugs are more efficacious in suppression of cough from laryngopharyngeal areas as compared to that from tracheobronchial areas of airways (Table 12.1).

C-fibre receptors These are sensitive to mechanical stimulation, cooling, chemical stimulation by capsaicin and phenylbiguanide.

Characteristic signs of laryngopharyngeal cough are active expirations and several fast and powerful inspiratory movements. The distinguishing feature of tracheobronchial cough lies in the presence of an inspiratory component, which is as strong as, or even stronger than, the active expiratory component (Fig. 12.11). From the pharmacological point of view, this type of cough is more resistant to cough suppressant agents. From our own results, we can conclude that the influence of antitussive agents varies very strongly. We found that some substances can suppress cough from laryngopharyngeal area more effectively, while other substances showed an inclination towards tracheobronchial cough suppression (Table 12.1). It is also necessary to say that laryngopharyngeal type of cough is more resistant to cough suppressants.

Tracheobronchial Tree : Tracheobronchial Type of Cough

There are three types of sensory nerve endings in tracheobronchial region of respiratory tract.

Rapidly adapting pulmonary stretch receptors (RARs) or 'irritant' receptors This type of receptors seems to play a very important role in cough reflex. RARs respond to mechanical and chemical stimuli (e.g. prostaglandin E_2, histamine, cigarette smoke). The most frequent cause of abnormal cough reaction is the presence of pathological processes in respiratory system, leading to increased irritability of afferent nerve endings or increased sensitivity to different stimuli. These conditions can be found during inflammatory diseases of upper and lower airways, i.e. to viral or bacterial presence. The drugs, that can normalise the pathophysiological processes in the airways can also suppress the cough reflex. Some representatives of these agents (benzonatate, droproprizine, glaucine, butamirate citrate, azipranon-R.U. 20201) produce anti-inflammatory, local anaesthetic, and bronchospasmolytic activities. In our experiments, we observed antitussive activity of these substances (Table 12.6).

Slowly adapting stretch receptors They are located in the membranous posterior wall of conducting airways within the smooth muscle. They are supposed to be important for the act of coughing. Benzonatate (Exangit, Tessalon) is the drug, that influences this type of receptors.

Tracheobronchial C-fibre receptors The stimulation of bronchial C-fibre receptors can cause cough as well as apnea and bronchoconstriction. Some stimuli used for activating C-fibre receptors can also activate RARs. Many cough inducing chemical stimuli (like bradykinin) may act directly on RARs, but they can also activate C-fibre receptors, to release tachykinins. These in turn will act on post-capillary venules with plasma extravasation and stimulation of adjacent RARs. The increase in interstitial liquid volume might affect the structure of epithelium with stimulation of branches of RARs.[101] Dry, non-productive cough associated with increased levels of bradykinin and substance P, in the respiratory tract is induced by angiotensin-converting enzyme inhibitors (ACEI). We confirmed in experimental conditions that long-lasting treatment

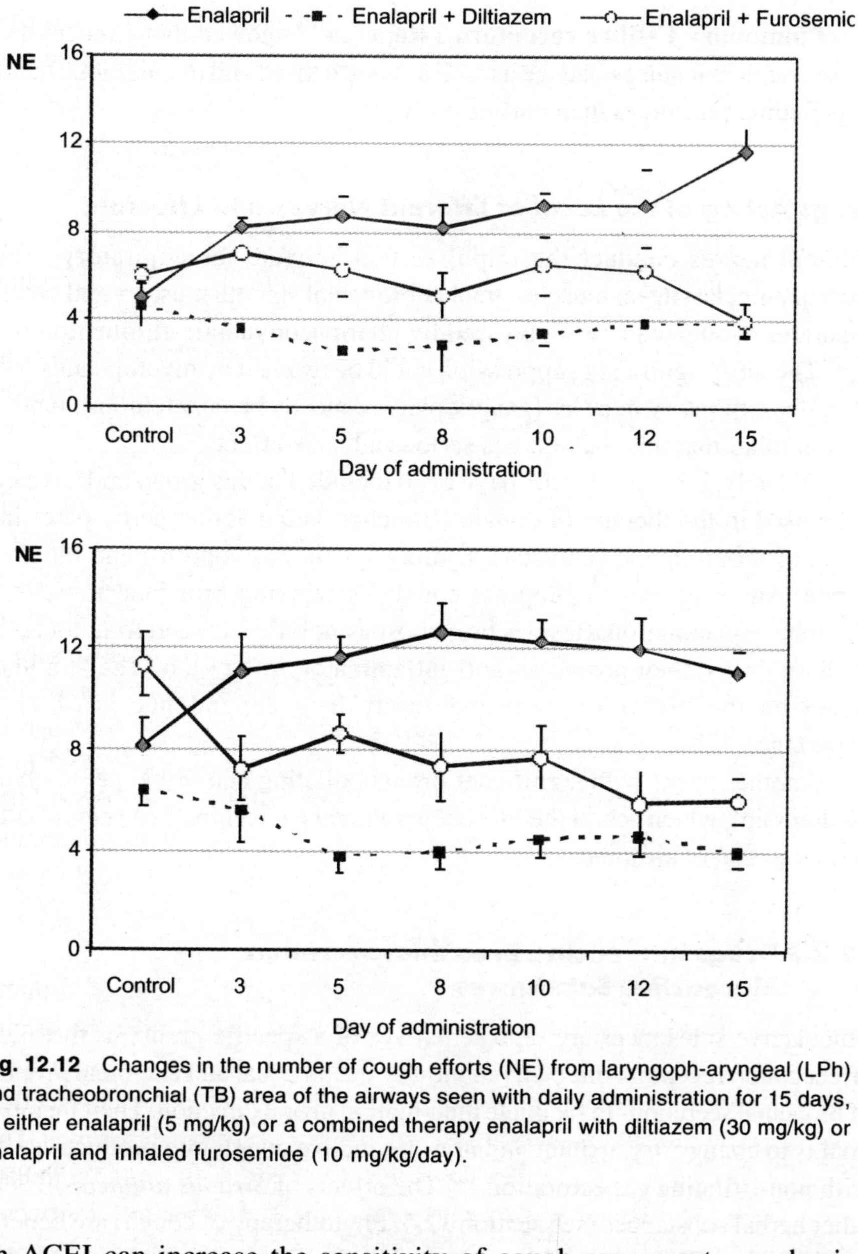

Fig. 12.12 Changes in the number of cough efforts (NE) from laryngoph-aryngeal (LPh) and tracheobronchial (TB) area of the airways seen with daily administration for 15 days, of either enalapril (5 mg/kg) or a combined therapy enalapril with diltiazem (30 mg/kg) or enalapril and inhaled furosemide (10 mg/kg/day).

with ACEI can increase the sensitivity of cough response to mechanical stimulus.[102] In addition to our results related to the management of ACEI cough, we found the possibility of restriction of this side effect by combined therapy with calcium channel blocker, diltiazem or by inhaled furosemide (Fig. 12.12).

Pulmonary C-fibre receptors Raj et al[103] showed that J receptors can cause cough in unanaesthetised as well as anesthetised and unconscious humans. This finding reinforces their earlier study.

Drugs Acting at the Level of Efferent Nerves and Effectors

Efferent nerves conduct the impulses that activate the expiratory skeletal musculature, laryngeal muscles, tracheobronchial smooth muscles and secreting apparatus. Cough can be suppressed by pharmacodynamic elimination of any part. The most significant suppression could be reached by myorelaxants, which block the expiratory muscles (ganglioplegics, mostly hexametonium). It must be kept in mind that this method has serious adverse effects.

Of lately, bronchodilators have been included in this group and have come to be used in the therapy of cough. Bronchodilating action participates in the effect of dropropizine (Ditustat), L-dropropizine (Levopront) and butamirate citrate (Sinecod), which suppress cough by relaxing bronchial muscles and facilitate expectoration. Besides bronchospasmolytic and secretomotor activity of these drugs, they posses an anti-inflammatory effect too. The stimulatory effect on the breathing centre without drug dependence is of greater importance.[1,104]

Another agent with significant bronchodilating activity is pentoxyverine (Sedotussin), which acts at the level of peripheral parasympathetic nerve endings similar to that of atropine.

12.2.3 Drugs Influencing Bronchial Secretion *Mucoactive Substances*

Mucoactive substances are representatives of a specific group, as they do not affect cough receptors directly, but modify the physical and chemical properties of bronchial secretions to facilitate their motion in oral direction. Their therapeutic goal is to change dry, irritant and non-productive cough into productive cough with non-irritating expectoration.[105] The effects of *Sirupus althaeae*[106,107] and other herbal substances (see section 12.5, Phytotherapy of cough) are beneficial in this respect. This group of drugs is used in clinical conditions for the treatment of cough with hypersecretion.[108]

Demulcerative and Hydrating Drugs

Demulcerative and hydrating drugs are substances with high molecular weight and water solubility without any pharmacological activity. They are used for the treatment of upper airway inflammation, sore throat and other diseases associated with dryness in mouth, irritation in throat and cough. Some examples are glycerin, synthetic cellulose derivatives, sugar syrup, and honey. The goal of this kind of treatment is to create a layer on the protective mucous membranes from irritant stimuli.[108,109] Many plants are rich in these kinds of agents.

12.3 COUGH AND INFLAMMATION

Inflammatory process in the airways increases mucus production (especially due to impaired mucociliary transportation) which could be one of the reasons for mechanical irritation. However, accumulated phlegm rich in inflammatory cells and mediators could be considered as a cough-provoking chemical stimulus.

Many inflammatory mediators may modulate cholinergic and sensory nerves in the airways through the activation of receptors on nerve terminals.[110] Sensory nerves in the airways contain several neuropeptides (tachykinins). The main members of this family are substance P (SP), neurokinin A (NKA) and neurokinin B (NKB), among which substance P is the best known. Stimulation of these nerves causes a constellation of responses known as neurogenic inflammation. Distribution of nerves containing substance P is close to that of RARs mediating cough in airways.[111] The most important enzyme for breakdown of SP in nerve fibres was discovered.[112] Neutral endopeptidase (NEP) is a key enzyme in the degradation of tachykinins in the airways. This enzyme is strongly expressed in epithelial cells.[113] In humans, aerosol of SP did not cause cough up to concentrations of 10^{-5} mol.l^{-1} in normal subjects, but it did in patients with upper respiratory tract infection.[114]

The attenuation of barrier function of airway epithelium is another factor involved in inflammation. This way the irritants can get to the nerve endings more easily. This process is aggravated by total destruction of epithelial cells, leading to loss of production of NEP.

Since damaged epithelium is not able to form neutral endopeptidase, during inflammation of airways, this may facilitate the penetration of substance. Fox[115] showed that SP causes cough by direct stimulation of RARs.[115] Tachykinins and SP showed an indirect activity resulting in cough reflex facilitation.[116] SP stimulates mucus secretion from submucosal glands and mediates increased plasma exudation and vasodilator response to tachykinins. Tachykinins also enhance cholinergic neurotransmission by facilitating acetylcholine release at cholinergic nerve terminals and by enhancing ganglion transmission.[117] In a variety of species including humans, tachykinins stimulate C-fibre receptors and rapidly adapting pulmonary stretch receptors and can cause cough.[118] Tachykinins may also interact with inflammatory and immune cells.

In addition to these mechanisms, tachykinins can increase sensitivity of the afferent nerve fibres in the genesis of cough due to underlying pathology. It is the presence of tachykinins (during airway inflammation) that produces a dry cough in response to tusssigenic stimuli which is the reason why it is not seen in healthy individuals. O'Connell[119] showed that cough reflex is 'upregulated' in persistent dry cough. This upregulation occurs at the level of afferent cough receptors in airways. By this the mechanism of action, certain important drugs lead to downregulation of the abnormally sensitive cough receptors.

It is possible that during disease, there is also decreased response of the afferent endings leading to the so-called ineffective type of cough.[7,120] The other reasons for this type of cough may be associated with central structure disorders, which take part in cough reflex regulation or a disorder of the effector mechanisms. The consequence of an ineffective cough can result in the increase in disease in the airways.[121]

Understanding the mechanisms underlying the genesis of the cough reflex, especially that during disease will enable an appropriate treatment. Cough, that arises to discharge the physiological role of cleaning the airways of accumulated secretions, phlegm, tissue detritus, dirt and foreign bodies which get into the airways, and the ciliary mechanisms, will not be influenced by pharmacological agents.[8,122] The best one can do is to reduce expectoration.[38,73] It must be kept in mind that only cough with under- lying disease will be influenced pharmacologically. We can suppress it or hold it to an acceptable level.

12.4 PHARMACOTHERAPY OF DIFFERENT TYPES OF COUGH

According to its cause and duration, cough can be divided into three categories: acute cough, lasting less than three weeks; subacute cough, lasting for three to eight weeks and chronic cough, lasting more than eight weeks. Since all types of cough are acute at the outset, it is the duration of cough that determines the spectrum of likely causes. On the basis of phlegm (mucus) production, cough can be dry, wet, or productive.[74] Painful cough is the name for pain-eliciting cough, which, sometimes represents concomitant symptoms of various pathological processes in the respiratory tract such as, bronchial asthma, chronic bronchitis, bronchogenic carcinoma gastro-oesophageal reflux. However, it could also have a psychogenic basis.[123] Cough can occur as a side-effect of other drugs treatment as for example, after administration of angiotensin-converting enzyme inhibitors (ACEI).[102,124]

12.4.1 Therapy of Acute Cough

Acute cough is mostly mild and lasts up to 21 days. It occurs during acute diseases of respiratory tract, caused especially by viral infections, common cold, acute bacterial sinusitis, exacerbations of chronic obstructive pulmonary disease (COPD), allergic rhinitis, rhinitis due to environmental irritants and pertussis. In its initial phase, cough may be non-productive (dry); but later, it can become productive. It may last for several days and then gradually weaken. This kind of cough need not be modulated therapeutically, as drugs would have no impact on the disease causing it.[125] Drugs are recommended if cough attacks occur too often or if cough is persistent and painful. In these situations drugs that suppress and lower the irritation of inflamed mucous membrane are used.[1,74,108]

Korppi et al[127] recommended that the use of antitussives in children should be restricted to such situations where their efficacy was proven, i.e. in the treatment of chronic non-productive cough.

For treatment of this form of cough, we recommend a combination of older-generation H_1 antihistamines and nasal decongestants (administration not more than 7 days). For patients who cannot take or tolerate this combination, it is possible to use intranasal ipratropium bromide (0.06% spray). Newer generation of antihistamines is ineffective for treating cough due to common cold. These agents are effective when cough is a symptom during histamine-mediated conditions such as allergic rhinitis. In this case, we can use nasal cromolyn and nasal forms of corticosteroids. Irwin and Madison[128] recommend the usage of antibiotic therapy for patients with exacerbations of COPD (if acute cough is accompanied by shortness of breath, wheezing or both), acute bacterial sinusitis, pneumonia and *Bordetella pertussis* infection. We suggest that antibiotic treatment should not be generalised but should be individualised. Its duration depends on symptom remission and normalisation of the patient's state of health.

12.4.2 Therapy of Subacute Cough

If cough lasts for 3 to 8 weeks, it is considered subacute. Treatment of this kind of cough is based on the elimination of the cause. Practically, it does not differ much from the treatment of chronic cough. For elimination of subacute form of cough, we use older generation of antihistamines combined with nasal decongestants, ipratropium bromide, bronchodilators from the group of beta-agonists, corticosteroids, antitussives, and target antibiotic treatment, if necessary.

12.4.3 Therapy of Chronic Cough

Chronic cough is defined as cough that lasts for more than three weeks.[129,130] Many physicians accept longer limit, six to eight weeks. This form of cough signals the possibility of serious diseases, such as chronic bronchitis, bronchial tumor, lung abscess or blood stasis in capillaries. According to Philp,[131] more than 90 per cent of cases of chronic cough are as a result of five common causes: smoking, postnasal drip, asthma, gastro-oesophageal reflux and chronic bronchitis. In general, specific therapy is preferred in the treatment of chronic cough (Table 12.7). The success of specific therapy depends on the correct diagnosis of cause or mechanisms, that evoke cough.[1,3,38,132] Kollarik and Undem.[133] showed that patients with chronic cough have a reduced threshold of cough elicitation and their afferent sensory fibres have become sensitized. The authors point out the role of transient receptor potential vanilloid-1 (TRPV-1) in these processes. We suppose that the agents influencing this type of receptor may be useful in the treatment of cough especially that which accompanies post-viral cough syndrome, chronic obstructive pulmonary disease and gastro-oesophageal reflux.

Symptomatic treatment of chronic cough (also called nonspecific therapy) is indicated only in cases where complications could represent a possible danger for the patient.[1,134] We prefer drugs from the group of non-narcotic antitussives with a peripheral site of action (Table 12.2). These drugs showed lower antitussive activity compared to codeine type agents, but their administration was not associated with adverse effects. From centrally acting drugs, we prefer agents from the group of synthetic morphine derivatives or clobutinol.

Table 12.7 Treatment of the chronic cough (Modified from Philip[131])

Cause	Therapy	Remarks
Cigarette smoking	Cessation of smoking cough within one month	Leads to a dramatic decrease in
Occupational exposure (e.g. dust, fumes, other irritants)	Reduction of exposure	Wearing a face mask, improving air circulation, a change of job may be necessary
Postnasal drip syndromes Non-allergic rhinitis	– Combination of older-generation of antihistamines and decongestants	Newer-generation of histamine antagonists are inferior in treating cough but avoid sedation.
	– Ipratropium (0.06%) nasal spray for 3 weeks	Mainly for patients who cannot take older-generation of antihistamines
	– Nasal steroids	Nasal steroids should be added, if cough is not controlled by antihistamine- decongestant medication or persist one to two weeks.
	– Vasoconstrictor e.g., oxymetazoline	Vasoconstrictor should not be used for more than 7 days.
Chronic bacterial sinusitis	– Antibiotics – Older-generation antihistamine-decon-gestant combination	If sinus infection is suspected, appropriate antibiotics may also be ordered. The selection and duration of antibiotic treatment is individual
Allergic rhinitis	– Avoidance of offending allergens – Newer-generation antihistamines	
Hypersensitivity that follows an upper respiratory infection (as in so-called cough variant asthma)	– Antihistamines, inhaled steroids–if unresponsive to treatment with antihista-mines, short-acting b_2 agonists, sodium nedocromil spray – antagonist of leukotrienes (Zafirlukast) – dextromethorphan or codeine	Present only a chronic, usually nonproductive cough, a positive result on metacholine challenge, physical examination out of periods with acute symptoms is essentially normal
Chronic bronchitis	– Discontinuation of smoking, – Avoidance of enviromental irritants and toxins – Preventive health measures (e.g. immunisations with pneumococcal vaccine, annual influenza vaccinations)	In this case we prefer the therapy of cough ipratropium, because it decreases mucus production, dilates the bronchi and is more effective in the therapy of cough than beta-agonists
	– Treatment of community-acquired respiratory infections	Antibiotics – macrolides, tetracyclines, flurochinolones thiotropium

Contd...

Cause	Therapy	Remarks
	– Postural drainage and hydration,	
	– Correction of malnutrition	
	– Inhaled corticosteroids/b_2 agonists, oral steroid therapy, if necessary	Roflumilast, Cilomilast, Erdosteine
	– Inhaled ipratropium	Thiotropium
	– Selective inhibitors of $PDE_{3,4}$	Roflumilast, Cilomlast
	– Mucolytics and expectorants	Erdosteine
Bronchial asthma	– Avoidance of allergens	Typical syndromes:
	– Prophylactic inhalation:	– dyspnoea
	– Sodium nedocromil	– coughing
	– b_2-agonist and/or	– wheezing
	– Steroid inhalers (6-8 weeks), in case if ineffective oral corticosteroids (Methylprednisolone)	Some times necessary long-term maintenance therapy with anti-inflammatory drugs. Methylprednisolone has the best pharmacokinetics and fewer side effects.
Drug induction: – Angiotensin-converting enzyme inhibitors (ACEI)	– Withdrawal of drug – Sulindac – Indometacin – Calcium channel blockers (e.g. nifedipine, dilthiazem) – Alternative class of drugs	The cough occurs in 5 to 20% of patients treated with ACEI
– Beta blockers	– Withdrawal of drug – Substitute a drug from a different class	Beta-blockers can cause increased airway resistance resulting from unopposed parasympathetic activity
Gastro-oesophageal reflux (GERD)	– H_2-receptor antagonists,	Ranitidine
	– High doses of proton-pump inhibitors, e.g. omeprazole,	Omeprazole, in a dose of 80.0 mg per day)
	– Prokinetic agent, e.g. metoclo-pramide, domperidone or cisapride before meals and at bedtime	Metoclopramide or cisapride may be added before meals and at bedtime, necessary to avoid eating or drinking for two hours before sleeping
	– Protective agent, e.g. sucralfate	Sucralfate may be helpful in a dose 1 g taken one our before meals
	– Anticholinergic drugs	As is necessary
	– Calcium channel blockers	As is necessary
	– Theophylline	As is necessary
	– Other muscle relaxants,	As is necessary
	– $GABA_B$-agonists	Baclofen
Psychogenic cough	– Anticholinergic drugs	Ipratropium, thiotropium
	– Aerosol form of lidocaine	Xylocaine
	– Benzonatate	Tessalon
	– Guaifenesine	Guajacuran
	– Benzodiazepines group	Diazepam
Tuberculosis	Antituberculotics	Isoniazid, Rifampicin, Ethambutol

12.4.4 Therapy of Non-Productive Cough

Dry, irritant non-productive cough significantly burdens the patient. Cough usually appears as rapid expulsion of air; it irritates tracheal as well as tracheobronchial mucous membranes. In this situation, cough must be suppressed by antitussives; of these, codeine is highly efficacious (Fig. 12.4). Adding expectorants may also help removing the irritants from the airways by increasing fluid content in the respiratory tract, and thus calming the airway mucous membranes.[1]

12.4.5 Therapy of Psychogenic Cough

Non-productive, irritating cough characterises psychogenic cough. Its incidence is very common in young people during pubescence. It may occur without any clear underlying reason.[35,136] Psychogenic cough does not respond to antitussives, and this cough is not present while eating or talking. But it may be accentuated if the patient becomes conscious of attracting attention by its presence. In the treatment of psychogenic cough, anticholinergic agents (ipratropium, thiotropium, oxytropium), local anaesthetics (lidocaine spray) and agents from the group of anxiolytics such as guaifenesin are used (Table 12.2). Even combinations of anxiolytics with antitussives like guaifenesin and butamirate citrate in Stoptussin.[1,73,74] are used. However, we found a strong cough-suppressive effect in benzodiazepine and phenothiazine derivatives (Table 12.5). These agents can also be used in the treatment of cough induced by psychogenic factors. In addition to their antitussive action they could also be used for their tranquilizing effect. But we have to be very careful while administering these drugs to patients who need to enforce expectoration. Special attention must be given to the use of diazepam in paediatric practice. In acute respiratory diseases associated with fever, it is used as a part of polyvalent therapy. Its administration can lead to suppression of breathing leading to phlegm collection and worsening of the child's condition. Adding psychotherapy can be useful too.

The current guidelines of British Thoracic Society do not recommend the combined use of benzodiazepine and opiate during flexible bronchoscopy.[72]

12.4.6 Therapy of Cough in Brochial Asthma and Cough-Variant Asthma

Bronchial asthma is often characterised by irritant, non-productive cough, which very often precedes the classical picture of asthma. In these cases, it is

Table 12.8 The cough-suppressing effects of some preparations with antitussive-expectorant activity (LPL, laryngopharyngeal; TB, tracheobronchial)

Trade name	*Composition*	*Antitussive activity (%)*	
		LPh	*TB*
STOPTUSSIN	guaifenesin + butamirate citrate	37	31.6
SOLUTAN	ephedrine + natrium iodatum + procaine+ plant extracts	40.4	47.2
SINECOD	butamirate citrate	67.3	47.3
IPECARIN	codeine, emetine, ephedrine, pilocarpine	36.1	44.7

recommended to use drugs from the group of beta$_2$-sympathomimetics that suppress cough even in allergic patients who has bronchial hyper-responsiveness.[137-140] Beta$_2$ sympathomimetics, similar to other broncho-dilators,[136] can reduce bronchial hyper-responsiveness, stimulate mucociliary clearance and increase water and ion flow into the bronchial lumen. This leads to forcing out the expectoration of viscous secretions.

Although cough may respond to a bronchodilator, inhaled (and sometimes oral) steroids are almost always necessary.[141] Cough-variant asthma can be difficult to control and after a 2-year follow-up, 80 per cent of patients still required inhaled steroids and 20 per cent were receiving daily oral prednisolone.[142]

In addition to these drugs, agents from the antihistamines group (sodium nedocromil) as immunoprophylactic agents as well as new agents from antagonists of leukotrienes.[143] We recommend zafirlukast, as it has better pharmacokinetic properties than montelukast, pranlukast and verlukast.

12.4.7 Productive Cough

Productive cough cannot be completely suppressed, retention of secretion will occur leading to other health problems for the patient or the development of pneumonia or atelectasis.[28,74,108] In some cases productive cough can be intense and occurs repeatedly. It will thereby burden the patient and disturb sleep. A reduction in the frequency and intensity of cough can be expected by administering expectorants or antitussive-expectorant agents, in this situation (Table 12.8). Mucoactive agents are very useful (bromhexine-Bromhexin, Bisolvon, ambroxol-

Table 12.9 Mucoactive substances

	Mucoactive substances	
Directly acting	Drugs destroying mucous polymers CIMEXYL, SOLMUCOL)	THIOLS - N-acetylcystein - (ACC, BRONCHOLYSIN, L- –Mesna (MISTABRON)
		Enzymes - Trypsin, chymotrypsin, streptokinase
		OTHER - Urea, citric acid, Hypertonic salt solutions, Inorganic iodides polymers
	Drugs modifying mucin biochemistry and mucus secretion	Carbocysteine (FENORIN, MUCOPRONT, MUCODYN)
	PAXIRASOL)	Bromhexine (BISOLVON, BROMHEXIN, FLEGAMINA,
		Erdostein (ERDOMED)
	Drugs modifying the adhesiveness of the gel layer	Ambroxol (AMBROBENE, AMBROSAN, RONCHOPRONT, MUCOSOLVAN)
		Tyloxapol (TACHOLIQUIN)
		Erdostein (ERDOMED)
Indirectly acting	Drugs modifying the sol layer and hydration	Water Sodium salts Potassium salts
	Volatile inhalants and balsams	Terpenes Phenol derivatives
	Drugs stimulating gastro-pulmonary reflex	Ammonium chloride Guaifenesin (GUAJACURAN) Ipecacuanha Sodium citrate
	Drugs modifying bronchial glands activity	Sympathomimetics Parasympathomimetics Corticosteroids Antihistamines

Mucosolvan, carbocysteine-Mucopront, erdostein-Erdomet), as they reduce phlegm viscosity (Table 2.9). Furthermore, it is advisable to add agents from the group of secretomotorics to the therapy, which act by induction of more effective phlegm expulsion from lower parts of the respiratory tract.[1,108] Many plant extracts and derivatives exert their antitussive effect by expectorant and mucolytic activity (see section 12.5 Phytotherapy of cough).

12.4.8 Painful Cough

With certain kinds of cough, patients feel a pain in throat or in the chest, especially behind the sternum. Painful cough is observed by pleuritis and lung cancer. The best therapy for suppression of cough in such cases is by a group of antitussives with analgesic activity.[144] Cough suppressive effect is also found in many analgesics (tilidine, tramadol, pentazocine and butorphanol). Often, the analgesic agents are prescribed for pain relief; they are able to suppress cough as well as reduce pain simultaneously.[35,145]

12.5 PHYTOTHERAPY OF COUGH

Phytotherapy has a very long tradition in the treatment of respiratory tract diseases. At times, when there were no reliable diagnostic instruments, the diagnosis as well as therapy were based on symptoms. A number of herbal preparations have been used in the therapy of cough. Recent trends of modern phytotherapy include specification of active substances responsible for therapeutic effect as well as quantification of their doses to enable rational treatment. The basic mechanism of action of herbal antitussives may be the same as that of traditional antitussives (central or peripheral cough suppression). The cough suppressive effect of herbal agents is connected with their local anaesthetic, spasmolytic, antibacterial and antiviral properties. The modulation of mucus production and quality is very important too. From pharmacological point of view, the following active substances are responsible for the antitussive and expectorant effect of herbal products.

12.5.1 Saponins

Saponins belongs to the group of herbal drugs with the best mechanism of action known to modulate cough parameters and phlegm quality. After oral administration of therapeutic doses, saponins *reflexly stimulate* the vagal nerves. This leads to increased phlegm secretion in the airways.[1] In addition, they stimulate the breathing and cough centre, resulting in frequent expectoration. However, higher doses of saponins can irritate the mucous membrane of stomach and intestines leading to emesis, diarrhoea and bleeding.

The best-known drugs containing saponins are Radix primulae, Herba thymi, Radix saponariae and Folium Hederae helicis. The administration of Hederae leaf-extract using double-blind trial, confirmed the ability to suppress cough reflex in patients with chronic bronchitis. The antitussive activity of Folium Hederae helix extract was comparable to cough-suppressive activity of ambroxol.[146] It is based on a high content of both saponins and flavonoids or tannins respectively.

12.5.2 Alkaloids

Alkaloids are herbal substances derived from amino acids. The mechanism of action of some alkaloids (emetin and cefalein) is similar to saponins, i.e. increasing phlegm secretion by reflex mechanisms. Both agents are present in the root of a South African plant *Uragoga ipecacuanhae*. After long-lasting administration or overdose, they can evoke arrhythmias, heart muscle impairment, and convulsions. Other antitussive active alkaloids, especially those originated from opium tincture, can interact with cough depression associated central receptor systems.

12.5.3 Flavonoids

There are several types of flavonoids and classified according to their basic structure, they are: flavanes (catechin), flavones (luteolin, apigenin, diosmin), isoflavones (genistein, daidazin), flavanols (rutin, quercetin, quercitrin, kaempferol, myricetin, hyperoside), flavanones (hesperidin, naringenin).[147] The relationship between flavonoids and cough reflex is mainly indirect and is connected to the stabilisation of vascular permeability, anti-inflammatory efficacy and influence on activity of the autonomic nervous system. Their biological effect is mainly related to stabilisation of vascular permeability and they thus render antioedematous and antihemorrhagic benefits. Flavonoids are powerful inhibitors of bacterial enzyme hyaluronidase, which is responsible for spreading bacterial toxins to the surrounding tissues.

Our experimental results demonstrate the protective effect of flavonoids (Provinol), isolated from red wine, on the tracheal smooth muscle response to bronchoconstrictor mediators and allergens in the model of ovalbumin-induced allergic asthma.[150] Antiflogistic and antiallergic effect of flavonoids is enhanced by concomitant administration of vitamin C.[151] Some flavonoids possess significant bacteriostatic effect on gram-positive and Gram-negative bacteria as well as on tuberclosis bacilli.[152,153]

Flavonoid properties together with antitussive-expectorant activity present in Hedera helix, Plantago lanceolata, Malva sylvestris, Polygonium aviculare,

Primula veris, Verbascum densiflorum and several others impart a curative effect in respiratory tract diseases.

12.5.4 Terpenoids

Terpenoids include a vast variety of natural chemical substances, and their classification is based on the number of structural units represented by mevalonic acid. Monoterpenoids, or essences, are vaporous agents which can irritate many tissues of the organism, including airway epithelium, by direct stimulation of secreting cells. Simultaneously, they can accelerate the movement of ciliar epithelium and have antibacterial and antiphlogistic effects.[154] The essence drugs include: Fructus anisi, Fructus foeniculi, Folium melissae, Herba seu Folium thymi. The therapeutically more effective ones are spring outgrowths of the coniferous trees, (e.g. *Pinus mugo, Pinus silvestris, Abies alba*). The adverse effects which can occur after administration of aetheric oils are nausea, allergic reactions, and renal parenchyma impairment.

12.5.5 Polysaccharides

Polysaccharides are divided into mucilages, gums and pectins. They have similar basic activity which is represented as the protection of sensory receptors on airway surface.

12.5.6 Mucilage

Inflammation of upper airways giving rise to a dry irritating cough is treated by using slime drugs. The best known are *Radix, Folium et Flos althaeae, Folium et Flos malvae, Folium plantaginis*. Slime consists of lyophillic colloids of water-soluble macromolecular polysaccharides, which depending upon the ratio creates either a thin sol or a gel. The slime in contact with the airway mucous membrane produces a protective layer on its surface, which diminishes the irritation of cough receptors (RARs) on myelinated fibres of vagal nerves, as well as irritation of nerve endings of non-myelinated C-fibres.[38] This leads to a decrease in the cough induced by inflammatory mediators or foreign bodies on the affected mucous membrane. The single, active polysaccharides are probably responsible for antitussive activity of slime. Polysaccharides show a significant cough suppressive effect which overlaps the effect of peripherally acting antitussives. Glucuronoxylans from herb *Rudbeckia fulgida* and the stem of *Mahonia aquifolium* showed immunomodulating activity on innate cellular and humoral immunity.[155-157] So far, no significant adverse effects were observed after administration of slime drugs.

12.5.7 Gums

Gums are hydrocolloids, translucent, amorphous substances that are produced by higher plants spontaneously after an injury. An effort has been made to distinguish between mucilage and gums on the basis that gums readily dissolve in water, whereas mucilages form slimy masses. Gums are typically heterogeneous in composition. Arabinose, galactose, glucose, mannose, xylose and various uronic acids are the most frequently observed components on hydrolysis of gums.[158] Herbal gums have significant antitussive effect after peroral administration.

12.5.8 Pectins

Pectins are hydrophilic colloid carbohydrates. The mechanism of their antitussive action is not precisely understood; but in experimental conditions, pectins isolated from citrus fruits (30%) showed (in dose of 50 mg/kg body weight) antitussive effect comparable to the effect of peripherally acting antitussives—prenoxdiazine (24%) and dropropizine (27%).[159]

12.6 Plant Compounds

Our experimental studies in the field of phytopharmacological research are focussed on detection and quantification of cough suppressive ability, especially of herbal substances from the group of polysaccharides. The following plant compounds showed the best efficacy in reducing cough parameters.

12.6.1 *Althaea officinalis L. (fam. Malvaceae)*

The root of marshmallow is used for soothing sore throats, laryngitis, tonsillitis, and cough.

Forms Marshmallow whole root, powdered root, root tea, syrup, complex extract of polysaccharides.

Active components The marmallow root contains up to 35 per cent slime (mucilage), 37 per cent starch, 10 per cent glucose, and the remaining 2 per cent is asparagin and betaine, pectin, flavonoids and minerals.

Therapeutic use *Althaea officinalis* is the main herb in the group from which mucilagenous drugs are isolated. The mucilage (or slime) consists of acid polysaccharide compounds containing predominantly arabinose, glucose, rhamnose, galactose and galacturonic acid. The slime drugs are used as obvious shield agents protecting the nerve endings and relieving pain. The protective action of marhamallow slime is also evident in inflamed and irritated mucous membranes of upper airways.

Here, they can act as antitussives. One of these substances is acid heteropolysaccharide rhamnogalacturonan, which forms approximately 30 per cent of the content of the slime. Nosalova et al[160] followed the antitussive activity of rhamnogalacturonan in experimental conditions and compared it with cough-suppressing effect of *Sirupus althaea* (a complex water and slime mucilage extract). Mechanical stimulation of laryngopharyngeal and tracheobronchial mucous areas of the airways was produced in conscious cats, using thin nylon fibre, induced cough. The cough parameters were recorded before and after intervals of 0.5, 1, 2 and 5 hours after administration of drugs.

In these experiments, rhamnogalacturonan caused a statistically significant decrease in the number of cough efforts and intensity of cough attacks (expiration and inspiration) from both laryngopharyngeal and tracheobronchial regions. Except for the intensity of cough efforts, administration of rhamnogalacturonan decreased all cough parameters. These findings are considered remarkable from a clinical point of view because they indicate that the tested compounds suppresses cough reflex but promote expectoration.

The antitussive activity of individual components of *A. officinalis* revealed a higher cough-suppressing effect of rhamnogalacturonan as compared to that of the water extract *Sirupus althaea* in the peripherally active antitussive agent dropropizine. Additionally, it was not as effective as the antitussive effect of the opioid, codeine.[161]

Side effects and interactions There were no significant adverse reactions observed after the administration of products containing marshmallow. Therefore, their use is recommended in pregnancy and paediatric practice. According to its principal mechanism of action, marshmallow mucilage can interfere with the absorption of other medicines within the digestive tract.

12.6.2 *Aloe vera (fam. Aloaceae)*

Aloe vera, one of the plants commonly used in traditional medicine, has been reported to possess a great variety of biological activities.

Forms *Aloe* is the dried latex (juice) of the leaves of *Aloe barbadensis Miller* (*A. vera Linné*).

Active components Aloe contains a number of anthraqinone glycosides, the principal one of which is barbaloin (Aloe-emodin anthrone C-10 glucoside). Free (nonglycosidal) Aloe-emodin and free and combined anthranol are also present. Except physiological active compounds (10–30%), Aloe contains inactive ingredients including large amounts (16–63%) of a resinous material plus volatile oil.[162]

More than 120 chemicals, especially terpenoids, anthraquinones, flavonoids, phenolic compounds and polysaccharides, were identified in aloe leaves.[163-165] The qualitative and quantitative determination of polysaccharide compounds is dependent on age and part of the plant.[166,167]

Therapeutic use Different types of chemical agents are coupled with remarkable pharmacological potency, including anti-proliferating efficacy,[168] wound healing,[169,170] positive effect on lipids and sugar metabolism[171] and anticancer and antimutagenic properties.[172]

Many pharmacodynamic properties of *A. vera* are fundamentally anti-inflammatory. Vazquez et al[173] showed that *A. vera* extracts decrease carrageenan-induced rat paw oedema and peritoneal neutrophil infiltration. It has also been shown that *A. vera* decreased production of inflammatory prostaglandins (PGE_2). An interesting fact is that *Aloe* contains a carboxypeptidase that is responsible for degradation of bradykinase. Undiluted fresh leaf juice of *A. vera* has a local anaesthetic analgesic, a bronchodilator, antiasthmatic and antibacterial activities. This agent inhibits histamine release and shows bradykinin antagonist activity.[174]

We believe that many of these activities are responsible for the suppression of the cough reflex. Polysaccharides from this plant are structurally similar to those from *Mahonia aquifollium*. A great reduction of the cough reflex parameters have been followed during application of a gel containing high level of acetylated mannans and glucanes. The cough suppressant ability of *A.* vera polysaccharides is lower than efficacy of the opioid agonist codeine, but much better than prenoxdiazine and dropropizine *A. vera*. (Fig. 12.13).

Side effects and interactions Dried aloe juice can provoke spasms of gastrointestinal tract (GIT), intestinal mucosa damage (irreversible),

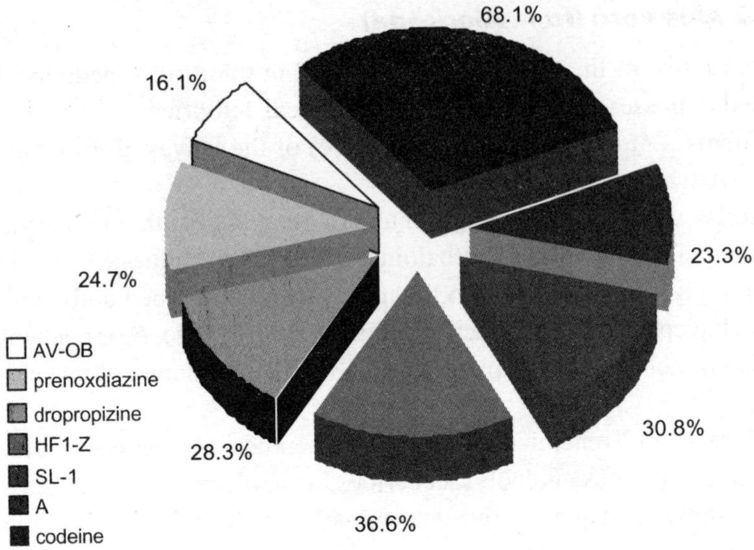

Fig. 12.13 Comparison of cough suppressive ability of polysaccharide substances isolated from different parts of *A.* vera leaves (A and HF1-Z from leaf gel; SL-1 from leaf epidermis—both in doses of 50 mg/kg) with those of commercially available products containing *A.* vera extract (Av-05) (50 mg/kg), an antitussive opioid (codeine, 10 mg/kg) and two non-opioid drugs (prenoxdiazine, 30 mg/kg and dropropizine,100 mg/kg).

haemorrhagic diarrhoea, nefrotoxicity (internal use) and contact dermatitis (topical use). Dried *Aloe* juice should not be used internally during pregnancy and lactation and should not be given to children younger than 12 years of age. It must not be recommended to patients with kidney disease, cardiac disease and bowel obstruction. Persons who are hypersensitive to *Aloe* should not use it topically.

Aloe taken internally may increase the effects of antidysrhythmics, cardiac glycosides, loop diuretics, systemic steroids and thiazide diuretics.[175]

12.6.3 *Arctium lappa* L. (fam. *Asteraceae*)

Arctium lappa or burdock has multiple branched stems, each of which is topped by crimson-violet flower heads producing 'burrs' that gave burdock its name.

Forms Dried root of the plant, infusion of root and leaves, polysaccharides extract are recommended for internal use. The burdock oil is often added to natural cosmetics.

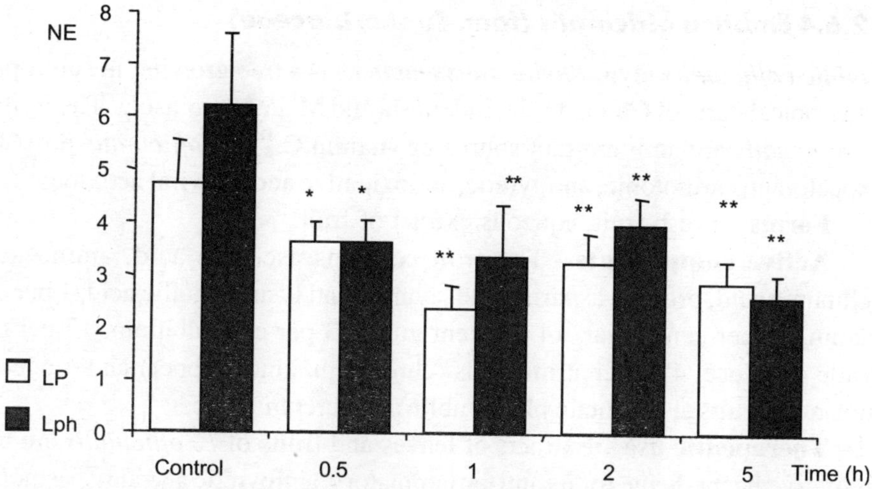

Fig. 12.14 Number of cough efforts (NE) recorded before and 0.5, 1, 2 and 5 hours after the application; LPh, Laryngopharyngeal; TB, tracheobronchial of a mixture of polysaccharides (LL-PS) in a dose of 100 mg/kg from *Arctium lappa* (aerial parts of plant). * P value lower than 0.05 ($p<0.05$); ** P Value lower than 0.01 ($p<0.01$)

Active components Polysaccharides, especially from the group of mucilage (69%),[176] and alkaloids are the main structural components. High content of insulin (up to 50%) is associated with a benefit of lipid and sugar metabolism.

Therapeutic use Anticancer, antimutagenic,[177] anti-inflammatory,[178] and antiviral[179] activities are related to high concentration of alkaloids, namely arctigenin.[180] Burdock root or whole plant extract is recommended in Chinese traditional medicine to treat upper respiratory infections. We observed cough depressant ability of polysaccharides and pure fructofuran from the root, too. Both substances can significantly decrease cough parameters from irritated regions of airways, especially those related to antitussive activity (Fig. 12.14).

Side effects and interactions High incidence of side effects, such as nausea (50%) and sedation for longer than 24 hours (100%), have been observed after adminstration of a high dose of a mixture of polysaccharides. Persons who are hypersensitive to Burdock should not use it. Burdock can increase hypoglycemic effect of antidiabetics and blood pressure lowering effect of antihypertensives (e.g. calcium channel blocker); and, therefore, its use must be avoided at the same time.[175]

12.6.4 *Emblica officinalis* (fam. *Euphorbiaceae*)

Emblica officinalis (syn. *Phyllanthus emblica*) is a tree growing in subtropical and tropical parts of China, India, Indonesia and Malaya peninsula. The fruits of *E. officinalis* are an important source of vitamin C.[181] *E. officinalis* possesses expectorant, cardiotonic, antipyretic, antioxidative and antiviral activities[182]

Forms Fresh fruit, aqueous extract of fruit.

Active components The fruit contains ascorbic acid, amino acids (glutamic acid, proline, aspartic acid, alanine and lysine), gallic acid, 1 per cent tannin, 35 per cent sugar, 14 per cent gum, 13 per cent albumin, 17 per cent crude cellulose, 4 per cent minerals (chromium, zinc, copper) and 4 per cent moisture. Fruits also contain phyllemblin and curcuminoides.

Therapeutic use Extracts of leaves and fruits of *E. officinalis* are used in Ayurvedic medicine for its anti-inflammatory, antipyretic and antispasmolytic activities. There are a few studies demonstrating the immunomodulatory effects of *E. officinalis*.[183] Other effects of this plant include protection against free radical damage induced during stress, anticancer and antimutagenic property and inhibition of lipid peroxidation, antibacterial, antiatherosclerotic and hypolipidemic activity. The water fraction of ethanol extract inhibited migration of human polymorphonuclears and platelets in relatively low concentration.[184]

Ethanol extract of *E. officinalis* exhibits significant antitussive activity tested in conscious cats by mechanical stimulation of laryngopharyngeal and tracheobronchial mucous areas of the airways.[185] Peroral dose 200 mg/kg body weight. of this substance was effective in decreasing cough parameters. Cough reduction after *E. officinalis* extract administration was lower than that of centrally acting codeine, but higher than the antitussive activity of non-opioid antitussives dropropizine and prenoxdiazine. It is supposed that this efficacy of *E. officinalis* is connected to inhibition of prostaglandin and leukotriene synthesis. Besides other pharmacological properties, which could take part in the antitussive effect of the extract plant, there are several other important properties such as the antioxidant, spasmolytic and antibacterial effects. It is probably the same as an irritant effect on the neural vagal endings of the gastrointestinal mucosal membranes, which stimulates the secretion of mucus in the respiratory tract.

Side effects and contraindication After administration of *E. officinalis* preparation, increased salivation and diuresis was observed. Overdose of therapeutic range can lead to emesis.

12.6.5 *Malva sylvestris L.* and *Malva mauritiana L.* (fam. Malvaceae)

The leaf tea is considered an expectorant and has been traditionally used for soothing sore throats, laryngitis, tonsillitis, and for the treatment of respiratory and digestive diseases.

Forms Flos, Folium and Herba malvae (mauritianae, sylvestris).

Active components The leaves of high mallow contain approximately 8 per cent mucilage (arabinose, glucose, rhamnose, galactose, xylose and glucuronic acid), small amounts of tannins and flavonoid sulphates.

The blossoms are composed of more than 10 per cent mucilage, which on hydrolysis affords traces of galactose, arabinose, glucose, rhamnose and galacturonic acid. The blossoms also contain high concentration of antioxidants including flavonoids and small amount of tannins. The flowers contain antocyan dye, made of malvidin 3,5 –diglucoside (malvin) and delphinidin.

Therapeutic use Experimental studies on mucous membranes showed that slime in water solution sticks to the mucous membrane and protects it from irritation.

The antitussive activity of slime from *Malva mauritiana* L. flowers is mediated by acid polysaccharide rhamnogalacturonan. Its major sugar components are L-rhamnose, D-galacturonic acid and D-galactose. The results of antitussive activity tests performed with mucilage and rhamnogalacturonan showed that both compounds suppress the cough reflex induced under experimental conditions. However, the administration of rhamnogalacturonan in dose of 50 mg/kg body weight. was associated with a 15 per cent higher antitussive activity as compared to slime.[186] Mucilage and rhamnogalacturonan caused statistically significant decrease of cough parameters mainly from laryngopharyngeal area of the airways.

The ability of mucilage and rhamnogalacturonan to suppress cough parameters was compared to those of drugs commonly used in clinical practice. The activity of both mucilage and its rhamnogalacturonan was lower than that of codeine, but higher than that of peripherally acting antitussives dropropizine and prenoxdiazine.

Side effects and contraindications As with marshmallow, no significant adverse effects associated with administration of *Malva sylvestris* or *Malva mauritiana* products were observed.

12.6.6 *Mahonia aquifollium (Pursh) Nutt. (fam. Berberidaceae)*

Mahonia aquifollium is evergreen, and it belongs to the most favourite of decorative garden trees. It is widespread in forests of some regions of North American Pacific coast.[187]

Forms Tincture with extract from the root or bark is used in traditional medicine for treatment of psoriasis.[188,189] Fresh fruits are known for their mild laxative effects.

Active components Numerous therapeutic benefits are related to high level of alkaloids, especially berberine, berbamine and oxyacanthine. Polysaccharides are less common.

Therapeutic use Tincture with extract of the root or bark is used in traditional (Chinese and Ayurvedic) medicine.[175,188,189] *Mahonia* (barberry) has been used as an antimicrobial agent against bacteria, fungi, viruses, helminths, and chlamydias. It antagonises the effects of *Vibrio cholerae* and *Escherichia coli* and decreases ventricular tachyarrhythmias. Reported antineoplastic activity (colon cancer) is related to inhibition of 5-lipo oxygenase and cyclooxygenase-2 also by berberine.[190,191]

Other alkaloids (berbamine and oxyacanthine) are responsible for anti-inflammatory as well as antinociceptive and antipyretic properties, which may be useful for rheumatism.[192] Vasodilatory and hypotensive effects have been found during experimental studies.[193]

Polysaccharide structural components, namely glucuronoxylan, are less common, but they showed immunomodulator efficacy.[194] We observed that herbal polysaccharides isolated from *Mahonia* have great cough suppressive activity. The effect of tested substances has been very prompt. We observed a noticeable reduction of cough parameters after 30 minutes of application of the tested agent.[195] Comparison with the activity of classic drugs, both narcotic and non-narcotic groups, revealed that *Mahonia* polysaccharide substances are less active than codeine, but twice more potent than clinically prescribed dropropizine and prenoxdiazine.

Side effects and contraindications After administration of *Mahonia*, GIT disturbances (diarrhoea, gastrointestinal discomfort), hypotension, cardiac damage, dyspnoea, confusion, disorientation and nephritis) can be seen. As it can cause spontaneous abortion, *Mahonia* should not be used during pregnancy.[175]

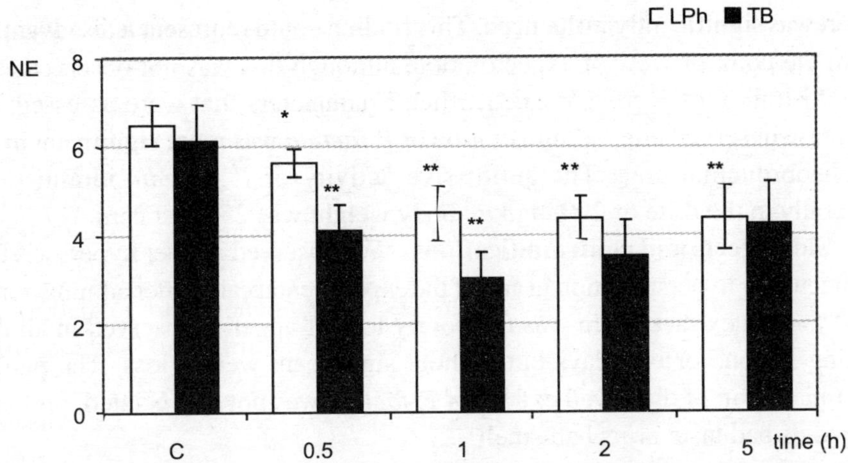

Fig. 12.15 Number of cough efforts (NE) recorded before and after 0.5 mins, 1, 2 and 5 hours, the administration of 200 mg/kg of *P. foetida*. LPh columns: mean values of cough parameters stimulation of laryngophary-ngeal area; TB. columns: mean values of cough parameters after stimulation of tracheobronchial area.

12.6.7 Paederia foetida (fam. Rubiaceae)

Paederia foetida (Bengali. *Gandhavadulia*; English Skunkvine) is a woody vine growing in the subtropical and tropical parts of Eastern and Southern Asia as well as in southern parts of USA (Florida).

Forms Extract of fruits, leaves.

Active components In *P. foetida*, various fatty acids were detected (nonanoic acid, capric acid, lauric acid, myristic acid, arachidic acid and palmitic acid). It also has higher concentration of conjugated dienoic acid and lower concentration of trieonic acid.[196]

Therapeutic use Extracts of leaves and fruits of *P. foetida* were used in Asia for its anti-inflammatory properties in the treatment of arthritis and for its antidiarrhoeal properties in the treatment of diarrhoea or dysentery. Other effects of this plant, include hepatoprotective effect[197] and anti-tumour-promoting effect of paederosid present in leaves,[198] antihelmintic effect,[199] and anti-inflammatory activity.[197,200,201]

We examined the antitussive activity of *P. foetida* in conscious cats by mechanical stimulation of laryngopharyngeal and tracheobronchial mucous areas of airways. We observed that *P. foetida* in dose of 200 mg.kg^{-1} body weight had good potency to inhibit cough. These effects were observed in decreasing both the number of efforts and intensity of attack. (Fig. 12.15) The intensity of maximal effort was significantly influenced. This finding could represent a disadvantage from the point of view of expectoration, although this was not observed after administration of *P. foetida* extract. In all parameters that were assessed, the decrease observed after administration of *P. foetida* was more significant in the tracheobronchial area. The antitussive activity of *P. foetida* administered perorally in the dose of 200 mg.kg^{-1} body weight was 25.3 per cent.

Side effects and contraindications We observed neither hypersecretion of mucus nor hypersalivation in any of the experimental cats. After administration of *P. foetida* extract, there was temporary loss of appetite observed in all cats lasting for one or two days but without significant weight loss. The peroral administration of dissolved extract of *P. foetida* was not appreciated, probably due to its bad taste or its bad smell.

12.6.8 *Salvia Officinalis (Fam. Lamiaceae)*

Salvia officinalis, also called sage, is typically found in countries around the Mediterranean Sea. In traditional medicine of many countries it is recommended treatment of mild inflammation of oral cavity, skin, stomach and intestine.

Forms Infusion of dried leaves tincture with leaves extract for external use and pure extract is often added to cosmetics.

Active components Essential oil is a compound of sage (2–6%), in which high levels of cis-thujone, alpha-humulene and 1,8-cineole have been found.[202] Diterpenes are biologically active fraction of methanolic aerial parts in Salvia extract. They have a powerful antioxidant capacity.[203] *Diterpene salvinorin* A, detected in high concentration in *Salvia divinorum*, has recently been shown to be a high-affinity and naturally occurring kappa-opioid receptor agonist.[204] Polysaccharide fraction of *Salvia*, rich in arabinogalactans, pectin and glucuronoxylan-related polymers, possess a significant immunomodulatory effect.[205] In these a high concentration of vitamins, especially group B, and catechol group of flavonoids have also been described.

Therapeutic use Cineol present in *Salvia* essence oil is useful for treatment of rheumatism. This substance, in the ointment form, can irritate skin, leading to a better vascular supply of the treated area. *Salvia* leaves are common compound of tea-mixtures recommended in respiratory tract diseases associated with cough, both productive and non-productive. Both groups of agents possess significant antibacterial activity; they enforce the airway mucous membrane gland secretion and promote expectoration. Antibacterial activity of essences is

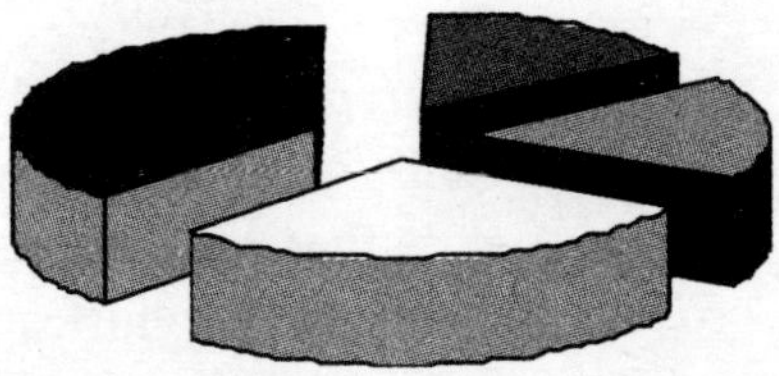

Fig. 12.16 Comparison of antitussive activity of *Salvia* polysaccharides (50 mg/kg.), codeine (10 mg/kg), dropropizine (100 mg/kg) and prenoxdi-azine (30 mg/kg) on mechanically induced cough.

the same as that of flavonoids. According to Perry et al,[206] essential oils with peroral administration, inhibit enzyme acetylcholinesterase in rat brain; and in healthy volunteers, essential oil administration produce a significant effect on cognition. *Salvia* extract may be recommended for the treatment of Alzheimer's disease. Dittmann et al[207] showed that the anti-inflammatory property of the plant is coupled with suppression of monoamino-oxidase (MAO) and inducible nitric oxide synthase (iNOS) enzyme functions.

Salvia extract showed great antitussive effect on experimental cough (Fig. 12.16). Significant decrease of the number of cough efforts, and intensity of cough attacks (in inspiration and expiration) from both laryngopharyngeal and tracheobronchial regions has been observed. Kappa-opioid receptor agonistic effect may be related to antitussive benefit as well as secretomotoric mechanism of essence oil including their anti-inflammatory property.

Contraindications and side effects No side effects related to the application of *Salvia* extract have been observed during experimental work. Allergic reactions to the high presence of essence oils in sensitive persons can occur. Overdose of terpenoides may lead to damage of liver or cardiovascular impairment.[208]

12.6.9 *Verbascum densiflorum Bertoloni* and *Verbascum phlomoides* L. (fam. Scrophulariaceae)

Verbascum densiflorum (syn. *V. thapsiforme Schrad.*), a large-flowered mullein, and *Verbascum phlomoides* L., an orange mullein, are biennial plants indigenous to countries in Europe, and in India, Egypt and Ethiopia. The leaves and flowers of mullein have been used traditionally for their demulcent, expectorant and astringent properties.

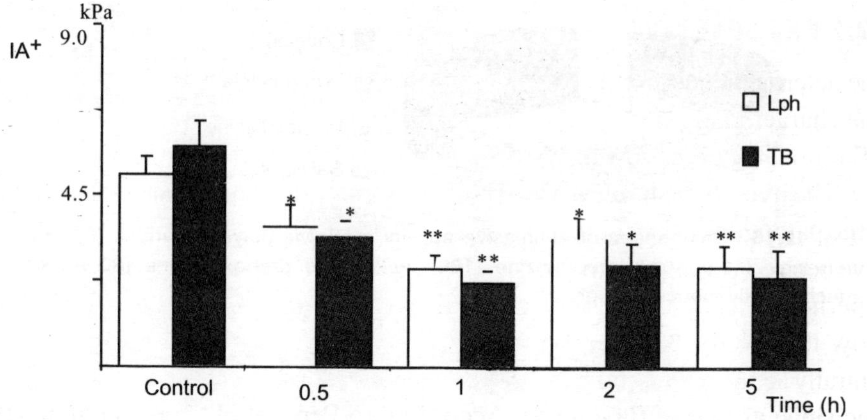

Fig. 12.17 Changes in cough intensity seen during expiration IA$^+$, before and seen after intervals of 0.5, 1, 2 and 5 hours, after the administration of 50 mg/kg of *Verbascum densiflorum* extract.

Forms Infusion, extract and tincture of the leaves and flowers.

Active components Mullein contains 3 per cent mucilage, iridoids, saponins, 1.5–4 per cent flavonoids, phenol-carboxylic acid, sterols and 11 per cent invert sugar.

Therapeutic use Saponins can increase the mucus secretion in the upper airways. Therefore, the drug is prescribed in dry inflammation of respiratory tract with non-productive cough. Our experiments showed a powerful ability of Verbascum extract to reduce experimental cough (Fig. 12.17).

A high content of flavonoids and slime, contribute to its expectorant properties. Slime makes a protective layer on the airway mucous membrane, and this leads to decreased mediator effect on cough receptors during inflammation.[209]

Mullein drug is usually combined with other expectorant and mucilagenous drugs containing essences and slime *Fructus anisi, Fructus foeniculi, Herba menthae piperitae, Herba thymi, Flos malvae sylvestris, Folium althaeae, Folium plantaginis*. Infusion of *Flos verbasci* has antiviral activity against influenza and herpes simplex viruses.[210]

Contraindications and side effects The contraindications and side effects of verbascum are not known. The leaf hairs of mullein can cause skin irritation in sensitive persons.

12.7 PERSPECTIVES OF COUGH THERAPY

The heterogeneous group of agents is connected with the future of cough therapy. The characteristic sign, is the ability of different drugs to inhibit the underlying inflammatory process, which can cause cough in certain conditions.

The hypothetical role of tachykinins (mainly substance P and neurokinin A) in the pathogenesis of cough has therapeutic implications. Antitussive properties have been consistently demonstrated for tachykinin-receptor antagonists in animal experiments, although evidence of efficacy in humans is limited. Various data show the role of NK_1 receptors and NK_2 receptors in antitussive activity of centrally acting antitussive agents NK_2 receptors might participate in the peripheral mechanism of action.

GABA is an inhibitory neurotransmitter found in the CNS and peripheral tissues, including the lungs. The GABA-agonists (gabalid and baclofen) inhibited cough in animals via a central mechanism.[26,27,211] In humans, low-dose oral baclofen inhibited cough, possibly via a peripheral mechanism.[212,213] Understanding the central and peripheral neural pathways will provide new targets for drug development.

According to recent research, potassium channels seem to be successful agents for cough therapy. This fact is based on the previous studies which demonstrated that the large conductance calcium-activated potassium (BK_{Ca} maxi-K) channel opener NS 1619 (benzimidazolone compound), and ATP sensitive-potassium channel opener,[214] inhibit citric acid-induced cough in experimental conditions.

The results of some authors[214,215] provide a basis for the potential use of ATP-sensitive potassium channel openers as peripherally acting non-narcotic antitussive drugs. Maxi-K activators take part in cough suppression at both the levels (peripheral and central).

Some years ago, ion channels belonging to the transient receptor potential (TRP) family were cloned. Since first types of receptors are activated by molecules with vanilloid moiety (heated to 52°C, protons and other lipid derivates), they have been named vanilloid receptor-1 (VR-1), and more recently renamed transient receptor potential vanilloid-1 (TRPV-1). It was demonstrated that these types of receptors play a role not only in physiological activation of cough reflex but also in an exaggerated cough response observed during certain pathological states. On this basis, it can be presumed that TRPV-1 receptor antagonists are of therapeutic value not only in the treatment of cough in patients with asthma and chronic obstructive pulmonary disease (COPD) but also in patients with other inflammatory diseases. These data were supported by that of Trevisari et al[216] which refer to a potent antitussive drug iodo-resiniferatoxin (I-RTX), which inhibits cough via TRPV-1 interaction. Therefore, blocking these channels may be a good strategy for an antitussive treatment.

A second family of receptors, that is sensitive to cold and menthol (CMR1), takes part in cough suppression with their own activation. Thus, their activation may prove to be useful as therapeutic agents.[45]

12.8 CONCLUSION

For treatment of pathological cough (postnasal drip, cough variant of bronchial asthma gastro-oesphageal reflux, sinusitis, etc.), we must concentrate on the causal therapy of cough.

REFERENCES

1. Korpas J, Nosalova G. Pharmacotherapy of the cough. Osveta, Martin, 1991.
2. Widdicombe JG. Neurophysiology of the cough reflex. European Respiratory Journal 1995;8:1193–202.
3. Bolser DC. Mechanisms of action of central and peripheral antitussive drugs. Pulmonary Pharmacology 1996;9:357–64.
4. Irwin RS. Quality of life in coughers. Abstract of 2nd International Symposium. Cough: Pharmacology and Therapy. London, October 2001.
5. Choundry NB, Fuller RW. Sensitivity of the cough reflex in patients with chronic cough. European Respiratory Journal 1992;5:296–300.
6. Eccles R. Codeine, cough and upper respiratory tract infection. Abstract of symposium Cough: Methods and Mechanism. London, 1996.
7. Korpas J, Tomori Z. Cough and other respiratory reflexes. Progress in Respiration Research, Vol. 12 Basel: S. Karger, 1979.
8. Nosalova G, Strapkova A, Korpas J, Crisciulo D. Objective assessment of cough suppressants under normal and pathological experimental conditions. Drugs Under Experimental and Clinical Research 1989;15:77–81.
9. Empey D W. Antitussive drugs. In: Munson PL, Mueller RA, Breese GR, editors. Principles of Pharmacology. ITP 1996;615–19.
10. Bucher K. Antitussive drugs. In: Physiological Pharmacology, Comprehensive treatice. Root WS, Hofman FG, editors. The Nervous System: Part B. New York, London: Academic Press 1965;2:p.486.
11. Hall RCW. Central nervous system effects of respiratory drugs. Drugs of Today 1985;21:405–26.

12. Irwin RS, Corrao WM, Pratter MR. Chronic persistent cough in the adult: the spectrum and frequency of causes and successful outcome of specific therapy. American Review of Respiratory Disease 1981;123:413–7.
13. Irwin RS, Pratter MR, Holland PS, Corwin RW, Hughes JP. Postnasal drip causes cough and is associated with reversible upper airway obstruction. Chest 1984;85:346–52.
14. Bucher K. Pathophysiology and pharmacology of cough. Pharmacological Reviews 1958;10:43–58.
15. Richardson PS. The principles of drug action on cough and on sputum characteristics. European Respiratory Journal 1980;61:67–79.
16. Sampson SR, Eyzaguirre C. Some functional characteristics of the mechanoreceptors in the larynx of the cat. Journal of Neurophysiology 1964;27:464–80.
17. Mills J, Sellick H, Widdicombe JG. Activity of lung irritant receptors in pulmonary microembolism, anaphylaxy and drug-induced bronchoconstrictions. Journal of Physiology 1969;203:337–57.
18. Widdicombe JG. Mechanism of cough and its regulation. European Respiratory Journal 1980;61:11–20.
19. Leith DE. Cough. In: Brain JD, Proctor DF, Reid LM, editors. Respiratory defense mechanisms: Part 2. New York, Basel: M Dekker Inc., 1977;p1216.
20. Peatfield AC. Mucus secretion and its role in defense reflexes. In: Hutas I, Debreczeni LA, editors. Advance in Physiological Sciences Respiration. Akademiai Kiado: Pergamon Press, 1981;10:519–28.
21. Jordan, D.: Central nervous mechanisms in cough. Pulmonary Pharmacology, 1996;9:389–92.
22. Jordan D. Central nervous control of the airways. In: Jordan D (ed). Central nervous control of autonomic function. London, Harwood Academic Press 1997;63–107.
23. Hedner T, Jonason J, Lundberg D. Respiratory effects of gamma-hydroxybutyric acid in anesthetized rats. Journal of Neurology and Transmission 1980;49:179–186.
24. Hedner J. Neuropharmacological aspects of central respiratory regulation: an experimental study in the rat. Acta Physiologica Scandinavica 1983;524:1–109.
25. Hedner J, Hedner T, Wessberg P, Jonason J. An analysis of the mechanism by which GABA depresses ventilation in the rat. Journal of Applied Physiology 1984;56:849–56.
26. Nosalova G, Varonos D, Papdopoulous-Daifotis Z. Cough and central GABA-ergic mechanism. Bratislava Medical Journal 1986a;85:526–32.
27. Nosalova G, Varonos D, Papdopoulous-Daifotis Z, Visnovsky P, Strapkova A. GABA-ergic mechanism in the central control of cough. Acta Physiologica Hungarica 1987;70:189–194.
28. Fox AJ. Modulation of cough and airway sensory fibres. Pulmonary Pharmacology 1996;9:335–42.
29. Bolser DC, Hey JA, Chapman RW. Influence of central antitussive drugs on the cough motor pattern. Journal of Applied Physiology 1999;86:1017–24.
30. Strapková A.: Pharmacological influencing of the cough reflex and reactivity of the airways. JLFUK Martin, 1995.
31. Nosalova G, Strapkova, A, Korpas J, Crisciulo, D. Objective assessment of cough suppressants under normal and pathological experimental conditions. Drugs Under Experimental and Clinical Research 1989;15:77–81.
32. Kamei J, Saitoh A, Morita K, Nagase H. Antagonistic effect of buprenorphine on the antitussive effect of morphine is mediated via the activation of m_1- opioid receptors. Life Sciences 1995;57:PL231–5.

33. Kamei J. Role of opioidergic and serotonergic mechanisms in cough and antitussives. Pulmonary Pharmacology 1996;9:349–56.
34. DeRuiter J. Narcotic analgesics: introduction. Principles of Drug Action 2; 2000.
35. Srapkova A, Nosalova G, Korpas J. Relationshipof antitussive and analgesic activity of various substances. Bratislava Medical Journal 1987;88:538–45.
36. Kamei J, Tanihara H, Kasuya Y. Antitussive effect of two specific kappa-opioid agonists, U-50,488H and U-62,066E, in rats. European Journal of Pharmacology 1990;187:281–6.
37. Brown C, Fezoui M, Selig WM, Schwartz CE, Ellis JL. Antitussive activity of sigma-1 agonists in the guinea pig. British Journal of Pharmacology 2004;141:233–40.
38. Nosalova G. Mechanism of action of the drugs influencing the cough reflex. Bratislava Medical Journal 1998;99:531–5.
39. Saitoh A, Ueno S, Kawai K, Natume K, Sakani S, Maeda M, Ohtaki M, Morita K, Kamei J, Endoh T, Nagase H. Antitussive effects of a novel d-opioid receptor antagonist, TRK-851. Abstract of 2nd International Symposium; Cough, London, 2001.
40. Kamei J, Tanihara H, Kasuya Y. Modulation of kappa-mediated antitussive activity in rats by delta-agonist. Research Communications in Chemical Pathology and Pharmacology 1992;76:375–8.
41. Kamei J, Iwamoto Y, Suzuki T, Misawa M, Nagase H, Kasuya Y. Antitussive effects of naltrindole, a selective delta-opioid receptor antagonist, in mice and rats. European Journal of Pharmacology 1993;249:161–5.
42. Kamei J, Iwamoto Y, Suyuki T, Misawa M, Nagase H, Kasuya Y. Involvement of delta 1-opioid receptor antagonism in the antitussive effect of delta-opioid receptor antagonists. European Journal of Pharmacology 1994;251:291–4.
43. Kotzer ChJ, Hay DWP, Dondio G, Giardina G, Petrillo P, Underwood DC. The antitussive activity of kappa-opioid receptor stimulation in guinea pigs. Journal of Pharmacology and Experimental Therapeutics 2000; 292:803–9.
44. Dhawan BN, Cesselin F, Raghubir R, Reisine T, Bradley PB, Portoghese PS, Hamon M. International Union of Pharmacology. XII. Classification of opioid receptors. Pharmacological Reviews 1996;48:567–52.
45. Belvisi MG, Geppetti P. Cough.7: Current and future drugs for the treatment of chronic cough. Thorax 2004;59:438–40.
46. Reinscheid RK, Nothacker HP, Bourson A, Ardati A, Henningsen R, Bunzow JR, Grandy DK, Langen H, Monsma FJJr, Civelli O. Orhanin FQ: a neuropeptide that activates an opioidlike G coupled receptor. Science 1995;270:792–4.
47. Fischer A, Forssman WG, Undem BG. Nociceptin induced inhibition of tachykinergic neurotransmission in guinea-pig bronchus. Journal of Pharmacology and Experimental Therapeutics 1998;285:902–7.
48. Karlsson JA, Lanner AS, Persson CG. Airway opioid receptors mediate inhibition of cough reflex bronchoconstriction in guinea pigs. Journal of Pharmacology and Experimental Therapeutics 1990;252:863–8.
49. Simon EJ, Hiller JMI. The opiate receptors. Annual Review of Pharmacology and Toxicology 1978;18:371–94.
50. Chau TT, Carter FE, Harris LS. Antitussive effect of the optical isomers of mu, kappa and sigma opiate agonists/antagonists in the cat. Journal of Pharmacology and Experimental Therapeutics 1983;226:108–13.
51. Rang HP, Dale MM, Ritter JM. Pharmacology. 4th edn. Churchill Livingstone 1999;p830.

52. Gilman AG, Goodman LS, Gilman A. Pharmacological basis of therapeutics. 6th edn. New York: MacMillian Publishing Co.,1990;p1905.
53. Terenius S. Endogenous peptides and analgesia. Annual Review of Pharmacology and Toxicology 1978;18:189–204.
54. Sarne Y, Fields A, Keren O, et al. Stimulatory effects of opioids on transmitter release and possible cellular mechanisms: overview and original results. Neurochemical Research 1996;21:1353–61.
55. Quock RM, Burkey TH, Varga E, Hosohata Y, Hosohata K, Cowell SM, Slate ChA, Ehlert FJ, Roeske WR, Yamamura HI. The kappa-opioid receptor: molecular pharmacology, signal transduction, and the determination of drugs efficacy. Pharmacological Reviews 1999;51:503–32.
56. Kamei J, Ogawa M, Kasuya Y. Monoamines and the mechanisms of action of antitussive drugs in rats. Archives Internationales de Pharmacodynamie et de Therapie 1987;290:117–27.
57. Kamei J, Ogawa M, Kasuya Y. Supersensitivity of 5, 7-dihydrotryptamine-treated rats to the respiratory depressant and antitussive effects of dihydrocodeine. European Journal of Pharmacology 1988;153:305–8.
58. O Connell F. Central pathways for cough in man-unanswered questions. Journal of Pulmonary Pharmacology and Therapeutics 2002;15:295–301.
59. Stone RA, Barnes PJ, Chung KF. Effect of 5-HT1A receptor agonist, 8-OH-DPAT, on cough responses in conscious guinea pig. European Respiratory Journal 1997;332:201–7.
60. Choundry NB, Studham J, Harland D, Fuller RW. Modulation of capsaicin induced airway reflexes in human, effect of monoamine oxidase inhibition. British Journal of Pharmacology 1993;35:173–81.
61. Nosalova G. Pharmacology of cough reflex. JLFUK Martin, 1991.
62. Birrell MA, Crispino N, Hele DJ, Patel HJ, Yacoub MH, Barnes PJ, Belvisi MG. Effect of dopamine receptor agonists on sensory nerve activity: possible therapeutic targets for the treatment of asthma and COPD. British Journal of Pharmacology 2002;136:620–8.
63. Li JQ, Jia YX, Yamaya M, Arai H, Ohrui T, Sekizawa K, Sasaki H. Neurochemical regulation of cough response to capsaicin in guinea pigs. Auton Autacoid Pharmacology 2002;22:57–63.
64. North RA. Opioid actions on ion channels. In: Hertz A, editor. Opioids: Handbook of Experimental Pharmacology. Berlin: Springer-Verlag, 1993;104.
65. Franova S, Nosalova G. Antitussive effect of diltiazem in experimental conditions. Bratislava Medical Journal 2004;105:203–6.
66. Strapkova A, Nosalova G, Korpas J. Relationship of antitussic and analgesic activity of various substances. Bratislava Medical Journal 1987;88:538–45.
67. Braga PC, Fossati A, Vimercati MG, Caputo R, Guffanti EE. Dextrorphan and dextromethorphan: comparative antitussive effects on guinea pigs. Drugs Under Experimental and Clinical Research 1994;20:199–203.
68. Chebib M, Johnston GAR. The ABC of GABA Receptors: A Brief Review. Clinical and Experimental Pharmacology and Physiology 1999;28:937–40.
69. Lum N. Oral cough and cold remedies—analysis of contraindications and precautions. On Continuing Practice 1991;18:2–8.
70. Schadel M, Romach MK, Sellers EM. Mania and cough syrup. Journal of Clinical Psychiatry 1993;54:173–4.
71. Hernandez SC, Bertolino M, Xiao Y, Pringle KE, Caruso FS, Kellar KJ. Dextromethorphan and its metabolite dextrorphan block alfa3beta4 neuronal nicotinic receptors. Journal of Pharmacology and Experimental Therapeutics 2000;293:962–7.

72. Stolz D, Chhajed PN, Leuppi JD, Brutsche M, Pflimlin E, Tamm M. Cough suppression during flexible bronchoscopy using combined sedation with midazolam and hydrocodone: a randomised, double blind, placebo controlled trial. Thorax 2004;59:773–6.
73. Nosalova G, Strapkova A, Korpas J, Kubec F. Guaifenesin as a component of new Czechoslovak antitussive-expectorant Stoptussin. Respiratory Pharmacology, Praha, Chemapol 1986;69–76.
74. Parvez L, Vaidya M, Sakhardande A, Subburaj S, Rajagopalan TG. Evaluation of antitussive agents in man. Pulmonary Pharmacology 1996;9:299–308.
75. Berkow R. The Merck Manual of Diagnosis and Therapy. 15th edn. Merck &´Co., Inc. Rahway, NJ 1987;pp1038,1088,1635.
76. Marks V, Cantor T, Mesko, D, Pullmann R, Nosalova G.: Differential diagnosis by laboratory medicine. Springer Verlag, 2002.
77. Yamada KA, Hamosh P, Gillis A. Respiratory depression produced by activation of GABA receptors in the hindbrain of the cat. Journal of Applied Psychology 1981;51:1278–86.
78. Morini A, L, impiego della clorpromazina nella terapia sintomatica della tosse. Rivista di Biologia 1956;70:1015–16.
79. Wirth L. Use of chlorpromazine in cough with particular reference to whooping cough. Military Medicine N.Y. 1958;22:195–6.
80. Nosalova G. Pharmacodynamic activities of antitussive agents. Martin 1977;163.
81. Nosalova G. Pharmacological influence on cough. Folia Medica Martiniana 1984;10:83–106.
82. Hosokawa T, Kamei J, Misawa M, Yanaura S, Hukuhara T. Effects of psychotropics on the periodic fluctuation in EEG synchronized with respiratory rhythms during cough reflex. Yakubutsu Seishin Kodo 1983;3:37–43.
83. Shioya T, Satake M, Kagaya M, Sano MA, Watanabe A, Fukui S, Sasaki M. Antitussive effects of the H1-receptor antagonist epinastine in patients with atopic cough (eosinophilic bronchitis). Arzneimittelforschung 2004;54:207–12.
84. Muether PS, Gwaltney JM Jr. Variant effect of first- and second-generation antihistamines as clues to their mechanism of action on the sneeze reflex in common cold. Clinical Infectious Diseases 2001;33:1483–8.
85. McLeod RL, Mingo G, O Reilly S, Ruck LA, Bolser DC, Hey JA. Antitussive action of antihistamines is independent of sedative and ventilation activity in the guinea pig. Pharmacology 1998; 57:57–64.
86. Dicpinigaitis PV, Gayle YG. Effect of the second-generation antihistamine, fexofenadine, on cough reflex sensitivity and pulmonary function. British Journal of Clinical Pharmacology 2003;56:501–6.
87. Ito N, Shioya T, Watanabe A, Sano M, Sasaki M, Miura M. Mechanism of the antitussive effect of azelastine in guinea pigs. Arzneimittelforschung 2002;52:441–7.
88. Kamei J, Morita K, Ohsawa M, Onodera K. Effects of epinastine on the antitussive and rewarding effects of dihydrocodeine in mice. Methods Find in Experimental and Clinical Pharmacology 1999;21:663–8.
89. Strapkova A, Nosalova G, Kovalcik V, Korpas J. The cough and antihistamines. Ceskoslovenska Fysiologie 1980;29:68.
90. Williams JG, Conaty JM, Townshend-Piala P. On the mechanism of histamine-induced bronchodilation in conscious guinea pigs. Agents and Action 1984;15:285–9.
91. Nosalova G, Strapkova A, Korpas J, Kovalcik V. Antihistamines and cough. Ceskoslovenska Fysiologie 1981;30:273–5.

92. Nosalova G, Strapkova A, Korpas J. Experimental cough and blocker of histaminic receptors. Bratislava Medical Journal 1983;79:286–92.
93. Bolser DC, DeGennaro FC, O Reilly S, Hey JA, Chapman RW. Pharmacological studies of allergic cough in guinea pig. European Journal of Pharmacology 1995;277:159–64.
94. Matsumoto S. Functional evidence of excitatory M-1 receptors in the rabbit airway. Journal of Pharmacology and Experimental Therapeutics 1997;281:531–9.
95. Fuller RW, Jackson DM. Physiology and treatment of cough. Thorax 1990;45:425–30.
96. Sant'Ambrogio G, Sant'Ambrogio FB. Sensory mechanism in cough. Role of laryngeal afferents in cough. Pulmonary Pharmacology 1996;9:309–14.
97. Widdicombe JG, Sant'Ambrogio G, Mathew OP. Nerve receptors of the upper airway. In: Mathew OP, Sant'Ambrogio G, editor. Respiratory function of the upper airway. New York, Marcel Dekker 1988;193–232.
98. Nosalova G, Strapkova A. Cough and local anesthetic effect of various substances. Ceskoslovenska Fyziologie 1989;38:165.
99. Sevecova D, Calkovska A. Pathophysiological mechanisms of meconium aspiration syndrome. Ceskoslovenska Pediatria 2002;57:183–186.
100. Sevecova D, Calkovska A, Drgova A, Javorka K. Surfactant lung lavage in rabbits with meconium aspiration—a pilot study. Acta Medica Martiniana 2002;2:9–14.
101. Widdicombe JG. Neurophysiology of the cough reflex. European Respiratory Journal 1995;8:1193–202.
102. Franova S, Nosalova G. ACE inhibitors and defense reflexes of the airways. Acta Physiologica Hungarica 1998;8:359–66.
103. Raj H, Bakshi GS, Tiwari RR, Anand A, Paintal AS. How does lobeline injected intravenously produce a cough? Respiratory Physiology & Neurobiology 2005;45;79–90.
104. Nosalova G, Strapkova A, Korpas J. Butamirate citrate action on cough components. Res Pharmac, Bratislava, Incheba 1984;45–53.
105. Strapkova A. Antioxidant activity of mucolytics. Farmaceuticky Obzor 2000;49:231–5.
106. Nosalova G, Strapkova A, Kardosova A, Capek P, Zathurecky L, Bukovska E. Antitussive action of extracts and polysaccharides of marshmallow *(Althaea officinalis L., var. Robusta).* Pharmazie 1992;47:224–6.
107. Nosalova G, Strapkova A, Kardosova A, Capek P. Antitussive activity of a rhamnogalacturonan isolated from the roots of *Althaea officinalis L., var. Robusta.* Journal of Carbohydrate Chemistry 1993;12:589–96.
108. Braga PC, Allegra L. Cough. New York: Raven Press, 1989.
109. Franova S, Kardosova A, Kostalova D. Herbal Polysaccharides in the therapy of cough. Bratislava Medical Journal 1998;99:108–10.
110. Barnes JP. Modulation of neurotransmission in airways. Physiological Reviews 1992; 72:699–729.
111. Hay DWP. Tachykinins and cough. Abstract of 2nd International Symposium. Cough: Pharmacology and Therapy, London 2001;25–27.
112. Sekizawa K. Role of substance P in cough. Abstract of symposium Cough: Methods and Mechanism. London 1996.
113. Barnes PJ. Neurogenic inflammation in the airways. Respiratory Physiology 2001;125:145–154.
114. Katsumata U, Sekizawa K, Inoue H, Sasaki H, Takishima T. Inhibitory actions of procaterol, a beta-2 stimulant, on substance P-induced cough in normal subjects during upper respiratory tract infection. Tohoku Journal of Experimental Medicine 1989;158:105–6.

115. Fox AJ. Modulation of airway receptors and cough. Abstract of symposium Cough: Methods and Mechanism. London, 1996.
116. Advenier C. Tachykinin antagonists and cough. Abstract of symposium Cough: Methods and Mechanism. London, 1996.
117. Watson N, Maclagan J, Barnes J.P. Endogenous tachykinins facilitate transmission through parasympathetic ganglia in guinea pig trachea. British Journal of Pharmacology 1993;109:751–9.
118. Widdicombe JG. Sensory mechanisms. Pulmonary Pharmacology 1996; 9: 383–387.
119. O'Connell F. Central pathways-unanswered questions. Abstract of 2nd International Symposium. Cough: Pharmacology and Therapy, London, 2001;25–7.
120. Laurence DR, Bennett PN, Brown MJ. Clinical Pharmacology. 8th edn. Edinburgh: Churchill Livingstone, 1997.
121. Nishino T, Tagaito Y, Isono S. Cough and other reflexes in irritation of the airway mucosa in man. Pulmonary Pharmacology 1996;9:285–93.
122. Sada E. The physiology of cough. International Pharmacy (FIP). Supplementum 1997;11:8–10.
123. Lavigne JV, Davis AT, Fauber R. Behavioral management of psychogenic cough. Alternative to the bedsheet and other aversive techniques. Pediatrics 1991;87:532–7.
124. Gajdos M, Huttova D. Angiotensin II AT_1 receptor blockers and diabetes mellitus. Cardiology 2002;11:535–40.
125. Irwin RS, Curley FJ, Benneti FM. Appropriate use of antitussives and protussives. Drugs 1993;46:80–91.
126. Kurz H. Antitussiva und Expektoranzien. Wissenschaftliche Verlagsgesellschaft mbH Stuttgart, 1989.
127. Korppi M, Laurikainen K, Pietikainen M, Silvasti M. Antitussives in the treatment of acute transient cough in children. Acta Pediatrica Scandinavica 1991;80:869–971.
128. Irwin RS, Madison JM. The diagnosis and treatment of cough. New England Journal of Medicine 2000;343:1715–21.
129. Irwin RS, Curley FJ, French CL. Chronic cough: the spectrum and frequency of causes, key components of the diagnostic evaluation, and outcome of specific therapy. American Review of Respiratory Disease 1990;141:640–7.
130. Cap P. Chronic persistent cough. Medicina 1999;4:7–8.
131. Philp EB. Chronic cough. American Family Physician 1997;56:1353–9.
132. Nosalova G. Tussis. Vademecum of Pediatrics. Osveta Martin 2001;1057–62.
133. Kollarik M. Undem BJ. Activation of bronchopulmonary vagal afferent nerves with bradykinin, acid and vaniloid receptor agonists in wild-type and TRPV1-/-mice. Journal of Physiology 2004;555:115–23.
134. Irwin RS, Boulet LP, Cloutier MM, Fuller RW, Gold PM, Hoffstein V, Ing AJ, McCool FD, OByrne P, Poe RH, Prakash UBS, Pratter MR, Rubin BK. Managing cough as a defense mechanism and a symptom. A consensus panel report of the American college of chest physicians. Chest 1998;114:1538–918.
135. Hutching HA, Eccles R, Smith AP, Jawad M. Voluntary cough suppression as an indication of symptom severity in upper respiratory tract infections. European Respiratory Journal 1993;6:1449–54.
136. Nosal S, Mikler J. Selected Chapters of Pediatrics. 5th edn. JLF UK Martin, 2000.
137. Banovcin P, Fedor M, Jakusova L, Rosslerova V, Mikler J, Nosal S.The effects of treatment with inhaled beclomethasone and sodium cromoglycate and their cessation on bronchial

responsiveness in asthmatic children. Abstracts of VIIIth Slovak-Poland Vojtek-Rudnik days of pediatric pulmonology, Rabka, 1995a;39–40.

138. Nosal S, Banovcin P, Mikler J, Fedor M, Jakusova L. Effect of Ventoline in the treatment bronchiolitis in children. Diagnostic and therapy in pediatric practice. JLFUK Martin, 1995.
139. Barnes PJ, Mueller R. Bronchodilators. In: Principles of Pharmacology. ITB 1996;585–98.
140. Hupka V, Kapellerova A, Raskova J. Bronchial hyperresponsiveness in children after mycoplasmic pneumonia. Studia Pneumologica et Phtiseologica 1996;56:19–21.
141. Nosal S, Vysehradska J, Mikler J, Banovcin P. Influencing interruption of steroid and cromolyn therapy on BHR and asthma bronchiale in children. Clinical Immunology and Allergology 1997;3:38.
142. Cheryian S, Greenberger PA, Patterson R. Outcome of cough variant asthma treated with inhaled steroids. Annales de Allergologie 1994;73:478–80.
143. Banovcin P, Zibolen M, Nosal S. Diagnostic and therapy in pediatric practice. JLFUK Martin, 1999.
144. Nosalova G, Strapkova A, Korpas J. Study of antitussive effect of analgesic tilidin. Bratislava Medical Journal 1985;84:653–8.
145. Strapkova A, Nosalova G, Korpas J. Antitussive effect of tramadol. Studia Pneumologica Phtiseologica 1988;48:377–83.
146. Meyer-Wegener J, Liebsher K, Hettich M, Kastner HG. Efeu versus Ambroxol bei chronisher bronchitis. Zeitschrift fur Allgemeinmedizin, 1993;69:61–6.
147. Mojzis J, Mojzisova G. Flavonoids and their biological activities. Vienala, Kosice 2001;11–13.
148. Mika K. Fytotherapy for doctors. Osveta, Martin, 1991;379.
149. Ruf JC. Wine and polyphenols related to platelet aggregation and atherosthrombosis. Drugs Under Experimental and Clinical Research 1999;25:125–31.
150. Varcholova L, Tobiasova Z, Franova S. The role of nitric oxide in bronchodilatory effect of provinol: the red wine polyphenolic compounds. Acta Medica Martiniana 2003;3/4:17–22.
151. Chang HW, Baek SH, Chung KW, Son KH, Kim HP, Kang SS. Inactivation of phospholipase A_2 by naturally occurring bioflavonoid, ochnaflone. Biochemical and Biophysical Research Communications 1994;205:843–9.
152. Takaisi-Kikuni NB, Schilcher H. Electron microscopy and microcalorimetric investigations of the possible mechanism of the antibacterial action of a defined propolis provenance. Planta Medica 1994;60:222–.
153. Kelly GE, Joannou GE, Reeder AY, Nelson C, Waring MA. The variable metabolic response to dietary isoflavones in human. Proceedings of the Society of Experimental Biology and Medicine 1995;208:40–3.
154. Burrow A, Eccles R, Jones AS. The effects of camphor, eucalyptus and menthol vapour on nasal resistance to airflow and nasal sensation. Acta Otolaryngologica 1983;96:157–61.
155. Bukovsky M, Kardosova A, Koscova H, Kostalova D. Immunomodulating activity of 4-O-methyl-D-glucurono-D-xylan from *Rudbeckia fulgida, var. sullivantii*. Biologia 1998;53:771–5.
156. Kostalova D, Kardosova A, Hajnicka V. Effect of *Mahonia aquifolium* stem bark crude extract and one of its polysaccharide componet on production of IL–8. Fytoterapia 2001;72: 802–6.
157. Ebringerova A, Kardosova A, Hromadkova Z, Malovikova A, Hribalova V. Immunomodulating activity of acidic xylans in relation to their structural and molecular properties. International Journal of Biological Macromolecules 2002;30:1–6.

158. Tyler VE, Brady LR, Robbers JE. Pharmacognosy. 9th edn. Philadelphia: Lea and Febiger, 1988;26–45.
159. Franova S, Nosalova G, Strapkova A, Capek P, Kardosova A. Pectins and antitussive activity. Ceskoslovenska Fyziologie 1995;44:30–1.
160. Nosalova G, Strapkova A, Kardosova A, Capek P, Zathurecky L, Bukovska E. Antitussive action of extracts and polysaccharides of marshmallow *(Althaea officinalis L., var. Robusta)*. Pharmazie 1992;47:224–6.
161. Nosalova G, Strapkova A, Kardosova A, Capek P. Antitussive activity of a rhamnogalacturonan isolated from the roots of *Althaea officinalis L., var. Robusta.* Journal of Carbohydrate Chemistry 1993;12:589–96.
162. Cupp MJ. Toxicology and Clinical Pharmacology of Herbal Products. Totowa, New Jersey: Humana Press, 2000.
163. Umano K, Nakahara K, Shoji A, Shibamoto T. Aroma chemicals isolated and identified from leaves of *Aloe arborescens Mill.Var.Natalensis Berger*. Journal of Agriculture and Food Chemistry 1999;47:3702–5.
164. Ding M, Ma S, Liu D. Simultaneous determination of hydroxyanthraquinones in Rh and experimental animal bodies by high-performance liquid chromatography. Analytical Science 2003;19:1163–5.
165. Rebecca W, Kayser O, Hagels H, Zessin KH, Madundo M, Gamba N. The phytochemical profile and identification of main phenolic compounds from the leaf exudates of *Aloe secundiflora* by high performance liquid chromatography-mass spectroscopy. Phytochemical Analysis 2003;14:83–6.
166. Lee KY, Wientraub ST, Yu BP. Isolation and identification of phenolic antioxidant from *Aloe barbadensis*. Free Radical Biology and Medicine 2000a;28:261–5.
167. Hu Y, Xu J, Hu Q. Evaluation of antioxidant potential of *Aloe vera (Aloe barbad miller)* extracts. Journal of Agriculture and Food Chemistry 2003;51:7788–91.
168. Vogler BK, Ernst E. *Aloe vera*: a systematic review of its clinical effectiveness. British Journal of General Practice 1999;49:823–8.
169. Mantle D, Gok MA, Lennard TW. Adverse and beneficial effects of plant extracts on skin and skin disorders. Adverse Drug Reactions and Toxicological Reviews 2001;20:89–103.
170. Choi SW, Son BW, Son YS, Park YI, Lee SK, Chung MH. The wound-healing effect of a glycoprotein fraction isolated from *Aloe vera*. British Journal of Dermatology 2001;145:535–45.
171. Reynolds T, Dweck AC. *Aloe vera* leaf gel: a review update. Journal of Ethnopharma-cology 1999;68:3–37.
172. Lee KH, Hong HS, Lee CH, Kim CH. Induction of apoptosis in human leukaemic cell lines K562, HL60 and U937 by diethylhexylphthalate isolated from *Aloe vera Linne*. Journal of Pharmacy and Pharmacology 2000b;52:1037–41.
173. Vazquez B , Avila G, Seguro D, Escalante B. Antiinflammatory activity of extracts from aloe vera gel. Journal of Ethnopharmacology 1996;55:69–75.
174. Ross IA. Medicinal Plants of the World. Totowa, New Jersey: Humana Press, 1999.
175. Skidmore-Roth L. Handbook of Herbs and Natural Supplements. St Louis, London, Philadelphia, Sydney, Toronto: Mosby, 2001.
176. Kato Y, Watanabe T. Isolation and characterization of xyloglucan from gobo *(Arctium lappa L.)*. Bioscience Biotechnology and Biochemistry 1993;57:1591–2.
177. Sato A. Studies on anti-tumor activity of crude drugs. I. The effects of aqueous extracts of some crude drugs in short-term screening test. Yakugaku Yasshi 1989;109:407–57.

178. Lin CC, Lu JM, Yang JJ, Chuang SC, Ujiie T. Anti-inflammatory and radical scavenge effects of *Arctium lappa*. American Journal of Chinese Medicine 1996;24:127–37.
179. Yao XJ, Wainberg MA, Parniak MA. Mechanism of inhibition of HIV-1 infection in vitro by purified extract of *Prunella vulgaris*. Virology 1992;187:56–62.
180. Sun WJ, Sha ZF, Gao H. Determination of arctiin and arctigenin in Fructus Arctii by reverse-phase HPLC. Yao Hsueh Hsueh Pao- Acta Pharmaceutica Sinica 1992;27:549–51.
181. Nandi P, Talukder G, Sharma A. Dietary chemoprevention of clastogenic effects 3,4-benzo(a)pyrene by *Emblica officinalis Gaertn*: fruit extract. British Journal of Cancer 1997; 76:1279–83.
182. Asmawi MZ, Kankaanranta H, Moilanen E, Vapaatalo H. Anti-inflammatory activities of *Emblica officinalis Gaertn*: leaf extracts. Journal of Pharmacology 1993;45:581–4.
183. Wagner H. Immunomodulatory agents from plants. Basel, Boston, Berlin: Birkhä user Verlag'Birkhä user Verlag, 1999.
184. Ihantola-Vomisto A, Summanen J, Kankaanranta H, Vuorela H, Asmawi ZM, Moilanen E. Anti-inflammatory activity of extracts from leaves of *Phyllanthus emblica*. Planta Medica 1997;63:518–24.
185. Nosalova G, Mokry J, Khan MTH. Antitussive activity of the fruit extract of *Emblica officinalis Gaertn* (*Euphorbiaceae*). Phytomedicine 2003;10:583–9.
186. Nosalova G, Capek P, Kardosova A, Strapkova A. Changes in cough reflex induced by administration of polysaccharides from flowers of *Malva mauritiana L.* Pharmaceutical and Pharmacological Letters 1994;3:245–8.
187. Clark LJ, Trelawny JG. Wild flowers of the Pacific Northwest. Sydney, British Columbia: Gray's Publishing Limited, 1976.
188. Muller K, Ziereis K, Gawlik I. The antipsoriatic *Mahonia aquifollium* and its active constituents: II. Antiproliferative activity against cell growth of human keratinocytes. Planta Medica 1995;61:74–5.
189. Wiesenauer M, Ludtke R. *Mahonia aquifollium* in patients with *Psoriasis vulgaris*- an intraindividual study. Phytomedicine 1996;3:231–5.
190. Muller K, Yiereis K. The antipsoriatic *Mahonia aquifollium* and its active constituents: I. Pro- and antioxidant properties and inhibition of 5-lipoxygenase. Planta Medica 1994;60:421–4.
191. Fukuda K, Hibiya Y, Mutoh M, Koshiji M, Akao S, Fujiwara H. Inhibition by berberine of cyclooxygenase-2 transcriptional activity in human colon cancer cells. Journal of Ethnopharmacology 1999;66:227–33.
192. Kupeli E, Kosar M, Yesilada E, Husnu K, Baser C. A comparative study on the anti-inflammatory antinociceptive and antipyretic effects of isoquinoline alkaloids from the roots of Turkish *Berberis* species. Life Sciences 2002;72:645–57.
193. Janbaz KH, Gilani AH. Studies on preventive and curative effects of berberine on chemical-induced hepatotoxicity in rodents. Fitoterapia J 2000;71:25–33.
194. Kardosova A, Ebringerova A, Alfoldi J, Nosalova G, Matakova T, Hribalova V. Structural features and biological activity of an acidic polysaccharide complex from *Mahonia aquifollium (Pursh Nutt)*. Carbohydrate Polymers 2004;57:165–76.
195. Kardosova A, Malovikova V, Patoprsty V, Nosalova G, Matakova T. Structural characterisation and antitussive activity of a glucuronoxylan from *Mahonia aquifolium (Pursh Nutt)*. Carbohydrate Polymers 2002;47:27–33.
196. Subrata DE, Dave KK, Bhavsar GC. Fatty acid compositions of *Gymnosporia montana* and *Paederia foetida* leaves. Indian Journal of Pharmaceutical Science 1993;55:110–2.

197. De S, Ravishankar B, Bhavsar GC. Evaluation of *Paederia foetida* for hepatoprotective and anti-inflammatory activities. Indian Journal of Natural Products 1993;9:7–11.
198. Kapadia GJ, Sharma SC, Tokuda H, Nishino H, Ueda S. Inhibitory effect of iridoids on Epstein-Barr virus activation by a short-term in vitro assay for anti-tumor promoters. Cancer Letters 1996;102:223–6.
199. Roychoudhury GK, Chakrabarty AK, Dutta B. A preliminary observation on the effects of *Paederia foetida* on gastro-intestinal helminthes in bovines. Indian Veterinary Journal 1970;47:767–9.
200. De S, Ravishankar B, Bhavsar GC. Investigation of the anti-inflammatory effects of *Paederia foetida*. Journal of Ethnopharmacology 1994;43:31–8.
201. Srivastava MC, Tewari JP, Kant V. Anti-inflammatory activity of an indigenous plant-*Paederia foetida (Gandhali)*. Indian Journal of Medical Science 1973;27:231–4.
202. Lima CF, Carvalho F, Fernandez E, Bastos ML, Santos-Gomes PC, Fernandes-Ferreira M, Pereira-Wilson C. Evaluation of toxic/protective effects of the essential oil of *Salvia officinalis* on freshly isolated rat hepatocytes. Toxicology in vitro 2004;18:457–65.
203. Janicsak G, Hohmann J, Zupko I, Forgo P, Redei D, Falkay G, Mathe I. Diterpenes from the aerial parts of *Salvia candelabrum* and their protective effects against lipid peroxidation. Planta Medica 2003;69:1156–9.
204. Chavkin C, Sud S, Jin W, Steward J, Zjawiony JK, Siebert DJ, Toth BA, Hufeisen SJ, Roth BL. Salvinorin A, an active component of the hallucinogenic sage *Salvia divinorum* is a highly efficacious kappa-opioid receptor agonist: structural and functional considerations. Journal of Pharmacology and Experimental Therapeutics 2004;308:1197–203.
205. Capek P, Hribalova V, Svandova E, Ebringerova A, Sasinkova V, Masarova J. Characterization of immunomodulatory polysccharides from *Salvia officinali L.* International Journal of Biological Macromolecules 2003;33:113–9.
206. Perry NS, Bollen C, Perry EK, Ballard C. *Salvia* for dementia therapy: review of pharmacological activity and pilot tolerability clinical trial. Pharmacology, Biochemistry and Behavior 2003;75:651–9.
207. Dittmann K, Gerhauser C, Klimo K, Hamburger M. HPLC-based activity profiling of *Salvia miltiorrhiza* for MAO A and iNOS inhibitory activities. Planta Medica 2004; 0:909–13.
208. Ulubelen A. Cardioactive and antibacterial terpenoids from some *Salvia* species. Phytochemistry 2003;64:395–9.
209. Blumenthal M, Goldberg A, Brinckmann J. Herbal Medicine: Expanded Commission E Monographs, American Botanical Council. Publ. by Integrative Medicine Communications, Newton, 2000;270–2.
210. Zgorniak-Nowosielska I, Grzybek J, Manolova N, Serkedjieva J, Zawlinska, B. Antiviral activity of *Flos verbasci* infusion against influenza and herpes simplex viruses. Archives of Immunology 1991;39:103–8.
211. Bolser DC, Aziz SM, DeGennaro FC, Kreutner W, Egan RW, Siegel MI, Chapman RW. Antitussive effects of GABAB agonists in the cat and guinea-pig. British Journal of Pharmacology 1993;110:491–5.
212. Dicpinigaitis PV, Dobkin JB. Antitussive effect of the GABA-agonist baclofen. Chest 1997;111:996–9.
213. Dicpignigaitis PV. Use of baclofen to suppress cough induced by angiotensin-converting enzyme inhibitors. Annals of Pharmacotherapy 1996;30:1242–5.
214. Morita K, Kamei J, An ATP-sensitive potassium channel opener as a peripherally acting antitussive. Abstracts of 2nd International symposium, London, 2001.

215. Morita K, Onodera K, Kamei J. Inhaled pinacidil, and ATP-sensitive K^+ channel opener, and mogusteine have potent antitussive effects in guinea pigs. Japan Journal of Pharmacology 2002;89:171–5.
216. Trevisari M, Milan A, Gatti R, Zanasi A, Harrison S, Fontana G, Morice AH, Geppetti P. Antittusive activity of iodo-resiniferatoxin in guinea pigs. Thorax 2004;59:769–72.

Index

A

B

C

D

E

F